Sleep and Circadian Rhythms in the ICU

Editor

VIPIN MALIK

CRITICAL CARE CLINICS

www.criticalcare.theclinics.com

Consulting Editor
RICHARD W. CARLSON

July 2015 • Volume 31 • Number 3

ELSEVIER

1600 John F. Kennedy Boulevard • Suite 1800 • Philadelphia, Pennsylvania, 19103-2899

http://www.theclinics.com

CRITICAL CARE CLINICS Volume 31, Number 3
July 2015 ISSN 0749-0704, ISBN-13: 978-0-323-39092-7

Editor: Patrick Manley
Developmental Editor: Casey Jackson

Critical Care Clinics (ISSN: 0749-0704) is published quarterly by Elsevier Inc., 360 Park Avenue South, New York, NY 10010-1710. Months of issue are January, April, July, and October. Business and Editorial Offices: 1600 John F. Kennedy Blvd., Suite 1800, Philadelphia, PA 19103-2899. Customer Service Office: 6277 Sea Harbor Drive, Orlando, FL 32887-4800. Periodicals postage paid at New York, NY and additional mailing offices. Subscription prices are $210.00 per year for US individuals, $503.00 per year for US institution, $100.00 per year for US students and residents, $255.00 per year for Canadian individuals, $630.00 per year for Canadian institutions, $300.00 per year for international individuals, $630.00 per year for international institutions and $150.00 per year for Canadian and foreign students/residents. To receive student/resident rate, orders must be accompanied by name of affiliated institution, date of term, and the signature of program/residency coordinator on institution letterhead. Orders will be billed at individual rate until proof of status is received. Foreign air speed delivery is included in all *Clinics* subscription prices. All prices are subject to change without notice. POSTMASTER: Send address changes to *Critical Care Clinics*, Elsevier Periodicals Customer Service, 11830 Westline Industrial Drive, St. Louis, MO 63146. **Customer Service: 1-800-654-2452 (US). From outside of the US, call 1-314-447-8871. Fax: 1-314-447-8029. E-mail: journalscustomerservice-usa@ elsevier.com (for print support) or journalsonlinesupport-usa@elsevier.com (for online support).**

Reprints. For copies of 100 or more of articles in this publication, please contact the Commercial Reprints Department, Elsevier Inc., 360 Park Avenue South, New York, NY 10010-1710. Tel.: 212-633-3874; Fax: 212-633-3820; E-mail: reprints@elsevier.com.

Critical Care Clinics is also published in Spanish by Editorial Inter-Medica, Junin 917, 1er A, 1113, Buenos Aires, Argentina.

Critical Care Clinics is covered in *MEDLINE/PubMed (Index Medicus), EMBASE/Excerpta Medica, Current Concepts/ Clinical Medicine, ISI/BIOMED,* and *Chemical Abstracts.*

Contributors

CONSULTING EDITOR

RICHARD W. CARLSON, MD, PhD
Chairman Emeritus, Director, Medical Intensive Care Unit, Department of Medicine,
Maricopa Medical Center; Professor, University of Arizona College of Medicine;
Professor, Department of Medicine, Mayo Graduate School of Medicine, Phoenix, Arizona

EDITOR

VIPIN MALIK, MD
Division of Pulmonary, Critical Care, and Sleep Medicine, National Jewish Health;
Assistant Professor of Medicine, Division of Pulmonary Sciences and Critical Care
Medicine, University of Colorado Denver, Denver, Colorado

AUTHORS

ALON Y. AVIDAN, MD, MPH
Professor of Neurology, Department of Neurology, UCLA; Director, UCLA Neurology
Clinic; Director, UCLA Sleep Disorders Center, David Geffen School of Medicine at UCLA,
Los Angeles, California

BETH Y. BESECKER, MD
Assistant Professor, Department of Internal Medicine, Division of Pulmonary, Allergy,
Critical Care, and Sleep Medicine, The Wexner Medical Center at The Ohio State
University, Columbus, Ohio

MARTHA E. BILLINGS, MD, MSc
Assistant Professor of Medicine, Division of Pulmonary Critical Care Medicine,
UW Medicine Sleep Center at Harborview, University of Washington, Seattle,
Washington

VERONICA BRITO, MD
Assistant Professor, Division of Pulmonary Critical Care and Sleep Medicine, Department
of Medicine, Baylor Scott & White Health, Texas A&M Health Science Center, Temple,
Texas

ANDREA CORTEGIANI, MD
Department of Biopathology, Medical and Forensic Biotechnologies (DIBIMEF), Section of
Anesthesiology, Analgesia, Emergency and Intensive Care, Policlinico "P. Giaccone,"
University of Palermo, Palermo, Italy

BENNETT P. DEBOISBLANC, MD
Professor of Medicine and Physiology, Section of Pulmonary and Critical Care Medicine,
Louisiana State University Health Sciences Center, New Orleans, Louisiana

XAVIER DROUOT, MD, PhD
CHU de Poitiers, Department of Clinical Neurophysiology, Hôpital Jean Bernard; Univ Poitiers, University of Medicine and Pharmacy; INSERM, CIC 1402, Equip Alive, CHU de Poitiers, Poitiers, France

DAWN ELIASHIV, MD
Professor of Neurology, Department of Neurology, UCLA; Co-Director, UCLA Seizure Disorders Center, David Geffen School of Medicine at UCLA, Los Angeles, California

SHEKHAR GHAMANDE, MD, FCCP, FAASM
Associate Professor, Division of Pulmonary Critical Care and Sleep Medicine, Department of Medicine, Baylor Scott & White Health, Texas A&M Health Science Center, Temple, Texas

CESARE GREGORETTI, MD
Department of Anesthesia and Intensive Care, Azienda Ospedaliero Universitaria "Città della Salute e della Scienza", Turin, Italy

PATRICK GREIFFENSTEIN, MD
Assistant Professor of Clinical Surgery, Section of Trauma and Critical Care Surgery, Louisiana State University Health Sciences Center, New Orleans, Louisiana

OCTAVIAN C. IOACHIMESCU, MD, PhD
Associate Professor of Medicine, Division of Pulmonary, Critical Care and Sleep Medicine, Department of Medicine, Emory University School of Medicine, Atlanta, Georgia

MUNA IRFAN, MD
Fellow in Sleep Medicine, Departments of Medicine and Neurology, Mayo Center for Sleep Medicine, Mayo Clinic and Foundation, Rochester, Minnesota

PETER JACKSON, MD
Division of Pulmonary and Critical Care Medicine, Department of Internal Medicine, School of Medicine, Oregon Health and Science University, Portland, Oregon

SHIRLEY F. JONES, MD, FCCP, FAASM
Assistant Professor, Division of Pulmonary Critical Care and Sleep Medicine, Department of Medicine, Baylor Scott &White Health, Texas A&M Health Science Center, Temple, Texas

AKRAM KHAN, MD
Associate Professor, Division of Pulmonary and Critical Care Medicine, Department of Internal Medicine, School of Medicine, Oregon Health and Science University, Portland, Oregon

DIONNE MORGAN, MBBS
Instructor, Department of Medicine, National Jewish Health, Denver, Colorado

MARK OLDHAM, MD
Department of Psychiatry, Yale-New Haven Hospital, New Haven, Connecticut

ROBERT L. OWENS, MD
Assistant Professor of Medicine, Division of Pulmonary and Critical Care Medicine, University of California, San Diego, La Jolla, California

LARA PISANI, MD
Department of Specialistic, Diagnostic and Experimental Medicine (DIMES), Respiratory and Critical Care, Sant'Orsola Malpighi Hospital, Alma Mater Studiorum, University of Bologna, Bologna, Italy

MARGARET A. PISANI, MD, MPH
Associate Professor of Internal Medicine, Section of Pulmonary, Critical Care and Sleep Medicine, Yale University School of Medicine, New Haven, Connecticut

SOLENE QUENTIN, MD
CHU de Poitiers, Department of Clinical Neurophysiology, Hôpital Jean Bernard; Univ Poitiers, University of Medicine and Pharmacy; INSERM, CIC 1402, Equip Alive, CHU de Poitiers, Poitiers, France

ALEJANDRO A. RABINSTEIN, MD
Professor of Neurology, Department of Neurology, Mayo Center for Sleep Medicine, Mayo Clinic and Foundation, Rochester, Minnesota

VITO MARCO RANIERI, MD
Department of Anesthesia and Intensive Care, Azienda Ospedaliero Universitaria "Città della Salute e della Scienza", Turin, Italy

SCOTT A. SANDS, PhD
Instructor in Medicine, Division of Sleep Medicine, Brigham and Women's Hospital, Harvard Medical School, Boston, Massachusetts; Department of Allergy, Immunology and Respiratory Medicine, Central Clinical School, Alfred Hospital, Monash University, Melbourne, Australia

BERNARDO SELIM, MD
Assistant Professor of Medicine, Department of Medicine, Mayo Center for Sleep Medicine, Mayo Clinic and Foundation, Rochester, Minnesota

ERIK K. ST. LOUIS, MD, MS
Associate Professor of Neurology, Departments of Medicine and Neurology, Mayo Center for Sleep Medicine, Mayo Clinic and Foundation, Rochester, Minnesota

SHEILA C. TSAI, MD
Associate Professor, Department of Medicine, National Jewish Health, Denver, Colorado; Associate Professor, Department of Medicine, University of Colorado Denver, Aurora, Colorado

SAIPRAKASH B. VENKATESHIAH, MD
Assistant Professor of Medicine, Division of Pulmonary, Critical Care and Sleep Medicine, Department of Medicine, Emory University School of Medicine, Atlanta, Georgia

JAMES VERMAELEN, MD
Fellow, Section of Pulmonary and Critical Care Medicine, Louisiana State University Health Sciences Center, New Orleans, Louisiana

NATHANIEL F. WATSON, MD, MSc
Professor, Department of Neurology, University of Washington, UW Medicine Sleep Center, Seattle, Washington

KAREN L. WOOD, MD
Associate Professor, Department of Internal Medicine, Division of Pulmonary, Allergy, Critical Care, and Sleep Medicine, The Wexner Medical Center at The Ohio State University, Columbus, Ohio

Contents

Since its first application in the late 1980s, noninvasive ventilation (NIV) has been the first-line intervention for certain forms of acute respiratory failure. NIV may be delivered through the patient's mouth, nose, or both using noninvasive intermittent positive pressure ventilation or continuous positive airway pressure. When applied appropriately, NIV may reduce morbidity and mortality and may avert iatrogenic complications and infections associated with invasive mechanical ventilation. This article provides physicians and respiratory therapists with a comprehensive, practical guideline for using NIV in critical care.

Restless legs syndrome is a common sensorimotor disorder characterized by an urge to move, and associated with uncomfortable sensations in the legs (limbs). Restless legs syndrome can lead to sleep-onset or sleep-maintenance insomnia, and occasionally excessive daytime sleepiness, all leading to significant morbidity. Brain iron deficiency and dopaminergic neurotransmission abnormalities play a central role in the pathogenesis of this disorder, along with other nondopaminergic systems, although the exact mechanisms are still. Intensive care unit patients are especially vulnerable to have unmasking or exacerbation of restless legs syndrome because of sleep deprivation, circadian rhythm disturbance, immobilization, iron deficiency, and use of multiple medications that can antagonize dopamine.

Congestive heart failure (CHF) is among the most common causes of admission to hospitals in the United States, especially in those over age 65. Few data exist regarding the prevalence CHF of Cheyne–Stokes respiration (CSR) owing to congestive heart failure in the intensive care unit (ICU). Nevertheless, CSR is expected to be highly prevalent among those with CHF. Treatment should focus on the underlying mechanisms by which CHF increases loop gain and promotes unstable breathing. Few data are available to determine prevalence of CSR in the ICU, or how CSR might affect clinical management and weaning from mechanical ventilation.

Sleep-disordered breathing in the perioperative setting poses an increase in both perceived and demonstrated challenges for health care providers. Some of these challenges relate to identifying patients at high risk for obstructive sleep apnea prior to surgery. Other management challenges include identifying the proper monitoring techniques, using the correct mix of pharmacologic and nonpharmacologic strategies to manage these patients, and identifying the proper and safe disposition strategy after surgery. Additional populations, such as pediatrics and the morbidly obese, are also highlighted, which may help address questions in populations that are frequently managed in the critical care setting postoperatively.

Sleep is disrupted in most patients hospitalized in the intensive care unit and the disturbances are even more profound in patients impacted by epilepsy. Nocturnal seizures must be differentiated from other common nocturnal events, such as delirium, parasomnias, and sedation. Many antiepileptic drugs produce undesirable side effects on sleep architecture that may further predispose patients to insomnia during the night and excessive sedation and hypersomnolence during the day. Failure to recognize, correctly diagnose, and adequately manage these disturbances may lead to more prolonged hospitalization, increased risk for nosocomial infections, poorer health-related qualify of life, and greater health care financial burden.

Sleep-disordered breathing (SDB) is a frequent presenting manifestation of neuromuscular disorders and can lead to significant morbidity and mortality. If not recognized and addressed early in the clinical course, SDB can lead to clinical deterioration with respiratory failure. The pathophysiologic basis of SDB in neuromuscular disorders, clinical features encountered in specific neuromuscular diseases, and diagnostic and management strategies for SDB in neuromuscular patients in the critical care setting are reviewed. Noninvasive positive pressure ventilation has been a crucial advance in critical care management, improving sleep quality and often preventing or delaying mechanical ventilation and improving survival in neuromuscular patients.

More than one-half million patients are hospitalized annually for traumatic brain injury (TBI). One-quarter demonstrate sleep-disordered breathing, up to 50% experience insomnia, and half have hypersomnia. Sleep disturbances after TBI may result from injury to sleep-regulating brain tissue, nonspecific neurohormonal responses to systemic injury, ICU environmental interference, and medication side effects. A diagnosis of sleep disturbances requires a high index of suspicion and appropriate testing. Treatment starts with a focus on making the ICU environment conducive to normal sleep. Treating sleep-disordered breathing likely has outcome benefits in TBI. The use of sleep promoting sedative-hypnotics and anxiolytics should be judicious.

Sedation in the intensive care unit (ICU) is a topic that has been frequently researched, and debate still exists as to what are the best sedative agents for critically ill patients. There is increasing interest in sleep and circadian rhythm disturbances in the ICU and how they may impact on outcomes. In addition to patient-related and ICU environmental factors that likely impact sleep and circadian rhythm in the ICU, sedative and analgesic medications may also play a role.

Delirium in the intensive care unit (ICU) is a common diagnosis, with an incidence ranging between 45% and 87%. Delirium represents a significant burden both to the patient and to the health care system, with a 3.2-fold increase in 6-month mortality and annual US health care costs up to $16 billion. In this review, the diagnosis, epidemiology, and risk factors for delirium in the ICU are discussed. The pathophysiology of delirium and evolving prevention and treatment modalities are outlined.

CRITICAL CARE CLINICS

ISSUE OF RELATED INTEREST

Sleep Medicine Clinics of North America, December 2014 (Vol. 9, No. 4)
Evaluation of Sleep Complaints
Clete Kushida, *Editor*
Available at: http://www.sleep.theclinics.com/

Preface

Sleep and Circadian Rhythms in the Intensive Care Unit

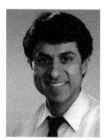

Vipin Malik, MD
Editor

Our knowledge of sleep physiology in critical care has grown over the last several decades. Nonetheless, several gaps remain, particularly those related to the mechanisms whereby sleep disruption influences the short- and long-term outcomes of critically ill patients. There is an urgent need to identify the deleterious effects of sleep disruption and various biomarkers that contribute to their pathogenesis in this patient group.

This issue of *Critical Care Clinics* discusses sleep and circadian rhythm disorders among critically ill patients, who generally have various coexisting acute and chronic medical conditions. Sedation and management of delirium are also reviewed.

The article by Dr Drouot and Dr Quentin specifically discusses sleep electroencephalographic patterns in the intensive care unit (ICU) and elaborates on atypical sleep and pathologic wakefulness. In the second article, Dr Billings and Dr Watson examine the causes, effects, and management of circadian disruption in critically ill patients. Circadian hormonal changes and effects of sleep disruption are discussed by Dr Morgan and Dr Tsai. An article by Dr Jones, Dr Brito, and Dr Ghamande is devoted to the pathophysiology, treatment, and critical care outcome of patients with obesity-hypoventilation syndrome. Dr Gregoretti, Dr Pisani, Dr Cortegiani, and Dr Ranieri provide a comprehensive and practical review of the use of noninvasive ventilation (NIV) in the ICU and the effect of NIV on sleep. The consequences of restless leg syndrome on sleep among critically ill patients are discussed by Dr Venkateshiah and Dr Ioachimescu, and the pathophysiology and management of central sleep apnea and Cheyne-Stokes respiration associated with congestive heart failure are discussed by Dr Sands and Dr Owens. In a separate article, Dr Wood and Dr Besecker cover the preoperative identification and intraoperative/postoperative management of patients with sleep disorders. Diagnosis and management of various epileptic forms with specific discussion of sleep-associated epilepsy are discussed by Dr Eliashiv and Dr Avidan.

Crit Care Clin 31 (2015) xiii–xiv
http://dx.doi.org/10.1016/j.ccc.2015.05.001
0749-0704/15/$ – see front matter © 2015 Published by Elsevier Inc.

criticalcare.theclinics.com

Specific management issues pertaining to sleep-disordered breathing associated with various neuromuscular disorders and traumatic brain injury are covered in two articles by Dr Irfan, Dr Selim, Dr Rabinstein, Dr Louis, and Dr Vermaelen, Dr Greiffenstein, Dr deBoisblanc. Finally, interactions between medications, sleep, and circadian rhythms in the ICU as well as the pathophysiology, prevention, and treatment modalities for ICU-associated delirium are discussed by Dr Oldham and Dr Pisani; Dr Jackson and Dr Khan, respectively.

I hope this issue of *Critical Care Clinics* provides the reader with a useful update on sleep and circadian disruption in the critical care setting.

I thank the authors for their excellent contributions to this issue and Casey Jackson and Patrick Manley for their editorial support.

Vipin Malik, MD
Division of Pulmonary, Critical Care
and Sleep Medicine
National Jewish Health
M323b, 1400 Jackson Street
Denver, CO 80206, USA

Division of Pulmonary Sciences
and Critical Care Medicine
University of Colorado Denver
Denver, CO 80204, USA

E-mail address:
malikv@njhealth.org

Sleep Neurobiology and Critical Care Illness

Xavier Drouot, MD, PhD[a,b,c,*], Solene Quentin, MD[a,b,c]

KEYWORDS

- Sleep alterations • Neurobiology • Sleep EEG pattern • Sleep organization
- Circadian rhythms

KEY POINTS

- Intensive care unit (ICU) patients experience severe sleep alterations, with reductions in several sleep stages, marked sleep fragmentation, low sleep continuity, and circadian rhythm disorganization.
- The numerous sources of these sleep alterations are associated with disruptions of sleep neurobiological processes and sleep dynamics that can alter sleep restorative functions.
- Understanding the neurobiology of sleep in the ICU is a major challenge for future sleep studies in critically ill patients.

INTRODUCTION

That critical illnesses and environmental factors in intensive care units (ICUs) are associated with sleep disturbances was recognized shortly after the first ICUs were created. Many studies documented objective lack of restorative sleep.[1–4] Sleep alterations in critically ill patients differ from sleep changes observed in ambulatory patients (such as patients with sleep apnea syndrome) in pathophysiology as well as the consequences of sleep loss.

The literature regarding consequences of sleep deprivation on health is growing rapidly but ICU patients are unlikely to avoid the biological and neurobehavioral repercussions of sleep loss. To appreciate all of the phenomena triggered by sleep loss in the ICU, it is important to understand the neurobiology of healthy sleep and the specific neurobiological derangements of sleep in critically ill patients.

Funding sources: None.

Conflicts of interest: None.

[a] CHU de Poitiers, Department of Clinical Neurophysiology, Hôpital Jean Bernard, 2 rue de la Milétrie, Poitiers 86000, France; [b] Univ Poitiers, University of Medicine and Pharmacy, 6 rue de la Milétrie, Poitiers 86000, France; [c] INSERM, CIC 1402, Equipe Alive, CHU de Poitiers, Cours Est J. Bernard, Poitiers 86000, France

* Corresponding author. CHU de Poitiers, Department of Clinical Neurophysiology, Hôpital Jean Bernard, 2 rue de la Milétrie, Poitiers 86000, France.

E-mail address: xavier.drouot@chu-poitiers.fr

Crit Care Clin 31 (2015) 379–391

http://dx.doi.org/10.1016/j.ccc.2015.03.001

criticalcare.theclinics.com

NEUROBIOLOGY OF THE NORMAL SLEEP CYCLE

In human beings, sleep is composed of non–rapid eye movement (NREM) sleep, which can be light NREM (stages 1 and 2) or deep sleep (stages 3 and 4). The distinction between wake and NREM sleep is made by visual analysis of a 30-second portion of an electroencephalogram (EEG): during waking, the EEG shows a mix of fast oscillations (>16 Hz) and alpha rhythm (8–12 Hz) of low amplitudes (<10 µV). During light NREM sleep (stages 1 and 2), the background EEG is characterized by slow theta oscillations (frequency between 4 and 7 Hz) and sleep spindle and K complexes. These latter regularly occur and provide the landmark of stage 2. During deep NREM sleep (also called slow wave sleep; stages 3 and 4), the EEG shows slow waves (0.5–2 Hz) of high amplitude (>75 µV). Rapid eye movement (REM) sleep is a particular sleep stage in which the EEG shows theta and alpha rhythms. Identification of REM sleep is based on the presence of rapid eye movements identified on electro-oculograms and complete chin muscle atonia. During REM sleep, the brain is highly active, and most dreams and nightmares occur during this stage.

Human sleep is monophasic, and is programmed to occur during nighttime. The sleep-wake cycle is accurately organized and controlled. A sleep deficit elicits a compensatory increase in the intensity and duration of sleep, and excessive sleep reduces sleep propensity. This process could be represented as a sleep-pressure regulation, which would maintain this pressure between an upper and a lower limit. Sleep homeostasis can be represented by the interaction of 2 main physiologic processes. The first process is known as process S, which increases during waking and declines during sleep. Electroencephalographic slow wave activity (SWA) corresponds with an indicator of sleep homeostasis and the level of SWA is determined by the duration of prior sleep and waking. The timing and propensity to fall asleep are also modulated by a circadian process. This second process is driven by the internal clock. This circadian rhythm is sensible to external factors that help to keep the sleep-wake cycle synchronized with night-day alternation. The main external synchronizing factors are light, physical activities, meals, and social interactions.

The quantity of sleep is acutely regulated, and sleep deprivation has many neurobiological consequences. On the day following 1 night without sleep, brain performances are severely decreased. The most visible behavior is an increased tendency to fall asleep, even when the person fights to remain awake. The night following the sleep deprivation is modified and a sleep rebound usually occurs. This sleep rebound triggers a lengthening of nighttime sleep, an increase in slow wave sleep, and an increase in REM sleep.

METHODS FOR SLEEP STUDY IN INTENSIVE CARE UNIT PATIENTS

Sleep can be assessed in terms of quantity (total sleep time and time spent in each sleep stage), quality (fragmentation, sleep EEG patterns), and distribution over the 24-hour cycle.

Full polysomnography (PSG) is the only reliable tool for measuring sleep, especially in patients with marked sleep disturbances. Accurate sleep scoring requires the recording of at least 3 EEG signals (preferentially F4-A1, C4-A1, O2-A1), 2 electro-oculography signals, and a submental electromyography (EMG) signal. Additional signals are usually recorded, such as nasal and oral airflow, thoracic and abdominal belts, electrocardiogram, and pulse oximetry. Sound and light levels should be measured, although these data are not obtained routinely.

SLEEP ELECTROENCEPHALOGRAM PATTERNS IN THE INTENSIVE CARE UNIT

Sleep scoring using either the system of Rechtschaffen and Kales[5] or the recently modified rules[6] poses a specific problem in critical care patients. A variable portion of the brains of critically ill patients does not generate the usual sleep EEG patterns and habitual markers of sleep.[7–11] The presence of theta and delta EEG activities during wakefulness, rapid fluctuations between EEG features of wake and NREM sleep, rapid eye movements during stage 2, and low-amplitude fast frequencies caused by sedation and delta burst arousal pattern are often observed.[8,12,13] In a study in conscious patients (Glasgow score >8) without neurologic disease who required mechanical ventilation for lung injury, 12 of 20 patients had abnormal sleep patterns[8]; among them, 7 patients showed EEG features of coma with reactive theta-delta activity and 5 had atypical sleep with virtually no stage 2 sleep and the presence of pathologic wakefulness (a combination of EEG features of slow wave sleep and behavioral correlates of wakefulness such as saccadic eye movements and sustained EMG activity). These 5 patients had worse acute physiology scores and received a higher mean benzodiazepine dose than the patients with disrupted but recognizable sleep patterns. In a similar group of 22 patients without sedation or neurologic disease,[9] only 17 patients (77.3%) had PSG recordings that could be scored. The remaining 5 patients had an EEG pattern of low-voltage mixed-frequency waves and variable amounts of theta-delta activity; all 5 developed sepsis during the study period, suggesting that sleep abnormalities were related to sepsis encephalopathy.[9]

In a recent study, Watson and colleagues[13] found major dissociations between EEG patterns and behavior in a group of 37 ICU patients. These dissociations consisted of abnormally slow EEG frequency in the theta range (3–7 Hz), a frequency that normally indicates sleep, or even delta range in some awake patients; In contrast, they observed low-amplitude, high-frequency beta EEG activity in patients who were in coma. Some patients who were awake and interactive with research personnel showed predominately theta activity (3–7 Hz), a frequency that normally indicates sleep. One patient, awake and able to follow simple instructions, was documented to have important delta activity, a finding that is normally associated with slow wave sleep. In contrast, unresponsive comatose patients were noted to have alpha activity present on PSG, which is an EEG frequency typically seen in the wake state. These observations led Cooper and colleagues[8] to propose new sleep states called pathologic wakefulness and atypical sleep.

Atypical Sleep and Pathologic Wakefulness

Several teams have deal in depth with the concept of atypical sleep and pathologic wakefulness. Drouot and colleagues[11] proposed a new classification based on the reports of Cooper and colleagues.[8] Drouot and colleagues'[11] study focused on ICU patients admitted for respiratory failure, treated with noninvasive ventilation, and who were not sedated nor taking drugs interfering with sleep physiology. The investigators proposed that atypical sleep and pathologic wake have to be used when patients clearly show alternation between 2 distinct vigilance states. Atypical sleep was defined as non-REM sleep without spindle or K complexes. In contrast, pathologic wakefulness was defined by the association of a global slowing of EEG frequencies (with a peak frequency ≤7 Hz) and an impaired EEG reactivity.[11] Watson and colleagues[13] emphasized Drouot and colleagues'[11] new classification by extending their findings in patients with higher severity of illness and receiving sedation. Investigators also incorporate the judicious EEG classification for coma developed by Young and colleagues.[14] In a similar way, Watson and colleagues[13] proposed a new algorithm that includes, as a first step, a comparison between patients' behavior and EEG patterns.

Pathophysiology of Atypical Sleep and Pathologic Wakefulness

Several factors may explain the EEG abnormalities seen in patients with atypical sleep. The first factor could be hypercapnia. In the Drouot and colleagues[11] study, several patients had hypercapnic respiratory failure, which is known to induce various abnormalities in brain function, ranging from mild hypovigilance to encephalopathy.[15–18] Similar EEG alterations have been reported in healthy awake individuals during hypercapnia.[19] However, arterial Pco_2 values did not differ between the group with atypical sleep/pathologic wakefulness and the group with normal sleep, suggesting that other factors could be involved in atypical sleep.[11] Sleep deprivation per se is known to alter EEG patterns during prolonged wakefulness and also during the subsequent recovery sleep. Sleep deprivation experiments showed linear decreases in alpha activity and increases in theta and delta activities on wakefulness EEGs.[20] The background EEG activity alterations in patients with atypical sleep/pathologic wakefulness were similar to those reported in healthy individuals subjected to sleep deprivation for 24 hours.[21,22] Recovery sleep following sleep deprivation is characterized by significantly decreased spindle[23] and K-complex densities.[24] Because ICU patients are exposed to sleep deprivation for several consecutive days or weeks,[25,26] atypical sleep may constitute a compensatory mechanism in which deep sleep predominates over light (stage 2) sleep to maximize sleep debt recovery. The association of hypercapnia and sleep deprivation in the genesis of atypical sleep has been suggested because spindle density (a marker of atypical sleep) decreases with increase of both SWA and arterial CO_2 levels.[27] Some patients with atypical sleep (with no spindle or very low spindle density) showed normal levels of arterial Pco_2. These patterns could have turned into atypical sleep because of a severe sleep deprivation.[27] However, whether hypercapnia inhibits spindle circuitry and K-complex generators or favor sleep stage associated with low spindle densities, such as slow waves sleep,[28] remains unknown.

Rapid Eye Movement Sleep in the Intensive Care Unit

Most of studies have reported that REM is commonly lacking in ICU patients.[3] However, REM sleep scoring can be difficult when submental muscle atonia, a hallmark of REM sleep, is lacking. REM sleep without atonia and dissociated REM sleep seems uncommon in ICU patients,[29] but these conditions have not been extensively studied. Whether loss of muscle atonia is related to pre-existing disease, medications, or the ICU environment remains to be established.[29] A study of ICU patients with Guillain-Barré syndrome showed a higher incidence of REM sleep abnormalities (including loss of atonia, short REM latency, and daytime REM sleep episodes) compared with ICU patients with paraplegia.[30]

Furthermore, hypercapnia can also produce a REM deficit. The amount of REM sleep was decreased in patients with hypercapnic respiratory failure.[31] However, contrasting results have been reported in experiments in rodents, which showed that hypercapnia increased the amount of REM sleep.[32]

In addition, most studies are transversal experiments and have performed a single PSG at a defined time during an ICU stay. Few studies have been published with longitudinal and repeated PSG, so the initial course of REM deprivation, and the presence and the timing of a potential REM rebound, are unknown, at least in medical ICUs. Some rare reports performed in surgical ICUs have shown an initial, severe REM sleep deficit, followed by an important rebound of REM sleep in the first week after surgery.[33–36]

SLEEP ORGANIZATION IN THE INTENSIVE CARE UNIT
Sleep Architecture

As mentioned in earlier, better analysis of sleep quantity and quality disturbances in ICU patients requires prolonged PSG that lasts at least 16 to 24 hours. Severe sleep-wake disorganization is a major characteristic of sleep in ICU patients. Loss of light/dark circadian synchronization and the prolonged inactive decubitus favor daytime sleep. Studies using long-duration recordings consistently showed abnormal sleep distribution over the 24-hour cycle, with as much as 50% of sleep occurring during the day.[8,9,25,37,38] All the studies found considerable interindividual variability in TST. For instance, TST ranged from 1.7 to 19.4 hours in one study.[9] Nevertheless, the results indicate that quantitative sleep deprivation is not consistently present.

Sleep stage distribution is substantially altered in ICU patients. Sleep stage 1, which normally constitutes less than 5% of TST, accounts for up to 60% of TST in critically ill patients.[8,9,25,33,34] Marked deficits in slow wave sleep (sleep stages 3 and 4) were documented in medical ICU patients and postsurgical patients.[25,33–36] REM sleep is often reduced or abolished,[8,25,39] especially during the first night following surgery.[33–36] Data on sleep stage 2 are conflicting. Sleep stage 2 was normal or increased in some studies[25,34,35,40] and decreased in other studies.[9,36,39] The discrepancies across studies preclude general conclusions.

In addition, differences in the time point of sleep recording may contribute to interindividual variability of sleep parameters. Surgical ICU patients best illustrate this fact because PSG can be performed at baseline (before surgery) and after anesthesia using a standardized regimen. The results showed marked reduction or elimination of slow wave sleep and REM sleep during the first 2 postoperative nights, with a significant rebound of REM sleep in the third or fourth postoperative night,[33–36,41] contrasting with little[35] or no rebound of slow wave sleep.[34,36] These results also highlight the need for longitudinal studies describing changes in sleep over time according to the reason for ICU admission and to disease severity.

Sleep Fragmentation

Concomitantly with sleep stage disorganization, ICU patients experience severe sleep fragmentation with arousals or awakenings. Studies of mechanically ventilated patients showed up to 79 arousals and awakenings per hour of sleep, leading to interruption of sleep every 46 seconds.[8,25,42]

Sleep Continuity

Based on Bonnet's[43] sleep continuity theory, which posits that at least 10 minutes of uninterrupted sleep are needed to serve a recuperative function, several investigators have deemed quantification of sleep continuity to be of interest. Recently, Drouot and colleagues[44] showed that, in nonsedated patients admitted for hypercapnic respiratory failure treated with noninvasive ventilation (NIV), the percentage of TST spent in short naps (ie, sleep episodes lasting between 10 and 30 minutes) was higher and the percentage of sleep time spent in sleep bouts (ie, sleep episodes lasting <10 minutes) was lower in patients with successful NIV compared with patients with NIV failure. Usual sleep quantification, such as TST, sleep stages composition, and sleep fragmentation, were not different between patients with good outcome compared with patients with poor outcome.

CIRCADIAN RHYTHMS AND MELATONIN IN INTENSIVE CARE UNIT PATIENTS

Not only sleep is disturbed, but more generally circadian rhythm. The latter can be assessed indirectly by measuring the oscillations in core body temperature, or directly by melatonin and melatonin metabolite assays.

In a study of 15 ICU patients, the circadian rhythm of core body temperature persisted, but the time of the acrophase showed marked intraindividual variability with shifts of several hours from day to day.[45] In a recent study, Gazendam and colleagues[46] found that acrophases were shifted (advanced or delayed) in 81% of patients, but that this shift was stable across days in each individual. In contrast, in a large cohort of 137 patients investigated after thoracic or vascular surgery, core body temperature showed no circadian rhythmicity in most patients during the first 3 postoperative days.[47]

The circadian rhythm generator, located in the suprachiasmatic nucleus, triggers melatonin production and release by the pineal gland. Melatonin levels start to increase around bedtime and peak at about 3 AM. The onset of melatonin secretion is a robust marker of circadian rhythms.[48] It can be investigated either by assaying serum melatonin concentrations or by determining the urinary 6-sulfatoxymelatonin (6-SMT) level, a surrogate marker for plasma melatonin in healthy subjects. Following the first report by Shilo and colleagues[49] of altered 6-SMT rhythm in ICU patients, several groups investigated melatonin production. One study showed striking abnormalities in urinary 6-SMT excretion in 16 of 17 ICU patients with sepsis, contrasting with normal excretion in 6 of 7 ICU patients without sepsis and in 18 of 23 controls.[50] In another study, the circadian rhythm of urinary 6-SMT concentration was altered in 12 of 16 ICU patients, and 6-SMT excretion was lower during periods with ventilation than during periods of spontaneous breathing.[51] In a recent study, a circadian rhythm of 6-SMT excretion was present in most (81%) patients, but only 4 subjects had normal timing, the others being phase delayed.[52] In addition, the circadian melatonin rhythm was altered in 7 of 8 ICU patients, with no correlation between melatonin levels and levels of sedation.[53]

Factors Interfering with Circadian Rhythms and Melatonin

Melatonin secretion can be influenced by numerous factors,[48] such as age, benzodiazepines, adrenergic compounds, β-blockers, opiates, light exposure, sedation, mechanical ventilation,[51] and sepsis.[50] The contribution of each of these factors in the melatonin release disturbances documented in ICU patients remains unclear.[54]

FACTORS RESPONSIBLE FOR SLEEP DISRUPTION IN THE INTENSIVE CARE UNIT

Numerous factors contribute to sleep disruption in ICU. Some of them are not specific to the ICU (eg, noise and light), although they are intense and frequent in the ICU. Some other conditions are more specifically met in the ICU and interfere with sleep neurobiology, such as continuous lighting, continuous bed rest, and sedation.

The Intensive Care Unit Environment

The level of noise is more than the World Health Organization recommendations in many ICUs,[55] making sleep difficult, and it was rated by patients as one of most sleep disruptive factors.[55,56] In a study involving completion of a questionnaire by patients recently discharged from the ICU, patients reported that vital sign assessments and phlebotomy were more disruptive than noise.[57] In a subsequent study using PSG and synchronized recordings of environmental noise in 22 ICU patients, episodes of noise were related to only 11.5% of all arousals and 17% of all awakenings.[9] Similarly, in another study, noise and patient-care activities explained only 30% of all arousals and awakenings; no causative factors were identified in the other cases.[25] However, because of the large number of peak sounds in the ICU (36.5 per hour of sleep in one study),[25] as well as the large number of arousals and awakenings in ICU patients (from 22 to 79 per hour of sleep),[8,25,42] a causal relationship between noise and arousal/awakening is difficult to ascertain.

Light Exposure

Continuous light exposure and the disappearance of the natural day-night rhythm in the ICU may alter the circadian clock. Nocturnal light intensities vary across ICUs but can exceed 1000 lux.[58,59] Because 100 lux is sufficient to affect melatonin secretion, nocturnal light exposure may modify circadian rhythms. In one recent study, light exposure at night was appropriate (median, <2 lux) but low during the day (median, 74 lux), further reducing day-night contrast.[40]

Loss of Physical Activity

Physical activity is a powerful zeitgeber (time cue), and greater diurnal activity is associated with larger variations in body temperature oscillations.[60] In bed rest experiments in which healthy individuals were asked to stay in bed for 36 hours, daytime naps were common, and sleep-onset REM occurred in up to 43% of naps and 80% of individuals.[61] In an elegant study[25] in which healthy volunteers stayed in bed in an ICU, most of the volunteers lost their circadian organization of sleep and slept during the day, suggesting that loss of activity per se may disrupt circadian rhythms and the sleep-wake cycle.

Effects of Drugs on Sleep

Many drugs used for light sedation or analgesia in the ICU influence sleep in healthy individuals and therefore could be causes of sleep disturbances.[62] Benzodiazepines are used to shorten sleep latency and facilitate sleep continuity. In healthy individuals, benzodiazepines lengthen sleep stage 2, increase TST, and decrease both slow wave sleep duration and REM sleep.[63,64] Tricyclic antidepressants and serotonin reuptake inhibitors increase slow wave sleep and block REM sleep.[65] In addition, tricyclic antidepressants and serotonin reuptake inhibitors may disrupt REM muscle atonia,[66] making this sleep stage difficult to recognize. Antipsychotics induce various sleep changes. Although haloperidol does not modify sleep architecture, olanzapine increases TST, slow wave sleep, and REM sleep, and risperidone only decreases REM sleep.[67] Anticonvulsants may alter the sleep architecture.[68–70] It should be emphasized that all neurotropic molecules may affect EEG patterns during sleep and wakefulness. Opioids reduce slow wave sleep and REM sleep.[71] In addition, abrupt drug discontinuation may elicit withdrawal reactions such as insomnia after discontinuation of sedatives.[72]

Sedation and Sleep Function

Some experiments suggested that propofol may subserve a function that overlaps with sleep function. In an elegant study, Tung and colleagues[73] showed that rats sedated with propofol during their habitual sleep period did not show signs of sleep deprivation (such as sleep rebound) in the following hours. In a second experiment, the restorative effect of natural sleep and 6-hour propofol anesthesia were compared in sleep-deprived rats. No differences were found between natural sleep and anesthesia regarding delta power, REM sleep, or NREM sleep, suggesting that sleep and anesthesia provided similar recovery from sleep deprivation.[74]

However, although propofol may mimic some NREM sleep functions, this does not extend to all sleep functions because propofol consistently suppresses REM sleep in humans.[75]

CONSEQUENCES OF SLEEP DISRUPTIONS ON SLEEP NEUROBIOLOGY
Prolonged Sleep Privation

Regarding the severity of sleep disruptions in the ICU, it is important to note that the sleep regimens imposed on ICU patients is different from those experienced by ambulatory patients, such as patients with sleep apnea syndrome. The critical illness and the environment trigger a severe state of prolonged sleep deprivation. Studies conducted in healthy volunteers have shown that chronic restriction to 4 hours of sleep per night produced a cumulative cognitive performance deficit.[76]

Biological Effect of Sleep Deprivation

The immune system has long been regarded as vulnerable to sleep deprivation. Numerous studies have established that sleep deprivation impairs cellular and humoral immune responses and alters cytokine production.[77] Sleep deprivation was followed by decreases in natural killer (NK) cell and lymphocyte counts in some studies[78] and by increases in others.[79] Counts of T-helper cells and NK cells decreased after 1 night, but increased after 2 nights without sleep.[78] Sleep restriction (4 hours of sleep for 6 nights) in healthy volunteers was followed by a blunted response to immunization after influenza vaccination.[80] These data suggest that sleep loss in ICU patients may decrease the strength of immune responses.

Sleep and Sepsis

There have been few studies of the relationship between sleep deprivation and sepsis. In rodents, Friese and colleagues[81] reported that the experimental fragmentation of sleep after sepsis was associated with an increased mortality. These data suggest that loss of natural increase of sleep triggered by severe infection could be detrimental to health. Whether this is also the case in humans remains to be investigated.

Neurophysiologic Consequences of Sleep Loss

Sleep deprivation may affect pulmonary mechanics and respiratory muscles. In several studies, sleep deprivation for 24 hours reduced both hypercapnic and hypoxic ventilatory responses by 19% in healthy individuals.[82–84] Inspiratory muscle endurance and maximal voluntary ventilation were decreased after 30 hours without sleep.[85] All these data were obtained in healthy individuals, and no study has investigated the effects of sleep deprivation on respiratory function in critically ill patients. If the physiologic alterations seen in healthy individuals also occur in critically ill patients, they may adversely affect weaning from assisted ventilation.

Neuropsychological and Behavioral Effects of Sleep Alterations

Sleep deprivation affects cognitive functions. Many experiments have shown that specific neurocognitive domains, including executive attention, working memory, and concentration, are particularly vulnerable to sleep loss, the result being cognitive slowing and response perseveration.[86] Prolonged sleep deprivation over several days have been shown to trigger perceptual distortions and hallucinations in healthy individuals.[87] All these effects may play a role in the occurrence of delirium in ICU patients.[88]

SUMMARY

ICU patients experience severe sleep alterations with reductions in several sleep stages, marked sleep fragmentation, low sleep continuity, and circadian rhythm disorganization. The numerous sources of these sleep alterations are associated with disruptions of sleep neurobiological processes and sleep dynamics that could alter sleep restorative functions. A crucial issue is how to objectively quantify this particular sleep, which is the step before imaging sleep protection strategies. Understanding the neurobiology of sleep in the ICU is a major challenge for future sleep studies in critically ill patients.

REFERENCES

1. Drouot X, Cabello B, d'Ortho MP, et al. Sleep in the intensive care unit. Sleep Med Rev 2008;12:391–403.
2. Parthasarathy S, Tobin MJ. Sleep in the intensive care unit. Intensive Care Med 2004;30:197–206.
3. Pisani MA, Friese RS, Gehlbach BK, et al. Sleep in the intensive care unit. Am J Respir Crit Care Med 2015;191:731–8.
4. Elliott R, McKinley S, Cistulli P. The quality and duration of sleep in the intensive care setting: an integrative review. Int J Nurs Stud 2011;48:384–400.
5. Rechtschaffen A, Kales A. A manual for standardized terminology, techniques and scoring system for sleep stages of human subjects. Washington, DC: Public Health Service, US Government Printing Office; 1968. p. 1–12.
6. Iber C, Ancoli-Israel S, Chesson A, et al. The AASM manual for the scoring of sleep and associated events: rules, terminology and technical specifications. 1st edition. Westchester (IL): American Academy of Sleep Medicine; 2007.
7. Bourne RS, Minelli C, Mills GH, et al. Clinical review: sleep measurement in critical care patients: research and clinical implications. Crit Care 2007;11:226.
8. Cooper AB, Thornley KS, Young GB, et al. Sleep in critically ill patients requiring mechanical ventilation. Chest 2000;117:809–18.
9. Freedman NS, Gazendam J, Levan L, et al. Abnormal sleep/wake cycles and the effect of environmental noise on sleep disruption in the intensive care unit. Am J Respir Crit Care Med 2001;163:451–7.
10. Watson PL. Measuring sleep in critically ill patients: beware the pitfalls. Crit Care 2007;11:159.
11. Drouot X, Roche-Campo F, Thille AW, et al. A new classification for sleep analysis in critically ill patients. Sleep Med 2012;13:7–14.
12. Watson PL, Ely EW, Malow B, et al. Scoring sleep in critically ill patients: limitations in standard methodology and the need for revised criteria. Crit Care Med 2006;34:A83.
13. Watson PL, Pandharipande P, Gehlbach BK, et al. Atypical sleep in ventilated patients: empirical electroencephalography findings and the path toward revised ICU sleep scoring criteria. Crit Care Med 2013;41(8):1958–67.
14. Young GB, McLachlan RS, Kreeft JH, et al. An electroencephalographic classification for coma. Can J Neurol Sci 1997;24:320–5.
15. Brochard L, Isabey D, Harf A, et al. Non-invasive ventilation in acute respiratory insufficiency in chronic obstructive bronchopneumopathy. Rev Mal Respir 1995;12:111–7 [in French].
16. Demedts M, Clement J, Schepers R, et al. Respiratory failure: correlation between encephalopathy, blood gases and blood ammonia. Respiration 1976;33:199–210.

17. Kilburn KH. Neurologic manifestations of respiratory failure. Arch Intern Med 1965;116:409–15.
18. Scala R, Naldi M, Archinucci I, et al. Noninvasive positive pressure ventilation in patients with acute exacerbations of COPD and varying levels of consciousness. Chest 2005;128:1657–66.
19. Halpern P, Neufeld MY, Sade K, et al. Middle cerebral artery flow velocity decreases and electroencephalogram (EEG) changes occur as acute hypercapnia reverses. Intensive Care Med 2003;29:1650–5.
20. Bonnet MH. Acute sleep deprivation. In: Kryger MH, Roth T, Dement WC, editors. Principles and practice of sleep medicine. Philadelphia: Elsevier Saunders; 2005. p. 51–66.
21. Naitoh P, Kales A, Kollar EJ, et al. Electroencephalographic activity after prolonged sleep loss. Electroencephalogr Clin Neurophysiol 1969;27:2–11.
22. Rodin EA, Luby ED, Gottlieb JS. The electroencephalogram during prolonged experimental sleep deprivation. Electroencephalogr Clin Neurophysiol 1962;14:544–51.
23. De Gennaro L, Ferrara M, Bertini M. Effect of slow-wave sleep deprivation on topographical distribution of spindles. Behav Brain Res 2000;116:55–9.
24. Sforza E, Chapotot F, Pigeau R, et al. Effects of sleep deprivation on spontaneous arousals in humans. Sleep 2004;27:1068–75.
25. Gabor JY, Cooper AB, Hanly PJ. Sleep disruption in the intensive care unit. Curr Opin Crit Care 2001;7:21–7.
26. Weinhouse GL, Schwab RJ. Sleep in the critically ill patient. Sleep 2006;29:707–16.
27. Quentin S, Thille A, Roche-Campo F, et al. Atypical sleep in ICU: role of hypercapnia and sleep deprivation. Am J Resp Crit Care Med 2014;189:A3615.
28. Wang D, Piper AJ, Wong KK, et al. Slow wave sleep in patients with respiratory failure. Sleep Med 2011;12:378–83.
29. Schenck CH, Mahowald MW. Injurious sleep behavior disorders (parasomnias) affecting patients on intensive care units. Intensive Care Med 1991;17:219–24.
30. Cochen V, Arnulf I, Demeret S, et al. Vivid dreams, hallucinations, psychosis and REM sleep in Guillain-Barre syndrome. Brain 2005;128:2535–45.
31. Roche-Campo F, Drouot X, Thille AW, et al. Sleep quality for predicting noninvasive ventilation outcome in patients with acute hypercapnic respiratory failure. Crit Care Med 2010;38:705–6.
32. Ioffe S, Jansen AH, Chernick V. Hypercapnia alters sleep state pattern. Sleep 1984;7:219–22.
33. Aurell J, Elmqvist D. Sleep in the surgical intensive care unit: continuous polygraphic recording of sleep in nine patients receiving postoperative care. Br Med J (Clin Res Ed) 1985;290:1029–32.
34. Kavey NB, Ahshuler KZ. Sleep in herniorrhaphy patients. Am J Surg 1979;138:683–7.
35. Knill RL, Moote CA, Skinner MI, et al. Anesthesia with abdominal surgery leads to intense REM sleep during the first postoperative week. Anesthesiology 1990;73:52–61.
36. Orr WC, Stahl ML. Sleep disturbances after open heart surgery. Am J Cardiol 1977;39:196–201.
37. Hardin KA, Seyal M, Stewart T, et al. Sleep in critically ill chemically paralyzed patients requiring mechanical ventilation. Chest 2006;129:1468–77.
38. Fanfulla F, Ceriana P, D'Artavilla Lupo N, et al. Sleep disturbances in patients admitted to a step-down unit after ICU discharge: the role of mechanical ventilation. Sleep 2011;34:355–62.

39. Broughton R, Baron R. Sleep patterns in the intensive care unit and on the ward after acute myocardial infarction. Electroencephalogr Clin Neurophysiol 1978;45: 348–60.
40. Elliott R, McKinley S, Cistulli P, et al. Characterisation of sleep in intensive care using 24-hour polysomnography: an observational study. Crit Care 2013;17:R46.
41. Johns MW, Large AA, Masterton JP, et al. Sleep and delirium after open heart surgery. Br J Surg 1974;61:377–81.
42. Parthasarathy S, Tobin MJ. Effect of ventilator mode on sleep quality in critically ill patients. Am J Respir Crit Care Med 2002;166:1423–9.
43. Bonnet MH. Performance and sleepiness as a function of frequency and placement of sleep disruption. Psychophysiology 1986;23:263–71.
44. Drouot X, Bridoux A, Thille AW, et al. Sleep continuity: a new metric to quantify disrupted hypnograms in non-sedated intensive care unit patients. Crit Care 2014;18:628.
45. Tweedie IE, Bell CF, Clegg A, et al. Retrospective study of temperature rhythms of intensive care patients. Crit Care Med 1989;17:1159–65.
46. Gazendam JA, Van Dongen HP, Grant DA, et al. Altered circadian rhythmicity in patients in the ICU. Chest 2013;144:483–9.
47. Nuttall GA, Kumar M, Murray MJ. No difference exists in the alteration of circadian rhythm between patients with and without intensive care unit psychosis. Crit Care Med 1998;26:1351–5.
48. Claustrat B, Brun J, Chazot G. The basic physiology and pathophysiology of melatonin. Sleep Med Rev 2005;9:11–24.
49. Shilo L, Dagan Y, Smorjik Y, et al. Patients in the intensive care unit suffer from severe lack of sleep associated with loss of normal melatonin secretion pattern. Am J Med Sci 1999;317:278–81.
50. Mundigler G, Delle-Karth G, Koreny M, et al. Impaired circadian rhythm of melatonin secretion in sedated critically ill patients with severe sepsis. Crit Care Med 2002;30:536–40.
51. Frisk U, Olsson J, Nylen P, et al. Low melatonin excretion during mechanical ventilation in the intensive care unit. Clin Sci (Lond) 2004;107:47–53.
52. Gehlbach BK, Chapotot F, Leproult R, et al. Temporal disorganization of circadian rhythmicity and sleep-wake regulation in mechanically ventilated patients receiving continuous intravenous sedation. Sleep 2012;35:1105–14.
53. Olofsson K, Alling C, Lundberg D, et al. Abolished circadian rhythm of melatonin secretion in sedated and artificially ventilated intensive care patients. Acta Anaesthesiol Scand 2004;48:679–84.
54. Bourne RS, Mills GH. Melatonin: possible implications for the postoperative and critically ill patient. Intensive Care Med 2006;32:371–9.
55. Elliott R, Rai T, McKinley S. Factors affecting sleep in the critically ill: an observational study. J Crit Care 2014;29:859–63.
56. Elliott RM, McKinley SM, Eager D. A pilot study of sound levels in an Australian adult general intensive care unit. Noise Health 2010;12:26–36.
57. Freedman NS, Kotzer N, Schwab RJ. Patient perception of sleep quality and etiology of sleep disruption in the intensive care unit. Am J Respir Crit Care Med 1999;159:1155–62.
58. Meyer TJ, Eveloff SE, Bauer MS, et al. Adverse environmental conditions in the respiratory and medical ICU settings. Chest 1994;105:1211–6.
59. Walder B, Francioli D, Meyer JJ, et al. Effects of guidelines implementation in a surgical intensive care unit to control nighttime light and noise levels. Crit Care Med 2000;28:2242–7.

60. Harma MI, Ilmarinen J, Yletyinen I. Circadian variation of physiological functions in physically average and very fit dayworkers. J Hum Ergol (Tokyo) 1982; 11(Suppl):33–46.
61. Nakagawa Y. Continuous observation of EEG patterns at night and daytime of normal subjects under restrained conditions. I. Quiescent state when lying down. Electroencephalogr Clin Neurophysiol 1980;49:524–37.
62. Schweitzer P. Drugs that disturb sleep and wakefulness. In: Kryger MH, Roth T, Dement WC, editors. Principles and practices of sleep medicine. 4th edition. Philadelphia: Elsevier; 2005. p. 499.
63. Achermann P, Borbely AA. Dynamics of EEG slow wave activity during physiological sleep and after administration of benzodiazepine hypnotics. Hum Neurobiol 1987;6:203–10.
64. Borbely AA, Mattmann P, Loepfe M, et al. Effect of benzodiazepine hypnotics on all-night sleep EEG spectra. Hum Neurobiol 1985;4:189–94.
65. Wilson S, Argyropoulos S. Antidepressants and sleep: a qualitative review of the literature. Drugs 2005;65:927–47.
66. Winkelman JW, James L. Serotonergic antidepressants are associated with REM sleep without atonia. Sleep 2004;27:317–21.
67. Gimenez S, Clos S, Romero S, et al. Effects of olanzapine, risperidone and haloperidol on sleep after a single oral morning dose in healthy volunteers. Psychopharmacology (Berl) 2007;190:507–16.
68. Bourne RS, Mills GH. Sleep disruption in critically ill patients–pharmacological considerations. Anaesthesia 2004;59:374–84.
69. Legros B, Bazil CW. Effects of antiepileptic drugs on sleep architecture: a pilot study. Sleep Med 2003;4:51–5.
70. Placidi F, Scalise A, Marciani MG, et al. Effect of antiepileptic drugs on sleep. Clin Neurophysiol 2000;111(Suppl 2):S115–9.
71. Cronin AJ, Keifer JC, Davies MF, et al. Postoperative sleep disturbance: influences of opioids and pain in humans. Sleep 2001;24:39–44.
72. Cammarano WB, Pittet JF, Weitz S, et al. Acute withdrawal syndrome related to the administration of analgesic and sedative medications in adult intensive care unit patients. Crit Care Med 1998;26:676–84.
73. Tung A, Lynch JP, Mendelson WB. Prolonged sedation with propofol in the rat does not result in sleep deprivation. Anesth Analg 2001;92:1232–6.
74. Tung A, Bergmann BM, Herrera S, et al. Recovery from sleep deprivation occurs during propofol anesthesia. Anesthesiology 2004;100:1419–26.
75. Kondili E, Alexopoulou C, Xirouchaki N, et al. Effects of propofol on sleep quality in mechanically ventilated critically ill patients: a physiological study. Intensive Care Med 2012;38:1640–6.
76. Van Dongen HP, Maislin G, Mullington JM, et al. The cumulative cost of additional wakefulness: dose-response effects on neurobehavioral functions and sleep physiology from chronic sleep restriction and total sleep deprivation. Sleep 2003;26:117–26.
77. Bryant PA, Trinder J, Curtis N. Sick and tired: does sleep have a vital role in the immune system? Nat Rev Immunol 2004;4:457–67.
78. Dinges DF, Douglas SD, Zaugg L, et al. Leukocytosis and natural killer cell function parallel neurobehavioral fatigue induced by 64 hours of sleep deprivation. J Clin Invest 1994;93:1930–9.
79. Born J, Lange T, Hansen K, et al. Effects of sleep and circadian rhythm on human circulating immune cells. J Immunol 1997;158:4454–64.

80. Spiegel K, Sheridan JF, Van Cauter E. Effect of sleep deprivation on response to immunization. JAMA 2002;288:1471–2.
81. Friese RS, Bruns B, Sinton CM. Sleep deprivation after septic insult increases mortality independent of age. J Trauma 2009;66:50–4.
82. Cooper KR, Phillips BA. Effect of short-term sleep loss on breathing. J Appl Physiol Respir Environ Exerc Physiol 1982;53:855–8.
83. Schiffman PL, Trontell MC, Mazar MF, et al. Sleep deprivation decreases ventilatory response to CO_2 but not load compensation. Chest 1983;84:695–8.
84. White DP, Douglas NJ, Pickett CK, et al. Sleep deprivation and the control of ventilation. Am Rev Respir Dis 1983;128:984–6.
85. Chen HI, Tang YR. Sleep loss impairs inspiratory muscle endurance. Am Rev Respir Dis 1989;140:907–9.
86. Durmer JS, Dinges DF. Neurocognitive consequences of sleep deprivation. Semin Neurol 2005;25:117–29.
87. Babkoff H, Sing HC, Thorne DR, et al. Perceptual distortions and hallucinations reported during the course of sleep deprivation. Percept Mot Skills 1989;68:787–98.
88. Watson PL, Ceriana P, Fanfulla F. Delirium: is sleep important? Best Pract Res Clin Anaesthesiol 2012;26:355–66.

Circadian Dysrhythmias in the Intensive Care Unit

Martha E. Billings, MD, MSc[a],*, Nathaniel F. Watson, MD, MSc[b]

KEYWORDS

- Critical care • Mechanical ventilation • Circadian rhythm • Melatonin

KEY POINTS

- Circadian abnormalities are widespread because of uniform sleep disruption and aberrant sleep architecture in the intensive care unit (ICU).
- Circadian dysrhythmias develop due to critical illness as well as the ICU environment and therapies (mechanical ventilation [MV], sedation).
- Sleep and circadian rhythms should be addressed by ICU providers as an aspect of care to restore health and physiologic homeostasis.
- Changes to the ICU environment, use of natural light, and administration of melatonin in the evening may improve circadian alignment.

INTRODUCTION
Circadian Physiology

All physiologic functions have an endogenous rhythm, which is modulated by neuro-endocrine signals and is regulated by the circadian clock. The rhythms are entrained to their natural environment by light, feeding, and other social cues with light being the most important factor. The principal clock resides in the suprachiasmatic nucleus (SCN) within the hypothalamus and serves as the master pacemaker for the individual. The SCN not only determines the timing of sleep and wakefulness but also regulates other circadian rhythms that are independent of sleep such as cortisol levels, core body temperature (CBT), and melatonin release.[1] The SCN coordinates the peripheral oscillators found in every organ and tissue via neurohormones and aligns these peripheral clocks to the central rhythm (**Fig. 1**).[2] On the cellular level, approximately 15% of gene expression as well as protein and lipid production are under circadian control, which are highly conserved across species.[3]

Disclosures: The authors report no commercial or financial conflicts of interest relevant to this article.
[a] Division of Pulmonary Critical Care Medicine, UW Medicine Sleep Center at Harborview, University of Washington, 325 Ninth Avenue, Box 359803, Seattle, WA 98104, USA; [b] Department of Neurology, University of Washington, UW Medicine Sleep Center, Seattle, WA 98104, USA
* Corresponding author.
E-mail address: mebillin@uw.edu

Crit Care Clin 31 (2015) 393–402
http://dx.doi.org/10.1016/j.ccc.2015.03.006
0749-0704/15/$ – see front matter © 2015 Elsevier Inc. All rights reserved.

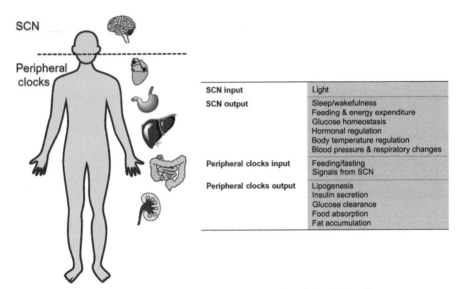

SCN

Peripheral clocks

SCN input	Light
SCN output	Sleep/wakefulness Feeding & energy expenditure Glucose homeostasis Hormonal regulation Body temperature regulation Blood pressure & respiratory changes
Peripheral clocks input	Feeding/fasting Signals from SCN
Peripheral clocks output	Lipogenesis Insulin secretion Glucose clearance Food absorption Fat accumulation

Fig. 1. The SCN is the master clock that regulates peripheral clocks in other organ systems and sets the circadian rhythm of temperature, sleep/wake, and metabolic, neuroendocrine and cardiovascular regulation via the peripheral clock output. (*From* Griffett K, Burris TP. The mammalian clock and chronopharmacology. Bioorg Med Chem Lett 2013;23:1929–34; with permission.)

Although circadian variation in blood pressure, CBT, urine output, lung function, metabolism, coagulation, and immune response is well established,[4] the clinical implications of this on disease manifestation and monitoring have been overlooked. The circadian pattern in heart attacks and asthma flares may reflect circadian changes in immune parameters such as cytokine release, leukocyte tissue migration, and T-helper response. Disease onset may also be timed by increases in sympathetic nervous system output resulting in bronchial constriction and higher blood pressure.[5] Asthmatic airways have greater circadian variability in peak flow. Lung inflammatory response to viruses and antigens may also be influenced by circadian factors.[6]

The circadian nature of physiology has profound implications for critical care. Circadian abnormalities can lead to derangements in physiologic homeostasis and affect critical illness. Patient assessments of temperature, blood pressure, metabolism, and lung function are often made disregarding circadian time, which limits comparability. Drug efficacy may differ depending on the timing of administration because immune response, metabolic function, hormones, and pharmacokinetics have circadian variation.[7] The developing field of chronopharmacology addressing this has not yet translated into the ICU. Furthermore, a patient with circadian abnormalities may be at greater risk for delirium, prolonged ICU stay, and morbidity.[8] Awareness of the intrinsic circadian rhythm of the patient in ICU has clinical relevance.

Circadian Disruption in the Intensive Care Unit

Sleep in the ICU is aberrant in timing, architecture, and amount. Studies using polysomnography (PSG) monitoring in the ICU show an absence of circadian sleep pattern with 50% of sleep in the daytime.[9] Perception of sleep by staff is inaccurate and typically grossly overestimated.[10] Sleep architecture is aberrant with rapid eye movement (REM) and slow wave (N3) sleep lacking and severe sleep fragmentation common.[11,12]

This pattern was observed in non–critically ill patients recovering from major noncardiac surgery in the surgical ICU, who underwent 24-h PSG monitoring for 2 to 4 days (**Fig. 2**).[10] This finding was replicated in 22 patients in medical ICU, 20 of whom were on MV but not on sedation.[13] This pattern has also been borne out in studies of children in the pediatric ICU, primarily patients with burn.[14]

Investigating sleep architecture in the ICU is challenging because of the encephalopathic electroencephalographic (EEG) pattern commonly seen in critically ill patients (**Fig. 3**). Differentiation of wake from sleep and staging sleep is nearly impossible with this pattern.[13,15,16] This EEG pattern is more prevalent in sepsis; it may predate septic physiology and resolve with improvement in sepsis.[13] Some have attempted alternative methods to stage sleep including spectral analysis of absolute delta activity.[15] Others have proposed a new scoring system to classify the atypical EEG patterns common to sedated, critical ill patients including polymorphic delta, burst suppression, and isoelectric pattern.[17]

Cause of Circadian Dysrhythmias in the Intensive Care Unit

The ICU environment is intrinsically detrimental to natural circadian rhythms (**Box 1**). Daylight is often obscured by lack of windows, and artificial lighting persists into the night. Studies measuring ambient light exposure do reveal dimness at night in the ICU[15] but with large variations as well as nighttime periods with light levels known to impact the circadian pacemaker.[18] Noises ranging from staff conversations to ventilator alarms are constant. Studies measuring noise in the ICU found mean levels exceeding Environmental Protection Agency recommendations for both day and night.[13] Other social circadian cues are absent, because feedings may be continuous and nursing and respiratory care continues 24 hours a day. Medications commonly administered in the ICU such as sedatives, analgesics, and vasoactive drugs may all affect sleep and circadian rhythms.[16,19] Physical symptoms of dyspnea, anxiety, and pain associated with critical illness and postoperative recovery may also compromise circadian rhythms and disrupt sleep (**Fig. 4**).

MV has been attributed to sleep and circadian rhythm disruption. MV ideally allows respiratory muscle rest and recovery by reducing work of breathing, improving gas exchange, and minimizing anxiety associated with dyspnea. However, with ventilator asynchrony and alarms, patients on MV have poor-quality sleep with frequent arousals

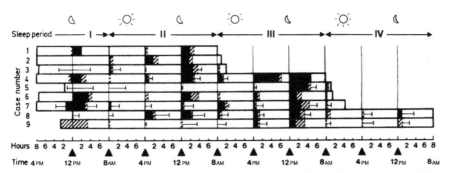

Fig. 2. Continuous PSG recording of patients in the surgical ICU showing lack of sleep consolidation, deprivation, and abnormal sleep architecture. (*From* Aurell J, Elmqvist D. Sleep in the surgical intensive care unit: continuous polygraphic recording of sleep in nine patients receiving postoperative care. Br Med J (Clin Res Ed) 1985;290:1031; with permission.)

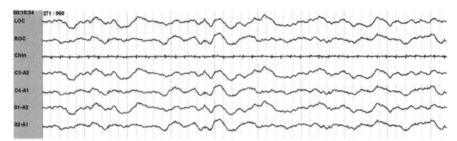

Fig. 3. Example 30-second epoch of encephalopathic EEG pattern seen in critically ill pa-tients, typically with sepsis and on sedation. (*From* Weinhouse GL, Watson PL. Sedation and sleep disturbances in the ICU. Crit Care Clin 2009;25:539–49, ix; with permission.)

as well as nonconsolidated and fragmented sleep.[20] Patients on MV also had much more daytime sleep, less slow wave sleep, and more fragmented sleep than healthy subjects in the same environment. In patients on MV, ICU factors such as noise and patient care did not seem to be major contributors to sleep disruption (17% noise arousal in patients on MV vs 68% in healthy subjects monitored in the ICU for 24 hours).[9] Multiple studies have investigated the impact of the mode of MV on sleep and circadian rhythm.[21–24] Pressure support (PS) mode during sleep was found to contribute to sleep disruption by causing relative hyperventilation and precipitating central apneas; this was reduced by adding dead space.[24] Proportional assist venti-lation (PAV) was found to be preferable to PS because it improved patient-ventilator synchrony.[22] As both PAV and PS can induce periodic breathing, most recommend resting on assist control at night to improve sleep quality and reduce arousals from central apneas.[20] For patients off sedation who have a tracheostomy in place with pro-longed weaning, MV during the night improved sleep quantity versus spontaneous breathing.[21] Thus respiratory support that does not induce hyperventilation or hypo-ventilation may improve sleep quality and help restore natural circadian sleep rhythm. In addition, MV and/or tracheostomy can treat any underlying obstructive sleep apnea that may disrupt sleep.

MV may not be the culprit of circadian misalignment. In long-term acute care facil-ities (LTACs), where residents are typically on long-term ventilator weans, abnormal-ities in circadian rhythm have not been observed. One study of 15 patients in LTAC recovering from critical illness found a normal circadian activity pattern via actigraphy, which was in phase with environmental cues and light level variation.[25] The

---

Box 1
Factors contributing to circadian disruption in the ICU

- Excessive artificial light/lack of natural light
- Noise
- Ventilator asynchrony and mode
- Patient care activity
- Psychosocial stress and physical pain
- Critical illness
- Medications

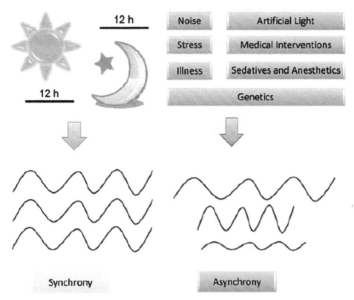

Fig. 4. Schematic of the effects of the ICU environment and illness on circadian alignment. (*From* Brainard J, Gobel M, Bartels K, et al. Circadian rhythms in anesthesia and critical care medicine: potential importance of circadian disruptions. Semin Cardiothorac Vasc Anesth 2015;19:54; with permission.)

environmental factors disrupting circadian rhythms in the ICU may not be present in LTACs. These patients are on MV, but typically have tracheostomies, do not receive continuous sedation, and have much lower nursing care needs than in the ICU. These patients are also not otherwise critically ill and may be able to participate in rehabilitation and be active in the daytime. The improved zeitgebers (eg, stimulus or cue that synchronizes the internal pacemaker) in LTACs, which include timed meals, rehabilitation therapy, light, and other social cues (and the patient's ability to respond to them), likely hasten the recovery from critical illness.

Abnormalities in Melatonin

Further circadian disruption may result from the intrinsic effects of critical illness, ICU medications, and environment on melatonin release. Circadian melatonin patterns have been noted to be abnormal in multiple studies in the ICU.[15,26–29] Most demonstrate a lack or attenuation of melatonin acrophase (peak) during the night compared with the day. Abolished serum circadian melatonin patterns, measured every 2 hours, were seen in 24 critically ill patients on continuous sedation; it was more pronounced in those with brain injury.[28] In a seminal study by Mundigler and colleagues,[29] septic patients in the ICU were found to lack a circadian pattern to melatonin secretion compared with nonseptic patients in the ICU. Melatonin levels as measured by 6-sulfatoxymelatonin (aMT6) excretion in the urine every 4 hours did not have a circadian rhythm in 16 of 17 septic patients compared with 7 nonseptic patients in the ICU, both groups receiving sedation. A more recent study investigating mechanically ventilated patients in the ICU did not replicate this finding among septic patients. However, investigators did find that most patients in the ICU had circadian melatonin misalignment. Patients exhibited primarily a phase delay pattern of their aMT6 excretion, which was not aligned with slow wave activity on EEG spectral analysis.[15] These studies were small observational studies (less than 25 patients) and subject to many potential confounders including use of sedation, vasoactive medications, type of illness and its severity, and light exposure. There are also many methodological differences in melatonin assays, sampling frequency, and duration perhaps accounting for the differences in results.

Critical illness and sepsis with the resulting neurohormonal dysregulation may also contribute to circadian dysrhythmias in the ICU. In a small study of 24 critically ill patients, researchers found no circadian pattern to cortisol release or cardiovascular parameters.[28] This result was not replicated in a much larger study that modeled circadian rhythm using ICU physiologic data from 14,705 patients. Variations in blood pressure and heart rate were found, although attenuated. However, this rhythm was lost in sepsis nonsurvivors, indicating that circadian cardiovascular variation is a potential biomarker of ICU survival in this group.[30]

CBT reaches its nadir in a circadian manner in the early morning.[1] The pattern persists even with febrile illness. CBT nadir can be used to identify the end of circadian night, and in patients in the ICU, the degree of CBT displacement from early morning is associated with illness severity.[31] These derangements in circadian rhythm are seen in experimental models of sepsis in humans and rats.[32,33] Furthermore, experimental response to endotoxin is modulated by circadian time.[34] Molecular studies demonstrate a link between immune response and circadian rhythm, with disruptions associated with disease.[35]

Management Goals

When treating patients in the ICU, providers should seek to enable consolidated sleep and restoration of circadian rhythm to both central and peripheral clocks. Primary to that goal is awareness of circadian rhythms including absence and misalignment. Unfortunately, evaluating sleep and circadian alignment is currently not feasible in the ICU outside of the research setting. Future investigation is needed to allow critical care teams to assess and enhance circadian alignment. Efforts should be made to enhance natural zietgebers (daylight, daytime activity off sedation, feeding, and other cues) to maintain rhythm entrainment and nighttime sleep.

Pharmacologic Strategies

- Melatonin
- Sedation minimization

Melatonin secretion is abnormal in timing and amplitude, with a blunting because of circadian rhythm derangement in the ICU. It is postulated that abnormalities in melatonin (as well as concomitant sleep deprivation) may contribute to ICU delirium.[36] Recent studies have assessed administering melatonin to help enhance circadian alignment and improve sleep. A small randomized control trial of patients undergoing tracheotomy in the ICU (nonsedated) showed improved nocturnal sleep with melatonin administration.[37] Melatonin has also been shown in animals to modulate immune response to endotoxemia, a model of sepsis.[38,39] Thus melatonin may be an underused tool in the ICU to promote healthy circadian rhythms with the potential to improve innate immunity.

Sedation, although it generates a state similar to sleep, is not equal to natural sleep, lacking circadian and ultradian pattern. Sleep provides a restorative function, essential for life. Benzodiazepines and opioids are known to reduce REM sleep and slow wave sleep (N3), the most restorative form of sleep.[19] Studies have found a lack of slow wave (N3) and REM sleep and only 2 to 3 hours of light sleep in patients in the ICU on continuous sedation who seemed to be sleeping.[40] Excess sedation may actually result in sleep deprivation and worsen circadian abnormalities. Excess sedation, primarily with anticholinergic agents and benzodiazepines, is associated with delirium, prolonged ICU length of stay, and prolonged days on MV. The effect of sedating medications in further reducing restorative slow wave (N3) sleep and REM sleep may augment this effect by contributing to relative sleep deprivation.[8,41] Consensus statements recommend minimizing sedation, eliminating continuous sedation to reduce delirium, and improve outcomes.[42] Allowing natural sleep and daytime alertness by reducing sedation may also improve circadian alignment.

Nonpharmacologic Strategies

- Diurnal daylight/blue light exposure
- Noise minimization, especially at night
- Meal time feeding/noncontinuous feeds

Light, blue spectrum (459–483 nm), is the most powerful entrainment signal, aligning intrinsic rhythm to the environment. Light can acutely suppress melatonin, regulate cortisol rhythm, and elevate body temperature and heart rate. Light has subjective benefits of improving alertness, improving mood and performance, and decreasing daytime sleepiness.[43] Exposure to daylight was found to reduce the odds of delirium among patients in the ICU.[44] Postoperative patients recovering from spinal surgery required less opioids in bright sunny rooms compared to dim rooms.[45] In a natural experiment, patients in the cardiac care unit recovering from myocardial infarction in sunny rooms had a shorter length of stay and lower mortality than those in dull rooms.[46] This result was not replicated in a study of patients with subarachnoid hemorrhage.[47] A recent larger study investigating the effect of light in the ICU found that outdoor light intensity did not affect measured light intensity at the ICU bed. Even in rooms with windows, there was limited diurnal variation and an overall low light intensity.[48] The hospital built environment, designing ICU rooms to allow exposure to natural daylight and window views from bed, may be another avenue to enhance circadian alignment. Further study on the effect of blue spectrum light on ICU outcomes is warranted.

Reducing nighttime noise that may disrupt sleep and further erode circadian rhythm may be another necessary ICU environment change. A simple intervention, using ear plugs, was found to reduce ICU delirium. Patients were randomized to wear ear plugs at night or not. Those wearing ear plugs had a lower odds of developing delirium and had subjectively better sleep.[49] White noise, acoustic foams to absorb noise in neonatal incubators, and implementing quiet times are other methods that have been shown to improve sleep.[50] The impact of noise reduction on circadian rhythm has not been evaluated.

Finally, implementing consistent meal times may improve circadian rhythm. Digestion, lipid metabolism, as well as liver and pancreatic function all have an intrinsic circadian rhythm. Traditional continuous tube feeds and parenteral nutrition abolish these natural rhythms and variations in bile acid synthesis, insulin secretion, and glycogen production, which typically occur primarily in the daytime. Nighttime is a period of fasting with gluconeogenesis and lipid catabolism. Circadian realignment may be enhanced by time-restricted feeding that parallels natural meal time during the day and fasting during the night. Time-restricted feeding may enhance peripheral metabolic entrainment.[2]

SUMMARY/DISCUSSION

The literature supports significant alteration in circadian rhythm in the ICU. There is evidence of misalignment, from the reduction in amplitude of melatonin acrophase and other circadian biomarkers to abolishment of rhythm. The evidence suggests some association between the degree of circadian pathology and critical illness severity. This result parallels that of animal model work showing circadian variation in immunity and response to illness. It is currently unclear if the circadian dysrhythmia is primarily intrinsic to critical illness or is a consequence of treatments including MV, sedative and vasoactive drugs, and the ICU environment. Most likely it is a combination of these factors. The research is still in its infancy because studies are just beginning to illuminate the role of circadian physiology on critical illness and recovery. Future research is required to enable clinicians to evaluate their patients' circadian rhythm or lack thereof at the bedside. Further investigations are needed to evaluate the efficacy of any interventions in improving circadian rhythm and the impact on ICU outcomes and long-term morbidity.

REFERENCES

1. Hastings M, O'Neill JS, Maywood ES. Circadian clocks: regulators of endocrine and metabolic rhythms. J Endocrinol 2007;195:187–98.
2. Sunderram J, Sofou S, Kamisoglu K, et al. Time-restricted feeding and the realignment of biological rhythms: translational opportunities and challenges. J Transl Med 2014;12:79.
3. Dallmann R, Viola AU, Tarokh L, et al. The human circadian metabolome. Proc Natl Acad Sci U S A 2012;109:2625–9.
4. Chan MC, Spieth PM, Quinn K, et al. Circadian rhythms: from basic mechanisms to the intensive care unit. Crit Care Med 2012;40:246–53.
5. Scheiermann C, Kunisaki Y, Frenette PS. Circadian control of the immune system. Nat Rev Immunol 2013;13:190–8.
6. Durrington HJ, Farrow SN, Loudon AS, et al. The circadian clock and asthma. Thorax 2014;69:90–2.
7. Dallmann R, Brown SA, Gachon F. Chronopharmacology: new insights and therapeutic implications. Annu Rev Pharmacol Toxicol 2014;54:339–61.
8. Weinhouse GL, Schwab RJ, Watson PL, et al. Bench-to-bedside review: delirium in ICU patients - importance of sleep deprivation. Crit Care 2009;13:234.
9. Gabor JY, Cooper AB, Crombach SA, et al. Contribution of the intensive care unit environment to sleep disruption in mechanically ventilated patients and healthy subjects. Am J Respir Crit Care Med 2003;167:708–15.
10. Aurell J, Elmqvist D. Sleep in the surgical intensive care unit: continuous polygraphic recording of sleep in nine patients receiving postoperative care. Br Med J (Clin Res Ed) 1985;290:1029–32.
11. Hilton BA. Quantity and quality of patients' sleep and sleep-disturbing factors in a respiratory intensive care unit. J Adv Nurs 1976;1:453–68.
12. Broughton R, Baron R. Sleep patterns in the intensive care unit and on the ward after acute myocardial infarction. Electroencephalogr Clin Neurophysiol 1978;45:348–60.
13. Freedman NS, Gazendam J, Levan L, et al. Abnormal sleep/wake cycles and the effect of environmental noise on sleep disruption in the intensive care unit. Am J Respir Crit Care Med 2001;163:451–7.
14. Kudchadkar SR, Aljohani OA, Punjabi NM. Sleep of critically ill children in the pediatric intensive care unit: a systematic review. Sleep Med Rev 2014;18:103–10.

15. Gehlbach BK, Chapotot F, Leproult R, et al. Temporal disorganization of circadian rhythmicity and sleep-wake regulation in mechanically ventilated patients receiving continuous intravenous sedation. Sleep 2012;35:1105–14.

16. Weinhouse GL, Watson PL. Sedation and sleep disturbances in the ICU. Crit Care Clin 2009;25:539–49, ix.

17. Watson PL, Pandharipande P, Gehlbach BK, et al. Atypical sleep in ventilated patients: empirical electroencephalography findings and the path toward revised ICU sleep scoring criteria. Crit Care Med 2013;41:1958–67.

18. Pulak LM, Jensen L. Sleep in the intensive care unit: a review. J Intensive Care Med 2014. [Epub ahead of print].

19. Weinhouse GL. Pharmacology I: effects on sleep of commonly used ICU medications. Crit Care Clin 2008;24:477–91, vi.

20. Ozsancak A, D'Ambrosio C, Garpestad E, et al. Sleep and mechanical ventilation. Crit Care Clin 2008;24:517–31, vi–vii.

21. Roche-Campo F, Thille AW, Drouot X, et al. Comparison of sleep quality with mechanical versus spontaneous ventilation during weaning of critically ill tracheostomized patients. Crit Care Med 2013;41:1637–44.

22. Bosma K, Ferreyra G, Ambrogio C, et al. Patient-ventilator interaction and sleep in mechanically ventilated patients: pressure support versus proportional assist ventilation. Crit Care Med 2007;35:1048–54.

23. Cabello B, Thille AW, Drouot X, et al. Sleep quality in mechanically ventilated patients: comparison of three ventilatory modes. Crit Care Med 2008;36:1749–55.

24. Parthasarathy S, Tobin MJ. Effect of ventilator mode on sleep quality in critically ill patients. Am J Respir Crit Care Med 2002;166:1423–9.

25. Koldobskiy D, Diaz-Abad M, Scharf SM, et al. Long-term acute care patients weaning from prolonged mechanical ventilation maintain circadian rhythm. Respir Care 2014;59:518–24.

26. Frisk U, Olsson J, Nylen P, et al. Low melatonin excretion during mechanical ventilation in the intensive care unit. Clin Sci (Lond) 2004;107:47–53.

27. Shilo L, Dagan Y, Smorjik Y, et al. Patients in the intensive care unit suffer from severe lack of sleep associated with loss of normal melatonin secretion pattern. Am J Med Sci 1999;317:278–81.

28. Paul T, Lemmer B. Disturbance of circadian rhythms in analgosedated intensive care unit patients with and without craniocerebral injury. Chronobiol Int 2007;24:45–61.

29. Mundigler G, Delle-Karth G, Koreny M, et al. Impaired circadian rhythm of melatonin secretion in sedated critically ill patients with severe sepsis. Crit Care Med 2002;30:536–40.

30. George ZC, Zhengbo Z, Mohammad G, et al. Modeling Circadian Rhythm Variations During Sepsis. B105 Sepsis: Care Models And Outcomes: American Thoracic Society 2014;189:A3795. [abstract].

31. Gazendam JA, Van Dongen HP, Grant DA, et al. Altered circadian rhythmicity in patients in the ICU. Chest 2013;144:483–9.

32. Baracchi F, Ingiosi AM, Raymond RM Jr, et al. Sepsis-induced alterations in sleep of rats. Am J Physiol Regul Integr Comp Physiol 2011;301:R1467–78.

33. Li CX, Liang DD, Xie GH, et al. Altered melatonin secretion and circadian gene expression with increased proinflammatory cytokine expression in early-stage sepsis patients. Mol Med Rep 2013;7:1117–22.

34. Alamili M, Bendtzen K, Lykkesfeldt J, et al. Pronounced inflammatory response to endotoxaemia during nighttime: a randomised cross-over trial. PLoS One 2014;9:e87413.

35. Arjona A, Silver AC, Walker WE, et al. Immunity's fourth dimension: approaching the circadian-immune connection. Trends Immunol 2012;33:607–12.
36. Bellapart J, Boots R. Potential use of melatonin in sleep and delirium in the critically ill. Br J Anaesth 2012;108:572–80.
37. Bourne RS, Mills GH, Minelli C. Melatonin therapy to improve nocturnal sleep in critically ill patients: encouraging results from a small randomised controlled trial. Crit Care 2008;12:R52.
38. Alamili M, Klein M, Lykkesfeldt J, et al. Circadian variation in the response to experimental endotoxemia and modulatory effects of exogenous melatonin. Chronobiol Int 2013;30:1174–80.
39. Alamili M, Bendtzen K, Lykkesfeldt J, et al. Melatonin suppresses markers of inflammation and oxidative damage in a human daytime endotoxemia model. J Crit Care 2014;29:184.e9–13.
40. Andersen JH, Boesen HC, Skovgaard Olsen K. Sleep in the intensive care unit measured by polysomnography. Minerva Anestesiol 2013;79:804–15.
41. Watson PL, Ceriana P, Fanfulla F. Delirium: is sleep important? Best Pract Res Clin Anaesthesiol 2012;26:355–66.
42. Barr J, Fraser GL, Puntillo K, et al. Clinical practice guidelines for the management of pain, agitation, and delirium in adult patients in the intensive care unit. Crit Care Med 2013;41:263–306.
43. Castro R, Angus DC, Rosengart MR. The effect of light on critical illness. Crit Care 2011;15:218.
44. Van Rompaey B, Elseviers MM, Schuurmans MJ, et al. Risk factors for delirium in intensive care patients: a prospective cohort study. Crit Care 2009;13:R77.
45. Walch JM, Rabin BS, Day R, et al. The effect of sunlight on postoperative analgesic medication use: a prospective study of patients undergoing spinal surgery. Psychosom Med 2005;67:156–63.
46. Beauchemin KM, Hays P. Dying in the dark: sunshine, gender and outcomes in myocardial infarction. J R Soc Med 1998;91:352–4.
47. Wunsch H, Gershengorn H, Mayer SA, et al. The effect of window rooms on critically ill patients with subarachnoid hemorrhage admitted to intensive care. Crit Care 2011;15:R81.
48. Castro RA, Angus DC, Hong SY, et al. Light and the outcome of the critically ill: an observational cohort study. Crit Care 2012;16:R132.
49. Van Rompaey B, Elseviers MM, Van Drom W, et al. The effect of earplugs during the night on the onset of delirium and sleep perception: a randomized controlled trial in intensive care patients. Crit Care 2012;16:R73.
50. Xie H, Kang J, Mills GH. Clinical review: the impact of noise on patients' sleep and the effectiveness of noise reduction strategies in intensive care units. Crit Care 2009;13:208.

Sleep and the Endocrine System

Dionne Morgan, MBBS[a], Sheila C. Tsai, MD[a,b],*

KEYWORDS

- Circadian rhythms • Sleep apnea • Endocrine abnormalities • Hormonal regulation
- Sleep disorders • Sleep deprivation • Critical illness • Critical care

KEY POINTS

- The endocrine system is influenced by both circadian rhythms and sleep-wake state.
- Hormonal abnormalities can contribute to sleep disruption and disorders.
- Sleep disorders can lead to hormonal dysregulation, resulting in endocrine abnormalities.
- Sleep fragmentation and deprivation are common in critically ill patients and may be associated with various hormonal disturbances.

INTRODUCTION

The endocrine system is a group of specialized organs or glands that secrete hormones directly into the circulation. These hormones are instrumental in growth, metabolism, and maintaining homeostasis. Similarly, sleep plays an important role in human homeostasis. Some hormonal secretion patterns are controlled mainly by the body's internal circadian pacemaker, located in the hypothalamus within the suprachiasmatic nucleus (SCN), whereas other hormones are primarily affected by the sleep-wake state. Sleep and the endocrine system are closely intertwined, with many hormonal secretions influenced by sleep. In addition, sleep quality and duration affect hormonal function such that sleep disorders and sleep fragmentation can contribute to endocrine abnormalities. Conversely, endocrine dysfunction can significantly affect sleep. In this article, the effect of sleep and sleep disorders on endocrine function and the influence of endocrine abnormalities on sleep are discussed. Sleep disruption and its associated endocrine consequences in the critically ill patient are also reviewed.

Disclosure statement: The authors do not have any commercial or financial conflicts of interest pertaining to this article.
[a] Department of Medicine, National Jewish Health, 1400 Jackson Street, A02, Denver, CO 80206, USA; [b] University of Colorado Denver, Aurora, CO 80045, USA
* Corresponding author.
E-mail address: tsais@njhealth.org

CIRCADIAN RHYTHM AND SLEEP-WAKE STATE CONTROL OF HORMONAL SECRETION

The primarily circadian-regulated hormones include those produced by the hypothalamic-pituitary axis, such as adrenocorticotropic hormone (ACTH) and cortisol, thyroid stimulating hormone, and melatonin. Growth hormone (GH), prolactin (PRL), and renin secretion are sleep related. Sleep, especially slow wave sleep (SWS), is associated with increased GH, growth hormone–releasing hormone (GHRH), and ghrelin levels.

Adrenocorticotropic Hormone and Cortisol

The hypothalamic-pituitary-adrenal axis (HPA) is primarily under circadian rhythm control. Cortisol and ACTH levels peak in the early morning and decline during the day. The primary circadian control is evidenced by the fact that daytime sleep does not significantly inhibit cortisol secretion. This diurnal variation in cortisol secretion persists even when sleep is altered and is not significantly affected by the absence of sleep or by sleep at an unusual time of day. The 24-hour periodicity of corticotropic activity is therefore primarily controlled by circadian rhythmicity.

However, secretion is also weakly modulated by the sleep-wake state. Sleep onset is normally associated with a decrease in cortisol secretion and nadir levels of cortisol and ACTH levels occur during the first part of sleep. Cortisol secretion is already low in the late evening, and sleep initiation results in prolongation of the low secretory state. At the end of sleep, morning awakening is associated with a burst of cortisol secretion. In sleep deprivation, the cortisol secretion pattern seems to be dampened such that the nadir of cortisol secretion is higher and the maximum morning cortisol level is lower than during nocturnal sleep.[1]

Melatonin

Melatonin release is controlled by the light-dark cycle and SCN through a series of complex polysynaptic pathways. It is produced and released from the pineal gland directly into the blood and cerebrospinal fluid. Melatonin levels start to increase in the evening and peak in the early morning. Melatonin is postulated to promote sleep by decreasing the firing rate of SCN neurons. Its production is suppressed by exposure to bright light.

Thyroid-Stimulating Hormone

Thyroid-stimulating hormone (TSH) is primarily under circadian control but is significantly influenced by the sleep-wake state. During daylight, TSH levels are low and stable. Starting in the early evening, TSH levels increase quickly and peak shortly before sleep onset. Sleep inhibits TSH levels from increasing further. Therefore, sleep has an inhibitory effect on TSH secretion, most notable during SWS. During the latter part of the sleep period, there is a progressive decline in TSH levels. The circadian effect on TSH secretion is predominant with some influence from sleep. For example, sleep deprivation results in higher TSH levels during the night because of the lack of sleep's inhibitory effect. But this inhibitory effect of sleep on TSH secretion seems to depend on time of day because daytime sleep does not seem to have this same suppressive effect on daytime TSH secretion.

Growth Hormone

GH secretion is largely influenced by sleep. The release of GH from the anterior pituitary gland is stimulated by hypothalamic GHRH and inhibited by somatostatin. In addition, ghrelin, a peptide produced by the stomach, acts as a potent endogenous stimulus for GH secretion by binding to the GH secretagogue receptor. GH secretion increases during sleep with less influence by the time of day. The sleep-onset GH pulse is the largest in men. Most GH secretion is associated with SWS (stage N3), although GH secretion also occurs in the absence of SWS. The amount of GH secretion closely correlates with the duration of stage N3 sleep. In older age, both N3 sleep and GH release decrease.

Prolactin

PRL secretion is strongly linked to sleep. Levels increase shortly after sleep, regardless of the time of day, although this stimulatory effect is greatest at night. During nocturnal sleep, the PRL levels peak around the middle of the sleep period. Awakenings associated with sleep disruption inhibit nocturnal PRL release. Therefore, the secretion of PRL is mainly sleep dependent.

In addition, a potential role of PRL in regulating rapid eye movement (REM) or SWS has been suggested because of a close temporal relationship between increased PRL secretion and SWS. However, this correlation is not as close as that seen with GH, and the normal secretory pattern of PRL does not decline with age despite a decline in SWS.

Gonadotropic Hormones

Gonadotropic hormone secretion seems to have both circadian rhythmicity and sleep influences. Gonadotropin-releasing hormone from the hypothalamus controls the secretion of luteinizing hormone (LH) and follicle-stimulating hormone (FSH) by the anterior pituitary. In men, LH is responsible for testosterone secretion, whereas FSH stimulates spermatogenesis. In women, the gonadotropins regulate the release of estrogen and progesterone and control the menstrual cycle.

The 24-hour patterns of gonadotropin release and gonadal steroid levels vary according to gender and the stage of life. There is a pulsatile increase in LH and FSH levels at sleep onset in children. As the child approaches puberty, the amplitude of the nocturnal pulses increases, which is one marker of puberty.

Testosterone production varies diurnally, but its production depends directly on sleep, with testosterone levels normally increasing at sleep onset. In young adult men, a notable diurnal rhythm in circulating testosterone levels exists, with minimal levels in the late evening and a clear nocturnal increase leading to maximal levels in the early morning. Approximately 3 hours of SWS is required, irrespective of whether it occurs during the day or at night, for peak testosterone production to occur, and levels remain stable thereafter while sleep is maintained. After waking, the plasma concentration of testosterone declines in proportion to the duration of time awake.[2] With sleep fragmentation experiments, the nocturnal increase in testosterone is attenuated, especially if no REM sleep is achieved.[3]

Renin-Angiotensin-Aldosterone System

Some circadian rhythmicity occurs in the renin-angiotensin-aldosterone system, with more urine flow and increased electrolyte excretion occurring during the day. Increased renin and aldosterone levels during sleep decrease urine output. In addition, plasma renin activity is synchronized with non-rapid eye movement (NREM)-REM cycles: higher levels occur during NREM sleep, and the lowest levels occur during REM sleep. Therefore, decreased urine flow and increased urine osmolality occurs during REM sleep. However, sleep deprivation decreases the usual elevation in aldosterone levels occurring during sleep, which results in increased sodium excretion.

Leptin and Ghrelin

Sleep plays an important role in energy balance. Both sleep and circadian rhythms control leptin secretion. Leptin is a hormone primarily secreted by adipocytes that promotes satiety and increases metabolism. Higher levels are noted in obese versus lean individuals suggesting possible leptin resistance. Levels fluctuate in response to caloric balance and increase at night. Leptin levels peak at night (around 2:30 AM) and nadir in the early afternoon (around 1 PM).[4] This nocturnal elevation of leptin level is thought to suppress hunger during sleep and may increase SWS.[5] When controlling for nutrition and activity, a shift in nighttime to daytime sleep results in leptin peaks during both day and night.[5,6]

Ghrelin is released primarily from the stomach, stimulates appetite, and promotes weight gain. Its release is controlled more by sleep-wake state than by circadian influences.[7] Ghrelin levels typically increase during the first half of the night and decrease in the second half, even when fasting. Ghrelin also enhances GH secretion and may stimulate SWS.[8]

Insulin and Glucose

A complex relationship between sleep, insulin, and glucose control also exists. Decreased glucose tolerance is noted during sleep, whether sleep occurs during the daytime or nighttime. This occurrence is thought to be related to decreased brain glucose use, decreased muscle use and tone, and anti-insulin effects of GH. Although decreased glucose metabolism occurs during NREM sleep, increased glucose metabolism occurs during REM sleep and wakefulness.[9]

Improved insulin sensitivity seems to occur at the end of sleep.[10] The improved glucose control at the end of the night is thought to be due to multiple factors, including increased metabolism during REM and wake time, greater body activity, augmented noninsulin-mediated glucose removal, and action by previously secreted insulin.[11,12]

EFFECTS OF ENDOCRINE ABNORMALITIES ON SLEEP

The previous section discussed normal hormonal secretion and the influence of sleep on hormonal balance. This section discusses endocrine disorders and their effect on sleep.

Acromegaly and Sleep Apnea

Acromegaly results from excessive GH production. In addition to notable physical findings, such as elongated digits and coarsening of features, several of other morphologic abnormalities can predispose to sleep apnea. These features include soft-tissue changes such as macroglossia, elongation and thickening of the soft palate, swelling and thickening of the pharyngeal walls, and thickening of the true and false vocal cords, which result in pharyngeal airway narrowing and an increased tendency of the airway to collapse.[13] Bony changes also contribute to this increased risk of obstructive sleep apnea (OSA): more vertical bony growth of the face results in posterior placement of the tongue, thus narrowing of the pharyngeal airspace. In addition, a more inferior position of the hyoid bone may contribute to upper airway instability.[14]

The relationship between sleep-disordered breathing and excessive GH production dates back to the late 1800s when Roxburgh and Collis linked acromegaly, snoring, and excessive daytime sleepiness.[15] More recent studies have demonstrated a high prevalence of sleep-disordered breathing in patients with acromegaly. An Australian study found a high prevalence of sleep apnea in acromegalic patients with approximately 60% of the patients with acromegaly having sleep apnea.[16] The same research group found that 33% of patients with acromegaly had central sleep apnea possibly due to increased hypercapnic ventilatory response.[17]

The prevalence of sleep apnea in those already treated for their acromegaly has been investigated. Although this percentage is lower than in untreated acromegalic patients, the prevalence remains high at more than 20%.[18] Surgical treatment of acromegaly may improve sleep-disordered breathing. Improvement in obstructive sleep apnea syndrome (OSAS) has been noted after transphenoidal hypophysectomy alone or transphenoidal hypophysectomy and radiation. However, uvulopalatopharyngoplasty has not been shown to improve OSA in these patients.[19] Treatment with octreotide has also been demonstrated to improve sleep-disordered breathing in patients with acromegaly. After 6 months of octreotide treatment, up to a 50% decline in respiratory events has been reported.[20,21] However, other studies have found that treatment of acromegaly does not result in resolution of the sleep-disordered breathing.[22,23] Furthermore, central sleep apnea seems to persist despite intracranial resection with or without radiation therapy.[23]

Thyroid Hormone and Sleep Disorders

Both hypothyroidism and hyperthyroidism can cause or exacerbate sleep disorders, such as OSAS, insomnia, and hypersomnia.

Symptoms of hypothyroidism overlap with those of OSA and may be difficult to distinguish. OSA may be a consequence of hypothyroidism. Up to 50% of hypothyroid patients have some degree of sleep-disordered breathing compared with 29% in the euthyroid control group.[24] Hypothyroidism can potentially cause or exacerbate OSAS for several reasons, including excess weight gain, reduction in ventilatory drive, thyroid myopathy, and abnormal mucopolysaccharide content in upper airway tissue. In addition, the presence of a goiter, independent of any concurrent hypothyroidism or hyperthyroidism, has occasionally been reported as a cause of OSAS due to mechanical constriction of the upper airway.

Evidence varies and is conflicting as to whether thyroid hormone supplementation improves sleep-disordered breathing. In some studies, thyroid hormone replacement has been shown to improve sleep-disordered breathing in hypothyroid patients with OSA.[25] In patients with sleep apnea and hypothyroidism, treatment of sleep apnea is recommended until thyroid replacement has been achieved because of reports of angina in patients initiated on thyroid replacement before management of sleep apnea. This angina resolves with initiation of continuous positive airway pressure (CPAP) therapy.[26] Fatigue and lack of energy are prominent features of hypothyroidism. In addition, the symptom of sleepiness has been noted quite commonly.[27]

Sleep propensity is increased even in patients with subclinical hypothyroidism.[28] Thyroid replacement therapy has been used with success in the management of sleepiness in patients diagnosed with idiopathic hypersomnia who were treated for subclinical hypothyroidism.[29] As such, patients with symptoms of hypersomnia should be evaluated for thyroid abnormalities.

Both hyperthyroidism and overdose of thyroid supplements have been associated with insomnia complaints.[30] Hyperthyroidism has been more typically associated with difficulty falling asleep rather than maintenance insomnia.[31] Thyroid excess may also contribute to restlessness with a higher prevalence of restless legs syndrome,[32] which in turn may exacerbate insomnia complaints.

Hypothalamic-Pituitary-Adrenal-Cortisol Axis Disorders and Sleep

Adrenal insufficiency, primarily due to deficient cortisol secretion, results in severe fatigue, sleepiness, and poor-quality sleep. These symptoms may persist even in patients who are on treatment.[33] Sleep-wake disorders have also been attributed to elevated cortisol levels. Furthermore, there has been a link between cortisol levels and chronic insomnia: higher nighttime levels are noted in patients with insomnia.[34,35] This relationship may be bidirectional but suggests that elevated cortisol levels may contribute to chronic insomnia.

There is limited information concerning a possible link between Cushing syndrome and an increased risk of OSAS. One study found that 18% of 22 subjects demonstrated an Respiratory Disturbance Index (RDI) of greater than or equal to 17.5.[36] In addition, there has been a link between exogenous corticosteroid therapy and sleep apnea.[37] Furthermore, well-known complications of corticosteroid therapy include issues with insomnia, in addition to other neuropsychiatric issues.[38]

Sex Hormones and Sleep Disturbances

Testosterone

Patients with low testosterone levels often note a lack of energy or fatigue. There is also a decline in sleep quality after middle age and with increasing age in men. This decline may be due in part to reduced testosterone levels in aging men.[39] Decreased testosterone may lead to increased fat mass, and there may be poorer sleep quality associated with obesity.[40,41] Weight loss may improve plasma testosterone levels in obese men.[42]

Although based largely on anecdotal evidence, exogenous testosterone has been considered to have a deleterious effect in OSA. Current guidelines suggest that it is contraindicated in the presence of untreated OSA.[43] In one study involving obese men with severe OSA and low plasma testosterone levels, testosterone supplementation, irrespective of baseline testosterone level, resulted in worsening of the oxygen desaturation index and nocturnal hypoxemia at 7 weeks but not at 18 weeks.[44] Testosterone supplementation may affect sleep in other ways. In one study of young men engaging in resistance exercises and taking anabolic steroids, there was a reduction in sleep efficiency and alteration of sleep architecture.[45]

Estrogen and progesterone

Several issues can potentially affect sleep in postmenopausal women such as alterations in mood, hot flashes, insomnia, and an increased prevalence of upper airway instability. The Wisconsin Sleep Cohort Study demonstrated that postmenopausal women are more frequently affected by respiratory instability. Postmenopausal women were more likely to manifest OSAS, even when corrected for body mass index (BMI) and age.[46] Hormonal therapy is often used to assist with insomnia associated with hot flashes in perimenopausal and postmenopausal women. Evidence suggests that administration of hormones can improve sleep quality in women. In one study, women who did not use hormone therapy reported more sleep difficulties than those on hormonal therapy.[47] The Sleep Heart Health Study examined the prevalence of an RDI greater or equal to 15 in women without and with hormonal therapy and found that there was 50% reduction in the elevated RDI rate in the hormone users.[48] Overall, these data suggest that hormonal therapy may be a useful adjunct, although not a replacement for therapies such as CPAP, in treating OSAS in postmenopausal women.

Melatonin Effects on Sleep

Melatonin plays a role in the regulation of human sleep. In addition to its direct sleep-facilitating effect, melatonin may improve sleep through a chronobiotic effect by entraining the circadian system to a desired sleep-wake cycle.[49,50] Exogenous melatonin decreases sleep latency, and the sustained release and transdermal formulations can increase total sleep time and sleep maintenance.[51–53] Exogenous melatonin, in 0.3-mg up to 5-mg doses, has also been shown to improve sleep efficiency in healthy people during the daytime when endogenous melatonin production is absent.[54] These results are consistent with the hypothesis that both exogenous and endogenous melatonin promote sleep by opposing the wake-promoting signal from the circadian clock. The intake of either low-dose (0.3 mg) or high-dose (5 mg) melatonin has a similar effect on sleep efficiency, indicating no additional benefit of exogenous melatonin concentrations more than the endogenous nighttime levels.[55] These findings also suggest that daytime melatonin intake may be useful for individuals, such as rotating shift workers, who need to obtain sleep during the daytime.

THE EFFECT OF SLEEP DISORDERS ON HORMONAL REGULATION
Sleep Deprivation

Sleep deprivation is common in industrialized countries. Insufficient sleep may occur as a result of voluntary sleep restriction, insomnia, or shift work. Decreased sleep is associated with increased risk for obesity, diabetes, and hypertension.

Adrenocorticotropic hormone and cortisol
Studies have shown that partial or complete sleep deprivation results in elevations of evening cortisol levels.[56] Conversely, sleep deprivation also results in a significant reduction of cortisol secretion the next day. This reduction in cortisol secretion seems to be related to an increase in SWS during the recovery night, which exerts an inhibitory effect on the HPA axis.[57] The impact of restricted sleep on the HPA axis seems to depend on the time of day. In addition, the amplitude of normal circadian rhythm decline in cortisol levels is reduced with insufficient sleep.[58]

Insulin and glucose metabolism
The interactions between sleep, circadian function, and glucose metabolism have also been evaluated.[59] Both sleep insufficiency and sleep fragmentation have been linked to abnormal glucose metabolism. It has been shown that sleep restriction affects glucose tolerance through a direct effect on insulin sensitivity. There is decreased insulin sensitivity associated with loss of sleep that is not compensated for by an increase in insulin release.[60] Subsequent studies in healthy human subjects involving sleep restriction and assessments of glucose metabolism have confirmed an approximately 20% reduction in insulin sensitivity without simultaneous increases in insulin levels, resulting in reduced glucose tolerance and, subsequently, an increased risk of diabetes.[61] In addition, the association of short sleep duration, usually less than 6 hours per night, with an increased risk of diabetes has been shown in multiple cross-sectional epidemiologic studies.[62]

Leptin, ghrelin, and appetite regulation
The duration of sleep plays an important role in the regulation of leptin and ghrelin levels in humans. Sleep loss may affect energy expenditure due its impact on the levels of leptin and ghrelin. Leptin and ghrelin exert opposing effects on appetite: leptin promotes satiety, whereas ghrelin promotes increased food intake and reduced fat metabolism. Several studies have shown that partial sleep deprivation is associated with significant decreases in leptin levels and conversely increases in levels of ghrelin. Although there is an increase in ghrelin levels after partial sleep restriction, the nocturnal increase in ghrelin levels is modestly reduced during acute total sleep deprivation.[7] Leptin levels decline with sleep restriction, although the nocturnal peak in leptin persists.[63] In a study of sleep deprivation in healthy adult men, while rigorously

controlling diet and activity, the decline in leptin levels was observed.[64] This decline in leptin levels correlates with increases in sympathetic nervous system activity, which suggests that increased autonomic activity might reduce leptin secretion. The association between sleep duration and leptin and ghrelin levels was observed in the Wisconsin Sleep Cohort Study. Limited total sleep time was associated with higher ghrelin and reduced leptin levels.[65] These findings would support the postulate that sleep deprivation may alter the ability of leptin and ghrelin to accurately signal caloric need and so lead to increased food intake due to an internal misperception of insufficient energy availability.

It is likely that the increased hunger and food intake are potential mechanisms by which sleep deprivation contributes to weight gain and obesity. In a study of healthy young male subjects, limiting sleep opportunity to only 4 hours versus 10 hours resulted in elevated daytime ghrelin and decreased daytime leptin levels. These changes were associated with both increased hunger and appetite.[64] In another trial, when subjects underwent 5 nights of insufficient sleep of only 5 hours per night, they had increased food intake and total daily energy expenditure. The increased food intake during the insufficient sleep schedule exceeded energy expenditure and so contributed to weight gain.[66]

Insomnia

Adrenocorticotropic hormone and cortisol

Investigators have studied the effect of chronic insomnia on the HPA axis and associated clinical consequences. In insomnia, higher nighttime cortisol levels have been noted. With chronic insomnia, there is an overall and sustained increase in ACTH and cortisol secretion, although maintaining the normal circadian pattern. It is possible that the chronic activation of the HPA axis places patients with insomnia at risk of significant medical morbidity.[67] Therapy for patients with insomnia may include sleep restriction combined with cognitive behavioral therapy. Lower cortisol levels occur during treatment, which confirms part of the proposed physiologic mechanisms behind insomnia. These data support the benefit of sleep restriction in contributing to a decrease in hyperarousal insomnia.[68]

Insulin and glucose metabolism

Studies in healthy volunteers have demonstrated that sleep fragmentation results in abnormal glucose metabolism, especially if there is associated suppression of SWS.[69] In addition, prospective population-based studies have linked poor sleep quality to incident diabetes. In one study, the risk of type 2 diabetes was found to be almost 3 times higher in subjects with insomnia, defined by a sleep duration less than 5 hours versus those with a longer sleep duration.[70,71]

Obstructive Sleep Apnea

Sleep-disordered breathing may have several adverse effects on the endocrine hormonal axes, especially with regard to glucose metabolism and insulin resistance.[72,73]

Insulin and glucose metabolism

The link between OSA and impaired glucose metabolism due to insulin resistance seems to occur independently of obesity. Patients with OSA have been shown to have higher fasting serum glucose and insulin resistance index, independent of adiposity. The severity of OSA is associated with increased insulin resistance.[74] Similarly, an increased apnea-hypopnea index has been associated with worsened glucose tolerance and insulin resistance independent of obesity.[75] It is postulated that the primary mechanism linking OSA to impaired glucose metabolism and diabetes may be a consequence of sleep fragmentation with diminished SWS. Sleep fragmentation is associated with elevated sympathetic nervous activity, which could lead to alterations in glucose metabolism.[69] It is possible that through mechanisms such as enhanced sympathetic activity, endothelial dysfunction, and impairment of peripheral vasodilation, insulin resistance may contribute to the metabolic syndrome.

The metabolic syndrome

The metabolic syndrome is a complex of metabolic disturbances diagnosed when 3 of the following 5 characteristics are present: abdominal obesity, increased serum triglyceride levels, low high-density lipoprotein (HDL) levels, elevated blood pressure, and elevated plasma glucose levels. Patients with OSA seem to be at higher risk of developing certain features of metabolic syndrome, specifically hypertension, insulin resistance, and type 2 diabetes. OSA has been independently associated with an increased prevalence of the metabolic syndrome.[76]

Even after adjusting for obesity, OSA has been associated with increased systolic and diastolic blood pressure, higher fasting insulin and triglyceride concentrations, decreased levels of HDL cholesterol, and increased cholesterol to HDL ratio. Therefore, it has been concluded that metabolic syndrome is more likely to be present in patients with OSA.[77] It is also likely that OSA and metabolic syndrome share similar pathophysiologic mechanisms. Patients with sleep apnea are often obese and have a heightened sympathetic drive, endothelial dysfunction, systemic inflammation, insulin resistance, hypercoagulability, and high plasma leptin levels, which are also secondary factors associated with metabolic syndrome.

Circadian Rhythm Disorders

Circadian misalignment occurs when the internal circadian clock is not properly aligned with the external environment, including light-dark, sleep-wake, and fasting-feeding cycles. This condition can occur acutely with jet lag or on a chronic basis with shift work, delayed sleep phase, or advanced sleep phase disorders. With nearly 20% of the working population in industrialized countries being shift workers,[78] the impact of shift work disorder can be quite significant. Night-shift work is an example of severe circadian misalignment, as workers are awake, active, and eating during their biological night and trying to sleep and fast during their biological day. Several studies have examined the effects of circadian misalignment on sleep and related hormones.

Adrenocorticotropic hormone, cortisol, and thyroid-stimulating hormone

The impact of delayed sleep phase syndrome (DSPS) on cortisol and TSH release has been investigated. One study showed that the hormonal rhythms were delayed in patients with DSPS, although there was no difference in total 24-hour secretions of TSH and cortisol when compared with controls. Based on these results, it would seem that the hormonal delay in DSPS is due more to the phase delay of the circadian clock rather than any overt hormonal dysfunction.[79]

Abnormally high cortisol levels have also been noted at the end of wake and start of sleep. Therefore, it has been postulated that the high cortisol secretion seen in circadian misalignment could contribute to insulin resistance and hyperglycemia.[80]

Insulin, glucose metabolism, and appetite regulation

Investigators have tested the different effects of phase advance and phase delay, compared with a daily 24-hour cycle, on sleep, energy expenditure, substrate oxidation, appetite, and related hormones in energy balance. They found that the primary effect of a phase shift, whether phase advanced or phase delayed, was a combined disturbance of glucose-insulin metabolism. Glucose concentrations were higher without any concomitant change in insulin concentrations.[81]

Acute circadian misalignment results in an increase in postprandial glucose and insulin levels with a concurrent decline in leptin levels. Similarly, low leptin levels are associated with appetite stimulation. An increase in appetite coupled with decreased energy expenditure could account for the increased risk of obesity noted in shift workers.[80]

There is considerable epidemiologic evidence that shift work is associated with increased risk for obesity, diabetes, and cardiovascular disease. Shift workers suffering from chronic sleep deprivation and circadian rhythm misalignment seem to be at an increased risk of type 2 diabetes.[82,83] Prospective studies have demonstrated this association. For example, in the Nurses' Health Study, researchers found that subjects who worked rotating night shifts had an increased risk for diabetes, even after adjusting for traditional diabetic risk factors, including BMI.[82] The risk was also noted to be higher in those with longer duration of shift work as compared with no shift work.

Evidence suggests that increased insulin resistance may be an intrinsic adverse effect of circadian rhythm misalignment on glucose metabolism, independent of sleep loss.[84] However, further prospective and interventional studies are needed to evaluate the role of circadian rhythm misalignment in the development and severity of type 2 diabetes.

Melatonin, gonadotropin, and oncogenic effect

Melatonin rhythms are also delayed in patients with DSPS, although the total 24-hour secretion of melatonin is similar to controls.[79] Shift workers may exhibit altered night-time melatonin secretion and reproductive hormone profiles that could increase their risk of hormone-dependent cancers. Several studies have been conducted to investigate the effect of circadian rhythm disruption on reproductive hormone production and nocturnal production of melatonin as a possible cause for breast cancer.[85] Melatonin is known to affect regulation of gonadal function because decreased concentrations, as seen in circadian rhythm misalignment, result in increased pituitary gonadotropin release, leading to testosterone or estrogen production.

Melatonin also has been found to have tumor suppressive properties. For example, in rodent models, pinealectomy was found to enhance tumor growth,[86] whereas exogenous melatonin administration has demonstrated anticancer activity.[87] Overall, the antitumor effect of melatonin may be due to its direct effect on hormone-dependent proliferation through interaction with nuclear receptors, an effect on cell cycle control, and possible increase in p53 tumor-suppressor gene expression.[85]

Disorders of Hypersomnia

Limited data exist regarding hypersomnia disorders and associated endocrine abnormalities. However, patients with narcolepsy are often obese and have been reported to be at increased risk of diabetes. Yet, there is a paucity of studies looking at the endocrine consequences of narcolepsy. In a case-control study, investigators studied glucose metabolism using the oral glucose tolerance test and assessed dynamic function of the HPA axis with the dexamethasone suppression test in narcoleptic patients.[88] The study showed that, independent of obesity, narcolepsy is not associated with impaired glucose metabolism. In addition, there was no alteration in dynamic HPA function, although the negative feedback response to dexamethasone was mildly enhanced in narcolepsy cases. Similarly, other studies using BMI-matched controls have not shown any increased risk of type 2 diabetes or impaired glucose metabolism, independent of BMI, in narcoleptic patients.[89,90]

SLEEP AND ENDOCRINE ABNORMALITIES IN CRITICALLY ILL PATIENTS

Sleep fragmentation and deprivation are common in critically ill patients and may be associated with various hormonal disturbances. Patients experience poor sleep quality characterized by frequent disruptions and loss of circadian rhythms because of factors such as environmental noise; light; patient care activities, such as vital signs checks, drug administration, and diagnostic testing; patient-ventilator dyssynchrony; and pain or discomfort. Although the total number of hours of sleep in a 24-hour period may be normal (7–9 hours), approximately 50% of the sleep time occurs as short periods of light sleep during the day.[91] In patients in the intensive care unit (ICU), there is an increased percentage of wakefulness and stage N1 sleep (40%–60%) with decreased amounts of N2 (20%–40%), N3 (10%), and REM sleep (10%).[92] Thus, there is a significant reduction in the total time spent in restorative N3 and REM sleep stages.

It has been shown that there is loss of the normal circadian secretion of melatonin in critical illness, especially in sepsis, which seems to occur independently of light exposure.[93,94] In one study of patients with sepsis, investigators found that despite the exclusion of exposure to ambient light in the ICU, there was loss of periodic excretion of the melatonin urinary metabolite 6-sulfatoxymelatonin.[95] In addition, this noncircadian release of melatonin seems to persist for several weeks after recovery from sepsis that may contribute to continued sleep disturbances after ICU discharge.

The disruption of sleep, particularly restriction of SWS, as is seen in critically ill patients, negatively affects glucose metabolism and results in blunted insulin secretion with decreased insulin sensitivity.[60,69] ICU-related sleep disruption could therefore contribute to and exacerbate glucose abnormalities in critical illness; this is of particular importance in the critically ill patient, who is susceptible to episodes of hyperglycemia and the adverse outcomes associated with inadequate glucose control.

Exogenous corticosteroid administration may exacerbate the poor sleep and sleep disruption that is seen in these critically ill patients. Similarly, cortisol and catecholamine levels along with indices of energy expenditure, such as oxygen consumption (V_{O_2}) and carbon dioxide production (V_{CO_2}), tend to increase in sleep deprivation. The persistent sleep disruption that occurs in the critically ill patient, especially in the setting of sepsis, intensifies this stress response.[56,60]

Furthermore, in the acute phase of critical illness, increased levels of GH and PRL are initially noted. This increase seems to occur regardless of sleep onset and is likely due to increased pituitary activity.[96] However, with prolonged critical illness, the normal pulsatile secretion of GH and PRL is impaired, which may be a consequence of the potent inhibitory effect of sleep deprivation on GH and PRL release.[96,97] This decrease in GH and PRL levels may play a role in critical illness muscle wasting and impaired immunity.

SUMMARY

This article discusses the interactions between sleep and endocrine function. The authors have demonstrated the importance of sleep quality and quantity on maintaining hormonal balance. Disrupting this balance can have significant health consequences. Abnormalities in the endocrine system, such as excess GH secretion or thyroid hormone production, can lead to significant sleep disruption, such as sleep apnea and insomnia, respectively. Treating these hormonal abnormalities can improve sleep. Similarly, poor-quality or insufficient sleep can have a major impact on hormonal balance. Considerable research supports the effect of poor sleep on insulin and glucose metabolism, as well as on appetite regulation. Growing evidence supports the adverse consequences of sleep restriction, insomnia, and circadian rhythm abnormalities on endocrine balance and overall health. Restoring sleep quantity and improving sleep quality may assist in hormonal regulation, which is of particular importance in the critically ill patient who experiences sleep fragmentation and deprivation with loss of circadian rhythms. Understanding the sleep disruption and endocrine imbalances that occur in critically ill patients supports the importance of sleep and the need to optimize sleep in this patient population.

REFERENCES

1. Van Cauter E, Blackman JD, Roland D, et al. Modulation of glucose regulation and insulin secretion by circadian rhythmicity and sleep. J Clin Invest 1991;88: 934–42.
2. Axelsson J, Ingre M, Akerstedt T, et al. Effects of acutely displaced sleep on testosterone. J Clin Endocrinol Metab 2005;90:4530–5.
3. Luboshitzky R, Herer P, Levi M, et al. Relationship between rapid eye movement sleep and testosterone secretion in normal men. J Androl 1999;20:731–7.
4. Sinha MK, Ohannesion JP, Heiman ML, et al. Nocturnal rise of leptin in lean, obese, and non insulin-dependent diabetes mellitus subjects. J Clin Invest 1996;97:1344–7.
5. Simon C, Grofier C, Schlienger JL, et al. Circadian and ultradian variations of leptin in normal man under continuous enteral nutrition: relationship to sleep and body temperature. J Clin Endocrinol Metab 1998;83:1893–9.
6. Saad MF, Riad-Gabriel MG, Khan A, et al. Diurnal and ultradian rhythmicity of plasma leptin: effects of gender and adiposity. J Clin Endocrinol Metab 1998; 83:453–9.
7. Dzaja A, Dalal MA, Himmerich H, et al. Sleep enhances nocturnal plasma ghrelin levels in healthy subjects. Am J Physiol Endocrinol Metab 2004;286:E963–7.
8. Weikel JC, Wichniak A, Ising M, et al. Ghrelin promotes slow-wave sleep in humans. Am J Physiol Endocrinol Metab 2003;284:E407–15.
9. Kern W, Offenheuser S, Born J, et al. Entrainment of ultradian oscillations in the secretion of insulin and glucagons to the nonrapid eye movement/rapid eye movement sleep rhythm in humans. J Clin Endocrinol Metab 1996;81:1541–7.
10. Levy I, Recasens A, Casamitjana R, et al. Nocturnal insulin and C-peptide rhythms in normal subjects. Diabetes Care 1987;10:148–51.
11. Boyle PJ, Scott JC, Krentz AJ, et al. Diminished brain glucose metabolism is a significant determinant for falling rates of systemic glucose utilization during sleep in normal humans. J Clin Invest 1994;93:529–35.
12. Van Cauter E, Polonsky KS, Scheen AJ. Roles of circadian rhythmicity and sleep in human glucose regulation. Endocr Rev 1997;18:716–38.
13. Colao A, Ferone D, Marzullo P, et al. Systemic complications of acromegaly: epidemiology, pathogenesis, and management. Endocr Rev 2004;25:102–52.
14. Hochban W, Ehlenz K, Conradt R, et al. Obstructive sleep apnoea in acromegaly: the role of craniofacial changes. Eur Respir J 1999;14:196–202.
15. Roxburgh F, Collis AJ. Notes on a case of acromegaly. Br Med J 1896;2:63–5.
16. Grunstein RR, Ho KY, Sullivan CE. Sleep apnea in acromegaly. Ann Intern Med 1991;115:527–32.
17. Grunstein RR, Ho KY, Berthon-Jones M, et al. Central sleep apnea is associated with increased ventilatory response to carbon dioxide and hypersecretion of growth hormone in patients with acromegaly. Am J Respir Crit Care Med 1994; 150:496–502.

18. Rosenow F, Reuter S, Deuss U, et al. Sleep apnoea in treated acromegaly: relative frequency and predisposing factors. Clin Endocrinol (Oxf) 1996;45:563–9.
19. Mickelson SA, Rosenthal LD, Rock JP, et al. Obstructive sleep apnea syndrome and acromegaly. Otolaryngol Head Neck Surg 1994;111:25–30.
20. Grunstein RR, Ho KKY, Sullivan CE. Effect of octreotide, a somatostatin analog, on sleep apnea in patients with acromegaly. Ann Intern Med 1994;121:478–83.
21. Herrmann BL, Wessendorf TE, Ajaj W, et al. Effects of octreotide on sleep apnoea and tongue volume (magnetic resonance imaging) in patients with acromegaly. Eur J Endocrinol 2004;151:309–15.
22. Pekkarinen T, Partinen M, Pelkonen R, et al. Sleep apnoea and daytime sleepiness in acromegaly: relationship to endocrinological factors. Clin Endocrinol (Oxf) 1987;27:649–54.
23. Pelttari L, Polo O, Rauhala E, et al. Nocturnal breathing abnormalities in acromegaly after adenomectomy. Clin Endocrinol (Oxf) 1995;43:175–82.
24. Pelttari L, Rauhala E, Polo O, et al. Upper airway obstruction in hypothyroidism. J Intern Med 1994;236:177–81.
25. Jha A, Sharma SK, Tandon N, et al. Thyroxine replacement therapy reverses sleep-disordered breathing in patients with primary hypothyroidism. Sleep Med 2006;7:55–61.
26. Grunstein RR, Sullivan CE. Sleep apnea and hypothyroidism: mechanisms and management. Am J Med 1988;85:775–9.
27. Krishnan PV, Vadivu AS, Alappatt A, et al. Prevalence of sleep abnormalities and their association among hypothyroid patients in an Indian population. Sleep Med 2012;13:1232–7.
28. Resta O, Carratù P, Carpagnano GE, et al. Influence of subclinical hypothyroidism and T4 treatment on the prevalence and severity of obstructive sleep apnoea syndrome (OSAS). J Endocrinol Invest 2005;28:893–8.
29. Shinno H, Inami Y, Inagaki T, et al. Successful treatment with levothyroxine for idiopathic hypersomnia patients with subclinical hypothyroidism. Gen Hosp Psychiatry 2009;31:190–3.
30. Lu CL, Lee YC, Tsai SJ, et al. Psychiatric disturbances associated with hyperthyroidism: an analysis report of 30 cases. Zhonghua Yi Xue Za Zhi (Taipei) 1995;56:393–8.
31. Sridhar GR, Putcha V, Lakshmi G. Sleep in thyrotoxicosis. Indian J Endocrinol Metab 2011;15:23–6.
32. Pereira JC Jr, Pradella-Hallinan M, Pessoa HL. Imbalance between thyroid hormones and the dopaminergic system might be central to the pathophysiology of restless legs syndrome: a hypothesis. Clinics 2010;65:547–54.
33. Aulinas A, Webb SM. Health-related quality of life in primary and secondary adrenal insufficiency. Expert Rev Pharmacoecon Outcomes Res 2014;14:873–88.
34. Seelig E, Keller U, Klarhöfer M, et al. Neuroendocrine regulation and metabolism of glucose and lipids in primary chronic insomnia: a prospective case-control study. PLoS One 2013;8:e61780.
35. Xia L, Chen GH, Li ZH, et al. Alterations in hypothalamus-pituitary-adrenal/thyroid axes and gonadotropin-releasing hormone in the patients with primary insomnia: a clinical research. PLoS One 2013;8:e71065.
36. Shipley JE, Schteingart DE, Tandon R, et al. Sleep architecture and sleep apnea in patients with Cushing's disease. Sleep 1992;15:514–8.
37. Berger G, Hardak E, Shaham B, et al. Preliminary prospective explanatory observation on the impact of 3-month steroid therapy on the objective measures of sleep-disordered breathing. Sleep Breath 2012;16:549–53.

38. Kenna HA, Poon AW, de los Angeles CP, et al. Psychiatric complications of treatment with corticosteroids: review with case report. Psychiatry Clin Neurosci 2011; 65:549–60.

39. Miller CM, Rindflesch TC, Fiszman M, et al. A closed literature-based discovery technique finds a mechanistic link between hypogonadism and diminished sleep quality in aging men. Sleep 2012;35:279–85.

40. Shi Z, Araujo AB, Martin S, et al. Longitudinal changes in testosterone over five years in community-dwelling men. J Clin Endocrinol Metab 2013;98:3289–97.

41. Resta O, Foschino Barbaro MP, Bonfitto P, et al. Low sleep quality and daytime sleepiness in obese patients without obstructive sleep apnoea syndrome. J Intern Med 2003;253:536–43.

42. Grossmann M. Low testosterone in men with type 2 diabetes: significance and treatment. J Clin Endocrinol Metab 2011;96:2341–53.

43. Hanafy HM. Testosterone therapy and obstructive sleep apnea: is there a real connection? J Sex Med 2007;4:1241–6.

44. Hoyos CM, Killick R, Yee BJ, et al. Effects of testosterone therapy on sleep and breathing in obese men with severe obstructive sleep apnoea: a randomized placebo-controlled trial. Clin Endocrinol 2012;77:599–607.

45. Venancio DP, Tufik S, Garbuio SA, et al. Effects of anabolic androgenic steroids on sleep patterns of individuals practicing resistance exercise. Eur J Appl Physiol 2008;102:555–60.

46. Young T, Finn L, Austin D, et al. Menopausal status and sleep-disordered breathing in the Wisconsin Sleep Cohort Study. Am J Respir Crit Care Med 2003;167:1181–5.

47. Sarti CD, Chiantera A, Graziottin A, et al. Hormone therapy and sleep quality in women around menopause. Menopause 2005;12:545–51.

48. Cistulli PA, Barnes DJ, Grunstein RR, et al. Effect of short-term hormone replacement in the treatment of obstructive sleep apnoea in postmenopausal women. Thorax 1994;49:699–702.

49. Burgess HJ, Revell VL, Molina TA, et al. Human phase response curves to three days of daily melatonin: 0.5 mg versus 3.0 mg. J Clin Endocrinol Metab 2010;95: 3325–31.

50. Sack RL, Brandes RW, Kendall AR, et al. Entrainment of free-running circadian rhythms by melatonin in blind people. N Engl J Med 2000;343:1070–7.

51. Sack RL, Hughes RJ, Edgar DM, et al. Sleep-promoting effects of melatonin: at what dose, in whom, under what conditions, and by what mechanisms? Sleep 1997;20:908–15.

52. Sharkey KM, Fogg LF, Eastman CI. Effects of melatonin administration on daytime sleep after simulated night shift work. J Sleep Res 2001;10:181–92.

53. Aeschbach D, Lockyer BJ, Dijk DJ, et al. Use of transdermal melatonin delivery to improve sleep maintenance during daytime. Clin Pharmacol Ther 2009;86: 378–82.

54. Wyatt JK, Dijk DJ, Ritz-De Cecco A, et al. Sleep facilitating effect of exogenous melatonin in healthy young men and women is circadian-phase dependent. Sleep 2006;29:609–18.

55. Zhdanova IV, Wurtman RJ. Efficacy of melatonin as a sleep-promoting agent. J Biol Rhythms 1997;12:644–50.

56. Leproult R, Copinschi G, Buxton O, et al. Sleep loss results in an elevation of cortisol levels the next evening. Sleep 1997;20:865–70.

57. Vgontzas AN, Mastorakos G, Bixler EO, et al. Sleep deprivation effects on the activity of the hypothalamic–pituitary–adrenal and growth axes: potential clinical implications. Clin Endocrinol 1999;51:205–15.

58. Guyon A, Balbo M, Morselli LL, et al. Adverse effects of two nights of sleep restriction on the hypothalamic-pituitary-adrenal axis in healthy men. J Clin Endocrinol Metab 2014;99:2861–8.
59. Reutrakul S, Van Cauter E. Interactions between sleep, circadian function, and glucose metabolism: implications for risk and severity of diabetes. Ann N Y Acad Sci 2014;1311:151–73.
60. Spiegel K, Leproult R, Van Cauter E. Impact of sleep debt on metabolic and endocrine function. Lancet 1999;354:1435–9.
61. Buxton OM, Pavlova M, Reid EW, et al. Sleep restriction for 1 week reduces insulin sensitivity in healthy men. Diabetes 2010;59:2126–33.
62. Knutson KL, Van Cauter E. Associations between sleep loss and increased risk of obesity and diabetes. Ann N Y Acad Sci 2008;1129:287–304.
63. Mullington JM, Chan JL, Van Dongen HP, et al. Sleep loss reduces diurnal rhythm amplitude of leptin in healthy men. J Neuroendocrinol 2003;15:851–4.
64. Spiegel K, Leproult R, L'Hermite-Baleriaux M, et al. Leptin levels are dependent on sleep duration: relationships with sympathovagal balance, carbohydrate regulation, cortisol, and thyrotropin. J Clin Endocrinol Metab 2004;89:5762–71.
65. Taheri S, Lin L, Austin D, et al. Short sleep duration is associated with reduced leptin, elevated ghrelin, and increased body mass index. PLoS Med 2004;1(3):e62.
66. Markwald RR, Melanson EL, Smith MR, et al. Impact of insufficient sleep on total daily energy expenditure, food intake, and weight gain. Proc Natl Acad Sci U S A 2013;110(4):5695–700.
67. Vgontzas A, Bixler EO, Lin HM, et al. Chronic insomnia is associated with nyctohemeral activation of the hypothalamic-pituitary-adrenal axis: clinical implications. J Clin Endocrinol Metab 2001;86(8):3787–94.
68. Vallières A, Ceklic T, Bastein CH, et al. A preliminary evaluation of the physiological mechanisms of action for sleep restriction therapy. Sleep Disord 2013;2013: 726372.
69. Tasali E, Leproult R, Ehrmann DA, et al. Slow-wave sleep and the risk of type 2 diabetes in humans. Proc Natl Acad Sci U S A 2008;105:1044–9.
70. Vgontzas AN, Liao D, Pejovic S, et al. Insomnia with short sleep duration and mortality: the Penn State cohort. Sleep 2010;33:1159–64.
71. Vgontzas AN, Liao D, Pejovic S, et al. Insomnia with objective short sleep duration is associated with type 2 diabetes: a population-based study. Diabetes Care 2009;32:1980–5.
72. Attal P, Chanson P. Endocrine aspects of obstructive sleep apnea. J Clin Endocrinol Metab 2010;95:483–95.
73. Yee B, Liu P, Phillips C, et al. Neuroendocrine changes in sleep apnea. Curr Opin Pulm Med 2004;10:475–81.
74. Ip MS, Lam B, Ng MM, et al. Obstructive sleep apnea is independently associated with insulin resistance. Am J Respir Crit Care Med 2002;165:670–6.
75. Punjabi NM, Sorkin JD, Katzel LI, et al. Sleep-disordered breathing and insulin resistance in middle-aged and overweight men. Am J Respir Crit Care Med 2002;165:677–82.
76. Svatikova A, Wolk R, Gami AS, et al. Interactions between obstructive sleep apnea and the metabolic syndrome. Curr Diab Rep 2005;5:53–8.
77. Coughlin SR, Mawdsley L, Mugarza JA, et al. Obstructive sleep apnoea is independently associated with an increased prevalence of metabolic syndrome. Eur Heart J 2004;25:735–41.
78. McMenamin T. A time to work: recent trends in shift work and flexible schedules. Mon Labor Rev 2007;3–15.

79. Shibui K, Uchiyama M, Kim K, et al. Melatonin, cortisol and thyroid-stimulating hormone rhythms are delayed in patients with delayed sleep phase syndrome. Sleep Biol Rhythms 2003;1:209–14.
80. Scheer F, Hilton M, Mantzoros C, et al. Adverse metabolic and cardiovascular consequences of circadian misalignment. Proc Natl Acad Sci U S A 2009;106: 4453–8.
81. Gonnissen H, Rutters F, Mazuy C, et al. Effect of a phase advance and phase delay of the 24-h cycle on energy metabolism, appetite, and related hormones. Am J Clin Nutr 2012;96:689–97.
82. Pan A, Schernhammer ES, Sun Q, et al. Rotating night shift work and risk of type 2 diabetes: two prospective cohort studies in women. PLoS Med 2011;8(12): e1001141.
83. Monk TH, Buysse DJ. Exposure to shift work as a risk factor for diabetes. J Biol Rhythms 2013;28:356–9.
84. Leproult R, Holmbäck U, Van Cauter E. Circadian misalignment augments markers of insulin resistance and inflammation, independently of sleep loss. Diabetes 2014;63:1860–9.
85. Davis S, Mirick DK. Circadian disruption, shift work and the risk of cancer: a summary of the evidence and studies in Seattle. Cancer Causes Control 2006;17: 539–45.
86. Tamarkin L, Cohen M, Roselle D, et al. Melatonin inhibition and pinealectomy enhancement of 7,12-dimethylbenz(a)anthracene-induced mammary tumors in the rat. Cancer Res 1981;41:4432–6.
87. Mocchegiani E, Perissin L, Santarelli L, et al. Melatonin administration in tumor-bearing mice (intact and pinealectomized) in relation to stress, zinc, thymulin and IL-2. Int J Immunopharmacol 1999;21:27–46.
88. Maurovich-Horvat E, Keckeis M, Zuzana Lattov Z, et al. Hypothalamo–pituitary–adrenal axis, glucose metabolism and TNF-alpha in narcolepsy. J Sleep Res 2014;23:425–31.
89. Beitinger PA, Fulda S, Dalal MA, et al. Glucose tolerance in patients with narcolepsy. Sleep 2012;35:231–6.
90. Engel A, Helfrich J, Manderscheid N, et al. Investigation of insulin resistance in narcoleptic patients: dependent or independent of body mass index? Neuropsychiatr Dis Treat 2011;7:351–6.
91. Cooper AB, Thornley KS, Young GB, et al. Sleep in critically ill patients requiring mechanical ventilation. Chest 2000;117:809–18.
92. Freedman NS, Gazendam J, Levan L, et al. Abnormal sleep/wake cycles and the effect of environmental noise on sleep disruption in the intensive care unit. Am J Respir Crit Care Med 2001;163:451–7.
93. Shilo L, Dagan Y, Smorjik Y, et al. Patients in the intensive care unit suffer from severe lack of sleep associated with loss of normal melatonin secretion pattern. Am J Med Sci 1999;317:278–81.
94. Perras B, Meier M, Dodt C. Light and darkness fail to regulate melatonin release in critically ill humans. Intensive Care Med 2007;33:1954–8.
95. Mundigler G, Delle-Karth G, Koreny M, et al. Impaired circadian rhythm of melatonin secretion in sedated critically ill patients with severe sepsis. Crit Care Med 2002;30:536–40.
96. Van den Berghe G. Novel insights into the neuroendocrinology of critical illness. Eur J Endocrinol 2000;143:1–13.
97. Vanhorebeek I, Langouche L, Van den Berghe G. Endocrine aspects of acute and prolonged critical illness. Nat Clin Pract Endocrinol Metab 2006;1:20–31.

Obesity Hypoventilation Syndrome in the Critically Ill

Shirley F. Jones, MD, FCCP, FAASM*, Veronica Brito, MD,
Shekhar Ghamande, MD, FCCP, FAASM

KEYWORDS

- Obesity hypoventilation syndrome • Critically ill • Hypercapnic respiratory failure
- Continuous positive airway pressure

KEY POINTS

- Obesity hypoventilation syndrome is a common but underrecognized cause of acute on chronic hypercapnic respiratory failure in the intensive care unit.
- The development of the obesity hypoventilation syndrome is multifactorial and is due to impairments in pulmonary function, ventilatory drive, sleep-disordered breathing, and hormonal regulation.
- Obesity, an awake $Paco_2$ greater than 45 mm Hg, and a serum bicarbonate level higher than 27 mEq/L are key diagnostic indicators of the disease.
- Positive airway pressure (PAP) (continuous PAP and noninvasive ventilation including bilevel PAP and more advanced modes) can successfully treat respiratory failure.
- Weight loss is critical in the management of obesity hypoventilation syndrome.
- Obesity hypoventilation is associated with significant morbidity and mortality.

INTRODUCTION

Obesity hypoventilation syndrome (OHS) is characterized as obesity and daytime hypoventilation in the absence of other causes of hypoventilation such as pulmonary disease, neuromuscular weakness, or chest wall disorders. A common presentation of OHS is in the critically ill patient who presents for acute on chronic hypercapnic respiratory failure. As the proportion of obese and morbidly obese individuals increases, intensive care unit (ICU) providers need heightened awareness of OHS and its complications, prognosis, and treatment modalities. An understanding of the how obesity affects pulmonary function and control of ventilation is needed. Continuous positive

Disclosures: None.
Division of Pulmonary Critical Care and Sleep Medicine, Department of Medicine, Baylor Scott &White Health, Texas A&M Health Science Center, 2401 South 31st Street, Temple, TX 76508, USA
* Corresponding author.
E-mail address: shjones@sw.org

airway pressure (CPAP), bilevel positive airway pressure (BPAP), and average volume-assured pressure support (AVAPS) are modes of noninvasive ventilation (NIV) used to manage respiratory failure in this population. Long-term strategies to address weight loss are important in the chronic management of the patient with OHS, and pharmacologic therapy plays a significant role in respiratory stimulation. OHS is associated with significant negative outcomes, particularly in the critically ill. This review serves to increase knowledge of the epidemiology, diagnosis, pathophysiology, treatment, and outcomes in patients with OHS.

EPIDEMIOLOGY

The exact prevalence of patients with OHS is unknown. Most studies examining the prevalence of OHS were conducted in sleep laboratories and clinics, estimating that 10% to 20% of patients with obstructive sleep apnea (OSA) have OHS.[1] According to data from the National Health and Nutrition Examination Survey in 2009-2010, 35.7% of United States adults are obese, with rates of obesity climbing fastest among the aging and men.[2] Rates of morbid obesity in the United States are increasing, with 5% of Americans having a body mass index (BMI; calculated as weight in kilograms divided by height in meters squared, ie, kg/m^2) greater than 40.[3] It can be assumed that rates of OHS will increase as the population of obese patients increases. An estimate of the prevalence of OHS in the general adult population of the United States is 1 in 300 to 1 in 600 adults.[4] The prevalence of OHS in hospitalized patients, and particularly the critically ill, is less known. In single study of consecutive adult hospitalized patients with a BMI of 35 or higher, OHS was present in 31%.[5] In the ICU, obese patients represent up to 50% of all patients,[6] and 8% of ICU admissions met criteria for OHS in a study at a single center.[7] However, the underdiagnosis and underreporting of OHS likely underestimates the true prevalence. Ethnic and geographic factors also affect OHS prevalence. For example, the prevalence of OHS was 2.3% among Japanese patients with OSA.[8] However, in a study conducted at a tertiary health care facility in Turkey, 3.4% of patients who underwent arterial blood gas analysis had evidence of hypoventilation, and OHS accounted for 24% of these subjects.[9]

PATHOPHYSIOLOGY

The progression from obesity to OHS is variable and multifactorial.[10,11] The prevalence of OHS correlates with the degree of obesity, severity of sleep-disordered breathing, and restrictive mechanics on lung function tests.[12–14]

Lung Mechanics

With obesity there is reduction in the functional residual capacity (FRC) and expiratory reserve volume (ERV).[15] These lung volumes are further reduced with OHS.[16] The fat distribution can affect lung volumes. A central pattern of obesity is seen with morbid obesity, with higher waist to hip ratio and larger neck circumference.[16] The central adiposity has been shown to correlate with lower forced vital capacity (FVC) and forced expiratory volume in 1 second (FEV_1) independent of the BMI.[17]

Data from anesthetized morbidly obese patients undergoing surgery suggests they have high pleural pressures throughout the chest. There is reduction in respiratory system compliance, primarily from lung compliance rather than chest wall compliance.[18] Compared with normal subjects, eucapnic obese individuals have a 20% lower respiratory system compliance, which drops further to almost 60% lower in OHS subjects[19]: high pleural pressures result in tidal breathing near their residual volume. Low lung volumes affect the respiratory mechanics unfavorably. At this point the airways are more prone to closure and the lungs are less compliant.[18] Resultant airway closure promotes air trapping and development of intrinsic positive end-expiratory pressure.[20] A supine position compounds the adverse lung mechanics in these patients regarding FRC, compliance, and airflow limitation.[21–23] Abdominal fat pushes against the diaphragm while supine, accounting for some of these changes.[21] Overall the work of breathing is increased in OHS subjects and worsens while supine.[24] Gas exchange is affected at low ERV and higher dead space, which occurs in obese subjects particularly in supine position.[25] Of note, the higher waist to hip ratio, more so than the BMI, also correlates with reduction in partial pressure of oxygen (Pao_2) and alveolar-arterial oxygen difference.[26] In addition, there is respiratory muscle fatigue in OHS in the face of increased work of breathing. The maximal voluntary ventilation is reduced in these subjects, and correlates with the level of hypercapnia.[27] This inadequacy of compensatory mechanism is of unclear etiology, although overstretching of the diaphragm, thickening of the diaphragm, and chronic hypoxia with hypercapnia have been proposed as plausible mechanisms.[28–30]

Sleep-Disordered Breathing

Most patients with OHS have OSA.[31,32] However, approximately 10% of patients have sleep-related hypoventilation without OSA.[10,31,32] The elevated apnea-hypopnea index (AHI) has been proposed as a mechanism for OHS development, but there are uncertainties with this hypothesis. In a meta-analysis the AHI was higher in patients with OSA who had hypercapnia when compared with eucapnic patients with OSA.[14] However, the difference in AHI between the groups was only 12 events per hour. In a conflicting report, Sin and colleaguebib33s[33] studied the modified hypercapnic ventilator response (cHCVR) in patients with and without OSA and did not find a correlation between the cHCVR and OSA, suggesting that sleep-disordered breathing did not lead to hypercapnia in patients with OSA. More recently, Macavei and colleagues[12] did not find the AHI to be an independent predictor of OHS.

Nocturnal hypercapnia resulting from OSA seems to be related to daytime hypercapnia, particularly with prolonged apneic periods and reduced time between apneic episodes.[34,35] This interval represents inadequate time for the minute ventilation to eliminate accumulated CO_2. The compensatory increase in serum bicarbonate must be unloaded during the nonsleep period to avoid blunting the effects on change in pH produced by change in partial pressure of CO_2 (Pco_2) on the brain chemoreceptors.[36] Raurich and colleagues[37] studied the CO_2 response in mechanically ventilated patients with OHS, and reported that patients with OHS with the highest serum bicarbonate had the most blunted CO_2 response. However, in patients who received acetazolamide, the serum bicarbonate was decreased and the CO_2 response improved.

Sustained hypoxia during sleep-disordered breathing in these patients contributes to the pathogenesis of OHS. Mokhlesi and colleagues[1] concluded from their meta-analysis that the time spent below 90% oxygen saturation at night was increased in subjects with OHS compared with eucapnic patients with OSA (56% vs 19%). This increase was reported to cause 24% variance in Pco_2,[17] and more recently was also confirmed to be significant in causing daytime hypercapnia.[12]

Ventilatory Drive

Obese subjects have been demonstrated to have higher oxygen consumption (Vo_2) and carbon dioxide production (Vco_2) which, compared with nonobese subjects, result in a higher minute ventilation with a higher neural drive to breathe.[22,38] Of note, the neural drive improves with weight loss in obese subjects.[39] Unlike eucapnic obese patients, those with OHS are unable to increase their neural drive, permitting daytime hypercapnia.[24,40,41] Patients with OHS have a blunted response to hypoxia and hypercapnia.[27,41–43] Increased serum bicarbonate contributes to the blunted response, as already discussed. Increased suboptimal tidal volume adds to the inadequate ventilatory response.[12,40] Furthermore, the ventilatory abnormalities in OHS are acquired[44,45] and can be corrected over time with use of positive airway pressure (PAP) therapy, independent of weight loss.[43,46,47]

Manuel and colleagues[48] recently proposed an "early OHS" terminology based on their data whereby they identified a group of patients with obesity but without daytime hypercapnia who had elevated serum bicarbonate. Despite not having daytime hypercapnia, their hypoxic ventilatory response was similar to patients with OHS and significantly worse than normal obese individuals. The investigators speculate that these patients might develop OHS if there were further deterioration. Although this is a single-center study without a longitudinal follow-up, intriguingly it suggests that sustained hypoventilation rather than intermittent hypoxia might be more relevant.

Until recently it was unclear whether moderate supplemental oxygen would affect patients with OHS in the same way as patients with chronic obstructive pulmonary disease (COPD). Hollier and colleagues[49] compared the responses of 14 patients with OHS with matched, nonobese healthy controls to exposure to fractions of inspired oxygen (Fio_2) of 0.28 and 0.5. In patients with OHS, hyperoxia (breathing at Fio_2 of 0.5) led to hypoventilation, increased dead space/tidal volume ratio (VD/VT), and a reduced pH. Of note, the VD/VT was reduced in both groups but the normal group was compensated by an increase in minute ventilation above baseline. In OHS patients there was a marked hypoventilation for first 5 to 10 minutes followed by a partial recovery of minute ventilation, which was insufficient to overcome the increase in VD/VT, which primarily arose from a reduction in tidal volume. An earlier study indicated a more marked increase in Pco_2 and reduction in minute ventilation in patients with an OHS breathing Fio_2 of 1,[50] indicating significant hyperoxia-induced respiratory depression.

Adipokines and Obesity Hypoventilation Syndrome

Adiposity can contribute to the pathogenesis of OHS via metabolic derangements. Leptin and adiponectin are adipokines released by adipose tissue. Leptin stimulates respiration, and leptin deficiency leads to hypoventilation.[51,52] Obese subjects demonstrate high leptin levels suggestive of resistance.[53] Leptin levels have been shown to be 50% higher in OHS than in controls.[54] Campo and colleagues[55] reported that hyperleptinemia in obese subjects reduces respiratory drive and hypercapnic response independent of the percentage of body fat. Similarly, serum leptin was found to be more strongly associated with hypercapnia than the degree of adiposity.[56] Hypoxia has been shown to stimulate leptin secretion, suggesting that increased leptin levels may be related to hypoventilation in OHS.[57] In fact, treatment of OHS with NIV did reduce leptin levels in a small group of patients.[58,59] The role of leptin in ventilatory control is still being elucidated. Adiponectin released by adipokines have an antiatherogenic effect, and the levels are reduced in obesity.[60] Hypoxia stimulates hypoxia-inducible factor 1α, thereby increasing leptin and reducing adiponectin levels.[61,62] Reduced adiponectin levels have been found in patients with OHS.[63]

CLINICAL PRESENTATION AND DIAGNOSIS

The initial presentation of OHS in critically ill patients is acute on chronic hypercapnic respiratory failure. Such patients tend to be severely obese, have severe OSA, and are usually drowsy. Cor pulmonale, facial plethora, enlarged neck circumference, rapid shallow respirations, a loud P2 on cardiac examination, and elevated jugular venous distention are findings on physical examination. If the patient has had a sleep study, the mean oxygen nadir during sleep is lower and time spent with oxygen saturation less than 90% is increased. In a study of patients with OHS the mean oxygen nadir was 65%, with a mean 50% of time with oxygen saturation less than 90%.[64] Approximately 90% of patients with OHS have concomitant OSA while the remainder has evidence of nonobstructive sleep hypoventilation, demonstrated by an increase in sleep partial pressure of CO_2 in arterial blood ($Paco_2$) or oxygen saturation 88% or less in the absence of obstructive events. Pulmonary function testing reveals a mild to moderate restrictive ventilatory defect and a severely reduced ERV without evidence of airflow obstruction. An awake arterial blood gas while on room air with a $Paco_2$ greater than 45 mm Hg is needed to confirm daytime hypoventilation. Daytime hypoxemia during wakefulness should also lead clinicians to suspect OHS.[1] It is important to recognize that OHS is a diagnosis of exclusion and exists in the absence of other causes of hypoventilation such as pulmonary disease, neuromuscular weakness, or chest wall disorders. The alveolar-arterial (A-a) gradient is usually normal and can differentiate pulmonary parenchymal disease as the cause of hypoventilation; however, owing to ventilation and perfusion mismatch in the lung bases of obese patients, it is not uncommon to have a modest elevation in A-a gradient.[65] Serum bicarbonate can be used as a screening test, with levels less than 27 mEq/L having a 97% negative predictive value.[1] A serum bicarbonate level of 27 mmol/L and higher gives sensitivity of 76.6% and specificity of 74.6%. A nadir oxygen saturation level (Spo_2) less than 80% is also an independent predictor of the diagnosis of OHS with a sensitivity of 82.8% and specificity of 5.5%.[66] Secondary erythrocytosis may be found on complete blood count. In the ICU, transcutaneous Pco_2 and end-tidal Pco_2 may also be useful in monitoring.[67]

Unfortunately OHS is often underdiagnosed, incorrectly diagnosed, and undertreated. Although Nowbar and colleagues[5] reported the prevalence of OHS among hospitalized patients with BMI of at least 35 as 30%, only 23% of these patients actually received the diagnosis of OHS and only 13% were discharged with recommendations for long-term treatment such as noninvasive or invasive ventilation. Marik and Desai[7] reported that of OHS patients admitted to the ICU, 75% had had multiple hospitalizations and had been diagnosed with asthma or COPD in the absence of supportive smoking history or pulmonary function testing. These findings indicate a lack of recognition and, hence, underdiagnosis of this disease. Marik and Desai[7] coined the term "malignant obesity hypoventilation syndrome" to describe patients admitted to the ICU with hypercapnic respiratory failure and multisystem organ dysfunction related to obesity. A BMI greater than 40 and a $Paco_2$ greater than 45 mm Hg with comorbid diseases of type 2 diabetes and metabolic syndrome were identified in all ICU patients, and 13% had a history of deep venous thrombosis.[7] In addition, 86% of patients were treated with diuretics for congestive heart failure. Echocardiographic findings of left ventricular hypertrophy, left ventricular dysfunction, and pulmonary hypertension were reported in most patients.[7] Eighteen percent of patients died during the index hospitalization, confirming the high mortality associated with the disease.[7]

TREATMENT

It is important to recognize that treatment of OHS in the critically ill patient should include acute management of respiratory failure but also consideration of long-term care strategies to deal with chronic respiratory failure, comorbid disease, and obesity. Management of acute respiratory failure includes invasive and noninvasive ventilatory strategies. Ventilation via PAP, oxygen, or both will more than likely be needed at home to manage chronic respiratory failure. Because pathophysiology centers on the detrimental effects of obesity, weight loss is prudent. Bariatric surgery and pharmacologic management of hypoventilation have varied success regarding certain measures and outcomes. Each approach is examined separately.

Positive Airway Pressure Therapy

CPAP, BPAP, and AVAPS have each been examined in OHS patients. The initial choice of PAP therapy in the critically ill OHS patient should be chosen after careful review of the clinical history and physical examination. Critically ill OHS patients may have contraindications to the use of PAP via a nasal or oronasal interface, and should instead be intubated and receive mechanical ventilation. Reasons for invasive mechanical ventilation would include mental obtundation, hemodynamic instability, multiorgan failure, and severe acidosis.[68] Additional important considerations in invasive airway management of critically ill obese patients include difficulty in intubation because of limited neck mobility and mouth opening in obese subjects,[69] and rapid oxygen desaturation when obese patients assume the supine position owing to an additional decrease in the FRC and ERV.[70] Successful intubation of the difficult airway in obese critically ill patients requires technical skill and familiarity with advanced techniques if needed.

At present there are no guidelines for pulmonary management of the critically ill OHS patient. Providers should keep in mind that much of the current knowledge of the effects of PAP on OHS were conducted in sleep laboratories in ambulatory patients and not in a critically ill population, nor exclusively in patients with OHS in the ICU. Gursel and colleagues[71] reported that higher positive end-expiratory pressure (PEEP) levels and longer times are needed to reduce Pco_2 in ICU obese patients in comparison with nonobese counterparts. There was no difference in the mode of NIV between obese and nonobese patients admitted to the ICU for acute hypercapnic respiratory failure; however, both pressure control and pressure support modes were used more frequently than AVAPS.[71]

Continuous positive airway pressure

As most patients with OHS have concomitant OSA, it seems reasonable to use CPAP in these patients. CPAP improves daytime hypercapnia,[72] can prevent obstructive events, and can reduce the work of breathing and expiratory flow limitation.[24] Reiterating that the effects of CPAP on OHS were conducted in sleep laboratories on ambulatory patients with OHS, providers should caution its use in critically ill OHS patients, as usually such patients present with acute hypercapnic respiratory failure, so a mode that promotes ventilation may be more suitable. Nevertheless it is important to address the effects of CPAP on OHS, particularly as management of this condition in the chronic setting is important. In a prospective study in severely obese patients with BMI of 50 or higher with OSA and with OSA and OHS matched for spirometry, BMI, and AHI, a single night of CPAP was able to effectively improve AHI and sleep measures in both groups. Higher CPAP pressures of 13.9 ± 3.1 cm H_2O were needed in the OHS group; however, 43% of OHS patients still had evidence of hypoxemia, with greater than 20% of total sleep time with Spo_2 less than 90% compared with 9% of those with OSA alone.[73] Higher levels of BMI and more total sleep time with Spo_2 less than 90% during the diagnostic polysomnogram was associated with this finding.[73] In a randomized trial of CPAP or BPAP in OHS patients without severe nocturnal desaturation (defined as Spo_2 <80% for >10 minutes or CO_2 retention >10 mm Hg despite optimal CPAP), change in daytime Pco_2, awake Spo_2, bicarbonate levels, and sleepiness were not different at 3 months in those who received CPAP or BPAP.[72] Probably just as important as the mode of PAP therapy is adherence to treatment. Mokhlesi and colleagues[74] reported that the use of CPAP or BPAP therapy for longer than 4.5 hours per day led to greater improvement in Pco_2 (7.7 vs 2.4 mm Hg) and Po_2 (9.2 vs 1.8 mm Hg) compared with less adherent use, with no between-group differences in CPAP or BPAP. In summary, then, CPAP can be used to treat OHS in most patients in the chronic setting. However, it must be emphasized that polysomnography with titration and follow-up is needed to determine which patients may require BPAP.

Bilevel positive airway pressure

BPAP delivered through an oronasal mask or nasal mask (also known as NIV) allows providers to set an expiratory positive airway pressure (EPAP) to alleviate the upper airway obstruction, which is important in addressing the OSA component of OHS, but also to set inspiratory positive airway pressure (IPAP) above the EPAP level to improve alveolar ventilation in patients with OHS. BPAP effectively improves Po_2 and reduces Pco_2 and pH in patients with OHS whether treatment is initiated in the acute or the ambulatory setting,[75] and improves the quality of life and ventilatory responsiveness to CO_2.[59,72,76] Although there is no universally accepted approach to titration of PAP in the sleep laboratory, a good rule of thumb is that the EPAP should be increased until there is resolution of obstructive events. Thus if the O_2 saturation remains persistently less than 90%, the IPAP should be added above the EPAP level. The difference between the IPAP and EPAP values generally needs to be 8 to 10 cm H_2O, and should be titrated to achieve oxygen saturation greater than 90%. Oxygen may need to be added and titrated despite improvement in ventilation in some patients. Unfortunately, for most ICUs this type of strategy is not used owing to the absence of polysomnography.

Taken together, the use of a strategy and protocol for noninvasive management in other forms of acute hypercapnic respiratory failure, such as COPD, may be useful in acute hypercapnic respiratory failure caused by OHS. It is well known that NIV improves outcomes in COPD[77]; however, the efficacy of this approach in acute hypercapnic respiratory failure caused by OHS remains unclear. In a prospective study of 716 consecutive patients with COPD and OHS admitted to an ICU,[78] the investigators used a protocol of initiating BPAP with IPAP 12 cm H_2O and increased pressure by 2 to 3 cm H_2O as tolerated. Initial EPAP of 5 cm H_2O was used, increasing by 1 to 2 cm H_2O if needed to improve hypoxemia or comfort, with supplemental oxygen to achieve an oxygen saturation of 92% or more or Pao_2 greater than 65 mm Hg. Similar outcomes of avoidance of intubation in comparison with COPD patients were reported.[78]

It is imperative that providers carefully monitor OHS patients who present with acute hypercapnic respiratory failure to determine response to NIV. Lemyze and colleagues[79] aimed to identify the determinant of NIV success or failure in morbidly obese patients with severe acute respiratory decompensation of OHS, irrespective of the cause of acute respiratory failure, in a single ICU. In 76 consecutive patients with BMI greater than 40, factors associated with NIV failure were pneumonia, high Sequential Organ Failure Assessment Score, and high Simplified Acute Physiologic Score 2 at admission. Such patients were admitted with hypoxic respiratory failure, had early NIV failure, and a significant mortality of 92% versus 17.5%. Factors associated with successful response to NIV included high Pco_2 at admission. Although a delayed response to NIV (defined as inability to decrease Pco_2 by 15% or raise pH to >7.3 in the first 2 hours) was observed in most patients, NIV was still successful.[79]

BPAP with spontaneous and spontaneous timed modes are available. In the spontaneous mode, the patient triggers the BPAP whereas in the spontaneous timed mode, a backup rate is ordered whereby if the patient fails to trigger the BPAP, the device delivers a machine-triggered cycle. Both modes are effective in the management of OHS, although the spontaneous mode is associated with an increase in respiratory events owing to the development of central and mixed events without a difference in transcutaneous Pco_2 between modes.[80]

Average volume-assured pressure support

AVAPS is a form of NIV that is adjunctive to BPAP, whereby tidal volume is set by the provider. In traditional bilevel pressure ventilation the tidal volume is pressure limited, in contrast to volume assurance by AVAPS. Although pressure-limited NIV has been shown to be better tolerated owing to its less varying peak inspiratory pressure, volume-assured NIV provides greater stability of the tidal volume.[81] Three studies have examined the outcomes of AVAPS in OHS, all of which, notably, excluded critically ill patients. Storre and colleagues[82] performed a randomized crossover trial in 10 patients with OHS (BMI >30 and $Paco_2$ ≥45 mm Hg) for which CPAP failed to reduce the transcutaneous Pco_2 level ($Ptcco_2$) to less than 45 mm Hg and reach a respiratory disturbance index of less than 10 events per hour. Sleep measures, health-related quality of life, the Severe Respiratory Insufficiency Questionnaire, and $Ptcco_2$ were measured and compared after 6 weeks of each modality. Although AVAPS led to significant improvements in $Ptcco_2$ compared with BPAP (-12.6 ± 12.2 vs -5.6 ± 11.8 mm Hg), this did not translate to improved clinical outcomes of sleep time, health-related quality of life, or severe respiratory insufficiency compared with BPAP. Perhaps this was due to variance in the peak inspiratory pressures leading to a higher respiratory disturbance index associated with AVAPS. In the second study, Murphy and colleagues[83] compared AVAPS with fixed pressure support in a randomized controlled trial including 50 patients with OHS. Both modalities improved the primary outcome of daytime $Paco_2$ at 3 months compared with baseline, but there was no between-group difference between fixed pressure support and AVAPS in daytime $Paco_2$ or health-related quality of life. Lastly, Janssens and colleagues[84] reported decreased objective total sleep time and subjective reports of lighter sleep with more awakenings with AVAPS in comparison with BPAP in a study of 12 patients with stable OHS. AVAPS, however, did significantly improve $Ptcco_2$ when compared with BPAP. At present there is no defined role for the use of AVAPS in stable OHS, although it can be considered in certain cases. Further research that includes studies with larger numbers of subjects and the inclusion of hospitalized patients is needed.

Bariatric Surgery

Many patients with obesity turn to bariatric surgery to bring about weight loss. Large population studies support that weight loss is associated with an improvement in the severity and likelihood of sleep-disordered breathing. A weight loss of 10% reduces the AHI by 26%.[85] In addition, weight loss can substantially improve outcomes in obese patients not only by reducing the severity of sleep-disordered breathing but also through improvement in respiratory mechanics, hypoxia, hypercapnia, and pulmonary function tests. Common types of bariatric surgical therapies include Roux-en-Y gastric bypass (RYGB), laparoscopic adjustable gastric banding (LAGB), laparoscopic sleeve gastrectomy, laparoscopic biliopancreatic diversion, and biliopancreatic diversion/duodenal switch, and achieve weight loss via malabsorption, restriction of food intake, and hormonal mechanisms. Bariatric surgery is considered for patients with a BMI of 40 or higher or 35 or higher for those with significant comorbidities, including obesity hypoventilation.[86] Whereas outcomes of bariatric weight-loss surgery are well known, its effects in strictly OHS patients are not. Nevertheless, in the largest prospective trial comparing bariatric surgery with controls, surgery led to a 23% reduction in the BMI compared with 0.1% in controls, with reductions in overall mortality and rates of obesity-related comorbidities.[87,88] Although bariatric surgery resulted in resolution of OSA in 63% of patients, it is equally important to recognize that despite significant amounts of weight loss, patients may still have OSA of moderate severity owing to the fact that patients are still moderately obese 10 years after surgery.[87] Furthermore, the greatest weight loss occurs within the first 2 years postoperatively, and some patients regain some of that weight. Hence, discontinuing the use of PAP devices without objective evidence of the resolution of sleep-disordered breathing is discouraged.

In addition to positive outcomes for sleep-disordered breathing, weight loss improves respiratory mechanics, blood gases, and pulmonary function tests. Pulmonary function improves in morbidly obese patients following laparoscopic RYGB and LAGB. FEV_1 increased to 112% and FVC to 109% of baseline value after just 3 months postoperatively,[89] although the number of subjects who met the criteria for OHS in this study is unknown. In addition, at 1 year SpO_2 improved from 88.3% to 96.2% following laparoscopic bariatric surgery in 11 patients with morbid obesity and OHS.[90]

Tracheostomy

Failure of an OHS patient to wean from mechanical ventilation or inability of NIV to achieve targeted clinical measures may necessitate the placement of tracheostomy. Following tracheostomy, OSA and daytime hypercarbia improve but may not completely resolve.[91,92] Furthermore, tracheostomy in morbidly obese patients is more challenging because of anatomic factors.[70] Of note, a trend toward higher 30-day mortality after tracheotomy in morbidly obese patients has been observed.[93]

Pharmacologic Therapy

As OHS patients have high serum bicarbonate levels, in theory acetazolamide, a carbonic anhydrase inhibitor, should reduce serum bicarbonate levels, thus promoting increased ventilation and lowering of Pco_2. In a study of 25 OHS patients receiving invasive mechanical ventilation in 2 ICUs, acetazolamide reduced serum bicarbonate levels by 8.4 ± 3.0 mmol/L alongside an increase in hypercapnic drive and ventilator response.[37] In 9 patients with OSA, acetazolamide reduced the AHI from 25 to 18 events per hour, but was unable to completely normalize the AHI.[94] The effect of medroxyprogesterone is mixed. Medroxyprogesterone did not reduce AHI in comparison with placebo in 10 patient s with OSA.[95] However, in 10 patients with OHS, its use was associated with reduction of Pco_2 by 13 mm Hg.[96] In a Cochrane Database review of drug therapy for OSA, the investigators concluded that there is currently insufficient evidence to recommend any systemic pharmacologic treatment for OSA, which is present in most patients with OHS.[97]

OUTCOMES

Nowbar and colleagues[5] described the outcomes of OHS patients in a comparison with obese patients hospitalized with acute illness. Patients with OHS were more likely to require hospital admission and mechanical ventilation, and showed a trend toward higher ICU admission. At 18 months they had higher mortality (18% vs 9%) than obese patients without hypercapnia. The adjusted relative risk of death in OHS was 4-fold higher than that for obese controls. Although there were no in-hospital deaths, most of the deaths occurred in the first 3 months following discharge. A smaller retrospective study[75] of patients using NIV for OHS, with 22 of the 54 patients initiated for acute hypercapnic respiratory failure, reported a low mortality, with only 1 death among the patients on NIV. About 22% of patients refused NIV, and there was 46% mortality in this population. This study from 2005 highlighted the adverse consequences of noncompliance with NIV in OHS patients, since when most studies have reported an increased use of NIV. Priou and colleagues[98] assessed the long-term outcomes of 130 consecutive patients with OHS patients on NIV, including 38 patients who were started on NIV in the ICU for acute respiratory failure. Over a 10-year period the mortality of these patients was 18.5% with an NIV discontinuation rate of 18.5%. Of note, treatment with oxygen was associated with higher mortality. Overall 5-year survival was 77.3%. This finding was similar to the results of Budweiser and colleagues[99] on 5-year survival in patients with OHS. A decrease in nocturnal Pco_2 and hemoglobin was associated with improved survival whereas hypoxemia, low pH, and elevated inflammation markers predicted worse survival. Carrillo and colleagues[78] prospectively studied the outcomes of acute hypercapnic respiratory failure caused by OHS (173 patients) versus COPD exacerbation (543 patients) when managed using NIV. The type of ventilator, duration of NIV, and complication rate were similar in both groups. Patients with OHS were older, but the severity scores were similar in both groups. Patients with OHS had lower rates of NIV failure, readmission to the ICU, and reduced in-hospital mortality (6% vs 18%). The 1-year survival was higher for OHS patients (odds ratio 1.83; 95% confidence interval 1.24–2.69; $P = .002$), but this did not retain significance after adjusting for confounding variables. In the report by Marik and Desai[7] describing a "malignant obesity hypoventilation syndrome," 61 patients with OHS (BMI >40) were admitted to the ICU with acute hypercapnic respiratory failure and had multiorgan dysfunction, with a high inpatient mortality of 18%. There was a high rate of NIV failure (39.7%), and 7 patients needed a tracheostomy. In 18 of the patients the end-expiratory esophageal pressure was 17 $\pm$ 2.9 cm H_2O, indicating the high work of breathing required to overcome the high pleural pressures. All of these patients were ventilated using airway pressure release ventilation, which has not been previously described. The investigators chose this to optimize lung recruitment and minimize sedation requirements. Another study compared the outcomes of 110 patients with OHS while on NIV with those of 220 patients with OSA using CPAP. Of interest, NIV was started following an episode of exacerbation in 70.3% of the patients from the OHS arm. Patients were matched for gender, age, and date of positive pressure therapy initiation. Patients with OHS had higher BMI (42.4 vs 34.9) but frequencies of diabetes mellitus, ischemic heart disease, and stroke were the same. After titration, the patients with OHS were more often on supplemental oxygen and the rate of lack of acceptance in the OHS cohort was 11.3%, contrasting with noncompliance and treatment withdrawal in 15.7% of patients with OSA on CPAP. This case-control study reported a 2-fold increased risk of 5-year mortality for those with OHS in comparison with those with OSA (15.5% vs 4.5%), and suggests that despite similar rates of noncompliance, the mortality remains higher for those with OHS than for those with OSA alone.[100]

SUMMARY

OHS is a common cause of acute on chronic hypercapnic respiratory failure in patients treated in the ICU. Understanding the mechanisms leading to this condition in obese individuals can positively affect the ability of clinicians to treat OHS. Both obesity and OSA are highly prevalent conditions in the adult population. It is estimated that 10% to

20% of patients with OSA also have OHS. OHS may be present in as many as 31% of obese patients admitted to the ICU, and obesity hypoventilation may be actually more prevalent than has been reported. Mechanisms for OHS include a restrictive respiratory physiology with a decreased FRC and ERV, lower respiratory system compliance, and the development of intrinsic PEEP. All of these factors are aggravated by a supine position, which increases hypercapnia and work of breathing. OSA per se may be implicated in the development of OHS when sustained hypoxia occurs. Patients with OHS have an impaired ventilatory drive, which can be improved with PAP therapy. Leptin, an adipokine, may lead to hypoventilation, and exists at higher levels in obese patients with OHS. Important diagnostic features of OHS include signs of cor pulmonale and hypoxemia in obese patients. An awake blood gas showing a $Paco_2$ greater than 45 mm Hg confirms the diagnosis. Other laboratory features include higher serum bicarbonate levels (>27 mEq/L). Both continuous and bilevel airway pressure therapy have been successfully used in the acute setting for OHS therapy, and certain presentations preclude their use (eg, multiorgan failure, obtundation). In general, patients with OHS need higher CPAP pressures than those with OSA. When used in the acute setting, bilevel pressures with an inspiratory to expiratory pressure difference of 8 to 10 cm H_2O are used and are titrated to achieve oxygen saturation greater than 90%. Engineered, more sophisticated modes of NIV can be applied to these patients in the acute setting. Different modalities can be set to use a backup rate while others can offer AVAPS. Pharmacotherapy has been attempted, but both acetazolamide and medroxyprogesterone lack substantial evidence of their effectiveness. Medical and surgical weight loss have been shown to improve hypoventilation in these patients and should be encouraged after the acute episode of respiratory failure has resolved, with patients being treated chronically with PAP therapy. Long-term mortality rates for OHS are higher than for patients with OSA, even when compliance to PAP therapy is similar. Mortality is higher for obese patients with OHS than for counterparts who do not have daytime hypercapnia. On the other hand, patients with OHS generally have a better survival than those with other causes of hypoventilation leading to respiratory failure, such as COPD.

REFERENCES

1. Mokhlesi B, Tulaimat A, Faibussowitsch I, et al. Obesity hypoventilation syndrome: prevalence and predictors in patients with obstructive sleep apnea. Sleep Breath 2007;11:117–24.
2. Ogden C. Prevalence of obesity in the United States 2009-2010. NCHS Data Brief 2012;82:1–8.
3. Ogden CL, Carroll MD, Curtin LR, et al. Prevalence of overweight and obesity in the United States. JAMA 2006;295:1549–55.
4. Littleton S, Mokhlesi B. The Pickwickian syndrome: obesity hypoventilation syndrome. Clin Chest Med 2009;30(3):467–78.
5. Nowbar S, Burkart KM, Gonzales R, et al. Obesity-associated hypoventilation in hospitalized patients: prevalence, effects and outcome. Am J Med 2004;116:1–7.
6. Akinnusi ME, Pineda LA, El Solh AA. Effect of obesity on intensive care morbidity and mortality: a meta-analysis. Crit Care Med 2008;36:151–8.
7. Marik PE, Desai H. Characteristics of patients with the "malignant obesity hypoventilation syndrome" admitted to an ICU. J Intensive Care Med 2013;28:124–30.
8. Harada Y, Chihara Y, Azuma M, et al. Obesity hypoventilation syndrome in Japan and independent determinants of arterial carbon dioxide levels. Respirology 2014;19(8):1233–40.

9. Bübül Y, Ayik S, Ozlu T, et al. Frequency and predictors of obesity hypoventilation in hospitalized patients at a tertiary health care institution. Ann Thorac Med 2014;9(2):87–91.

10. Berger KI, Ayappa I, Chatr-Amontri B, et al. Obesity hypoventilation syndrome as a spectrum of respiratory disturbances during sleep. Chest 2001;120:1231–8.

11. Perez de Llano LA, Kesten S. Clinical heterogeneity among patients with obesity hypoventilation syndrome: therapeutic implications. Respiration 2008;75:34–9.

12. Macavei VM, Spurling KJ, Loft J, et al. Diagnostic predictors of obesity-hypoventilation syndrome in patients suspected of having sleep disordered breathing. J Clin Sleep Med 2013;9:879–84.

13. Laaban JP, Chailleux E. Daytime hypercapnia in adult patients with obstructive sleep apnea syndrome in France, before initiating nocturnal nasal continuous positive airway pressure therapy. Chest 2005;127:710–5.

14. Kaw R, Hernandez AV, Walker E, et al. Determinants of hypercapnia in obese patients with obstructive sleep apnea: a systematic review and metaanalysis of cohort studies. Chest 2009;136:787–96.

15. Jones RL, Nzekwu MM. The effects of body mass index on lung volumes. Chest 2006;130:827–33.

16. Resta O, Foschino-Barbaro MP, Bonfitto P, et al. Prevalence and mechanisms of diurnal hypercapnia in a sample of morbidly obese subjects with obstructive sleep apnea. Respir Med 2000;94:240–6.

17. Lazarus R, Sparrow D, Weiss ST. Effects of obesity and fat distribution on ventilatory function: the normative aging study. Chest 1997;111:891–8.

18. Behazin N, Jones SB, Cohen RI, et al. Respiratory restriction and elevated pleural and esophageal pressures in morbid obesity. J Appl Physiol (1985) 2010;108:212–8.

19. Sharp JT, Henry JP, Sweany SK, et al. The total work of breathing in normal and obese men. J Clin Invest 1964;43:728–39.

20. Pankow W, Podszus T, Gutheil T. Expiratory flow limitation and intrinsic positive end-expiratory pressure in obesity. J Appl Physiol (1985) 1998;85:1236–43.

21. Pelosi P, Croci M, Ravagnan I. Total respiratory system, lung, and chest wall mechanics in sedated-paralyzed postoperative morbidly obese patients. Chest 1996;109:144–51.

22. Steier J, Jolley CJ, Seymour J, et al. Neural respiratory drive in obesity. Thorax 2009;64:719–25.

23. Yap JC, Watson RA, Gilbey S. Effects of posture on respiratory mechanics in obesity. J Appl Physiol (1985) 1995;79:1199–205.

24. Lee MY, Lin CC, Shen SY, et al. Work of breathing in eucapnic and hypercapnic sleep apnea syndrome. Respiration 2009;77:146–53.

25. Chlif M, Keochkerian D, Choquet D, et al. Effects of obesity on breathing pattern, ventilatory neural drive and mechanics. Respir Physiol Neurobiol 2009;168:198–202.

26. Zavorsky GS, Hoffman SL. Pulmonary gas exchange in the morbidly obese. Obes Rev 2008;9:326–39.

27. Javaheri S, Colangelo G, Lacey W, et al. Chronic hypercapnia in obstructive sleep apnea-hypopnea syndrome. Sleep 1994;17:416–23.

28. Sharp JT, Druz WS, Kondragunta VR. Diaphragmatic responses to body position changes in obese patients with obstructive sleep apnea. Am Rev Respir Dis 1986;133:32–7.

29. Farkas GA, Gosselin LE, Zhan WZ, et al. Histochemical and mechanical proper-ties of diaphragm muscle in morbidly obese Zucker rats. J Appl Physiol (1985) 1994;77:2250–9.
30. Jonville S, Delpech N, Denjean A. Contribution of respiratory acidosis to dia-phragmatic fatigue at exercise. Eur Respir J 2002;19:1079–86.
31. Kessler R, Chaouat A, Schinkewitch P, et al. The obesity-hypoventilation syn-drome revisited: a prospective study of 34 consecutive cases. Chest 2001; 120:369–76.
32. Olson A, Zwillich C. The obesity hypoventilation syndrome. Am J Med 2005;118: 948–56.
33. Sin DD, Jones RL, Man GC. Hypercapnic ventilatory response in patients with and without obstructive sleep apnea: do age gender, obesity and daytime PaCO(2) matter? Chest 2000;117:454–9.
34. Berger KI, Ayappa I, Sorkin IB, et al. CO(2) homeostasis during periodic breath-ing in obstructive sleep apnea. J Appl Physiol (1985) 2000;88:257–64.
35. Ayappa I, Berger KI, Norman RG, et al. Hypercapnia and ventilatory periodicity in obstructive sleep apnea syndrome. Am J Respir Crit Care Med 2002;166: 1112–5.
36. Gifford AH, Leiter JC, Manning HL. Respiratory function in an obese patient with sleep-disordered breathing. Chest 2010;138:704–15.
37. Raurich JM, Rialp G, Ibáñez J, et al. Hypercapnic respiratory failure in obesity hypoventilation syndrome: CO(2) response and acetazolamide treatment effects. Respir Care 2010;55:1442–8.
38. Bahamman A. Acute ventilatory failure complicating obesity hypoventilation: update on a 'critical care syndrome'. Curr Opin Pulm Med 2010;16:543–51.
39. El-Gamal H, Khayat A, Shikora S, et al. Relationship of dyspnea to respiratory drive and pulmonary function tests in obese patients before and after weight loss. Chest 2005;128:3870–4.
40. Lopata M, Onal E. Mass loading, sleep apnea, and the pathogenesis of obesity hypoventilation. Am Rev Respir Dis 1982;126:640–5.
41. Sampson MG, Grassino K. Neuromechanical properties in obese patients during carbon dioxide rebreathing. Am J Med 1983;75:81–90.
42. de Lucas-Ramos P, de Miguel-Díez J, Santacruz-Siminiani A, et al. Benefits at 1 year of nocturnal intermittent positive pressure ventilation in patients with obesity-hypoventilation syndrome. Respir Med 2004;98:962–7.
43. Lin C. Effect of nasal CPAP on ventilatory drive in normocapnic and hypercapnic patients with obstructive sleep apnoea syndrome. Eur Respir J 1994;7:2005–10.
44. Javaheri S, Colangelo G, Corser B, et al. Familial respiratory chemosensitivity does not predict hypercapnia of patients with sleep apnea-hypopnea syndrome. Am Rev Respir Dis 1992;145:837–40.
45. Jokic R, Zintel T, Sridhar G, et al. Ventilatory responses to hypercapnia and hyp-oxia in relatives of patients with the obesity hypoventilation syndrome. Thorax 2000;55:940–5.
46. Berthon-Jones M, Sullivan CE. Time course of change in ventilator response to CO_2 with long-term CPAP therapy for obstructive sleep apnea. Am Rev Respir Dis 1987;135:144–7.
47. Han F, Chen E, Wei H, et al. Treatment effects on carbon dioxide retention in patients with obstructive sleep apnea-hypopnea syndrome. Chest 2001;119:1814–9.
48. Manuel AR, Hart N, Stradling JR. Is raised bicarbonate, without hypercapnia, part of the physiological spectrum of obesity-related hypoventilation? Chest 2015;147:362–8.

49. Hollier CA, Harmer AR, Maxwell LJ, et al. Moderate concentrations of supplemental oxygen worsen hypercapnia in obesity hypoventilation syndrome: a randomized crossover study. Thorax 2014;69:346–53.
50. Wijesinghe M, Williams M, Perrin K. The effect of supplemental oxygen on hypercapnia in subjects with obesity-associated hypoventilation: a randomized crossover clinical study. Chest 2011;139:1018–24.
51. Atwood C. Sleep-related hyperventilation: the evolving role of leptin. Chest 2005;128:1079–81.
52. Kalra S. Central leptin insufficiency syndrome: an interactive etiology for obesity, metabolic and neural diseases and for designing new therapeutic interventions. Peptides 2008;29:127–38.
53. Levy P, Pépin JL, Arnaud C, et al. Intermittent hypoxia and sleep-disordered breathing: current concepts and perspectives. Eur Respir J 2008;32:1082–95.
54. Phillips BG, Kato M, Narkiewicz K, et al. Increase in leptin levels, sympathetic drive, and weight gain in obstructive sleep apnoea. Am J Physiol Heart Circ Physiol 2000;279:H234–7.
55. Campo A, Frühbeck G, Zulueta JJ, et al. Hyperleptinemia, respiratory drive and hypercapnic response in obese patients. Eur Respir J 2007;30:223–31.
56. Phipps PR, Starritt E, Caterson I, et al. Association of serum leptin and hypoventilation in human obesity. Thorax 2002;57:75–6.
57. Grosfeld A, Zilberfarb V, Turban S, et al. Hypoxia increases leptin expression in human PAZ6 adipose cells. Diabetologia 2002;45:527–30.
58. Yee BJ, Cheung J, Phipps P, et al. Treatment of obesity hypoventilation syndrome and serum leptin. Respiration 2006;73:209–12.
59. Redolfi S, Corda L, La Piana G, et al. Long-term non-invasive ventilation increases chemosensitivity and leptin in obesity hypoventilation syndrome. Respir Med 2007;101:1191–5.
60. Higashiura K, Ura N, Ohata J, et al. Correlations of adiponectin level with insulin resistance and atherosclerosis in Japanese male populations. Clin Endocrinol 2004;61:753–9.
61. Hosogai N, Fukuhara A, Oshima K, et al. Adipose tissue hypoxia and obesity and its impact on adipocytokine dysregulation. Diabetes 2007;56:901–11.
62. Chen B, Lam KS, Wang Y, et al. Hypoxia dysregulates the production of adiponectin and plasminogen activator inhibitor-1 independent of reactive oxygen species in adipocytes. Biochem Biophys Res Commun 2006;341:549–56.
63. Borel JC, Roux-Lombard P, Tamisier R, et al. Endothelial dysfunction and specific inflammation in obesity hypoventilation. PLoS One 2009;4:e6733.
64. Mokhlesi B. Obesity hypoventilation syndrome: a state of the art review. Respir Care 2010;55(10):1347–62.
65. Rochester DS, Arora NS. Respiratory failure in obesity. In: Mancini M, Lewis B, Contaldo F, editors. Medical complications of obesity. London: Academic Press; 1980. p. 183.
66. Bingol Z, Pihtili A, Cagatay P, et al. Clinical predictors of obesity hypoventilation syndrome in obese subjects with obstructive sleep apnea. Respir Care 2015. [Epub ahead of print].
67. Piper AJ, Gonazalez-Bermejo J, Janssens J. Sleep hypoventilation diagnostic considerations and technological limitations. Sleep Med Clin 2014;9:301–13.
68. Mokhlesi B, Kryger MH, Grunstein RR. Assessment and management of patients with obesity hypoventilation syndrome. Proc Am Thorac Soc 2008;5:218–25.
69. Foster G. Principles and practice in the management of obesity. Am J Respir Crit Care Med 2003;168:274–80.

70. El-Solh A. Clinical approach to the critically ill, morbidly obese patient. Am J Respir Crit Care Med 2004;169:557–61.

71. Gursel G, Aydogdu M, Gulbas G, et al. The influence of severe obesity on non-invasive ventilation (NIV) strategies and response in patients with acute hypercapnic respiratory failure attacks in the ICU. Minerva Anestesiol 2011;11:17–25.

72. Piper AJ, Wang D, Yee BJ. Randomised trial of PCP vs bilevel support in the treatment of obesity hypoventilation syndrome without severe nocturnal desaturation. Thorax 2008;63:395–401.

73. Banerjee D, Yee BJ, Piper AJ. Obesity hypoventilation syndrome hypoxemia during continuous positive airway pressure. Chest 2007;131:1678–84.

74. Mokhlesi B, Tulaimat A, Evans AT, et al. Impact of adherence with positive airway pressure therapy on hypercapnia in obstructive sleep apnea. J Clin Sleep Med 2006;2:57–62.

75. Perez de Llano LA, Golpe R, Piquer MO, et al. Short term and long term effects of nasal intermittent positive pressure ventilation in patients with obesity hypoventilation syndrome. Chest 2005;128:587–94.

76. Chouri-Pontarollo N, Borel JC, Tamisier R, et al. Impaired objective daytime vigilance in obesity-hypoventilation syndrome: impact of noninvasive ventilation. Chest 2007;131:148–55.

77. Keenan SP, Sinuff T, Burns KE. Clinical practice guidelines for the use of noninvasive positive-pressure ventilation and non-invasive continuous positive airway pressure in the acute care setting. CMAJ 2011;183:E195–214.

78. Carrillo A, Ferrer M, Gonzalez-Diaz G, et al. Noninvasive ventilation in acute hypercapnic respiratory failure caused by obesity hypoventilation syndrome and chronic obstructive pulmonary disease. Am J Respir Crit Care Med 2012;186:1279–85.

79. Lemyze M, Taufour P, Duhamel A, et al. Determinants of noninvasive ventilation success or failure in morbidly obese patients in acute respiratory failure. PLoS One 2014;9:e97563.

80. Contal O, Adler D, Borel JC, et al. Impact of different backup respiratory rates on the efficacy of noninvasive positive pressure ventilation in obesity hypoventilation syndrome a randomized trial. Chest 2013;143:37–46.

81. Schonhofer B, Sonneborn M, Haidl P, et al. Comparison of two different modes for noninvasive mechanical ventilation in chronic respiratory failure: volume versus pressure controlled device. Eur Respir J 1997;10:184–91.

82. Storre JH, Suethe B, Fiechter R, et al. Average volume-assured pressure support in obesity hypoventilation a randomized crossover trial. Chest 2006;130:815–21.

83. Murphy PB, Davidson C, Hind MD, et al. Volume targeted versus pressure support non-invasive ventilation in patients with super obesity and chronic respiratory failure: a randomised controlled trial. Thorax 2012;67:727–34.

84. Janssens J, Metzger M, Sforza E. Impact of volume targeting on efficacy of bi-level non-invasive ventilation and sleep in obesity hypoventilation. Respir Med 2009;103:165–72.

85. Peppard PE, Young T, Palta M, et al. Longitudinal study of moderate weight change and sleep-disordered breathing. JAMA 2000;284:3015–21.

86. Mechanick J, Youdim A, Jones DB, et al. Clinical practice guidelines for the perioperative nutritional, metabolic, and nonsurgical support of the bariatric surgery patient—2013 update: cosponsored by American Association of Clinical Endocrinologists, the Obesity Society, and American Society for Metabolic & Bariatric Surgery. Surg Obes Relat Dis 2013;9(2):159–91.

87. Sjöström L, Lindroos AK, Peltonen M, et al. Lifestyle, diabetes, and cardiovascular risk factors 10 years after bariatric surgery. N Engl J Med 2004;351:2683–93.
88. Sjöström L. Review of key results from the Swedish Obese Subjects (SOS) trial—a prospective controlled intervention study of bariatric surgery. J Intern Med 2013;23:219–34.
89. Nguyen NT, Hinojosa MW, Smith BR. Improvement of restrictive and obstructive pulmonary mechanics following laparoscopic bariatric surgery. Surg Endosc 2009;23(4):808–12.
90. Lumanchi F, Marzano B, Fanti G, et al. Hypoxia and hypoventilation syndrome improvement after laparoscopic bariatric surgery in patients with morbid obesity. In Vivo 2010;24:329–31.
91. Kim SH, Eisele DW, Smith PL. Evaluation of patients with sleep apnea after tracheotomy. Arch Otolaryngol Head Neck Surg 1998;124:996–1000.
92. Rapoport DM, Garay SM, Epstein H, et al. Hypercapnia in the obstructive sleep apnea syndrome. A reevaluation of the "Pickwickian syndrome". Chest 1986;89:627–35.
93. Darrat I, Yaremchuk K. Early mortality rate of morbidly obese patients after tracheotomy. Laryngoscope 2008;118(2):2125–8.
94. Tojima H, Kunitomo F, Kimura H, et al. Effects of acetazolamide in patients with the sleep apnoea syndrome. Thorax 1988;43:113–9.
95. Cook WR, Benich JJ, Wooten SA. Indices of severity of obstructive sleep apnea syndrome do not change during medroxyprogesterone acetate therapy. Chest 1989;96:262–6.
96. Sutton FD, Zwillich CW, Creagh CE. Progesterone for outpatient treatment of Pickwickian syndrome. Ann Intern Med 1975;83:476–9.
97. Mason M, Welsh EJ, Smith I. Drug therapy for obstructive sleep apnoea in adults. Cochrane Database Syst Rev 2013;(5):CD003002.
98. Priou P, Hamel JF, Person C, et al. Long-term outcome of noninvasive positive pressure ventilation for obesity hypoventilation syndrome. Chest 2010;138:84–90.
99. Budweiser S, Riedl SG, Jörres RA, et al. Mortality and prognostic factors in patients with obesity hypoventilation syndrome undergoing noninvasive ventilation. J Intern Med 2007;261:375–83.
100. Castro-Anon O, Pérez de Llano LA, De la Fuente Sánchez S, et al. Obesity-hypoventilation syndrome: increased risk of death over sleep apnea syndrome. PLoS One 2015;10:e0117808.

Noninvasive Ventilation in Critically Ill Patients

Cesare Gregoretti, MD[a],*, Lara Pisani, MD[b], Andrea Cortegiani, MD[c],
Vito Marco Ranieri, MD[a]

KEYWORDS

- Noninvasive ventilation • Acute respiratory failure • Critically patients

KEY POINTS

- Noninvasive ventilation (NIV) is widely used in the critical care area and it is the first-line intervention for certain forms of acute respiratory failure.
- Explore the results of clinical studies on NPPV is very important to avoid drawbacks and to reduce the rate of failure during its application.
- Understanding principle of functioning of ventilator and modes will lead the operator to choose the best approach for his/her patients.

INTRODUCTION

Noninvasive ventilation (NIV) refers to the delivery of noninvasive intermittent positive pressure ventilation (NPPV) or noninvasive continuous positive airway pressure (CPAP) through the patient's mouth, nose, or both via an external interface. In contrast with conventional invasive mechanical ventilation (IMV) delivered via endotracheal tube or tracheostomy, NIV does not interfere with the patient's native upper airways and overall it does not impair glottis function. It may reduce the patient's effort and improve gas exchange while preserving the ability to swallow, cough, and speak. In addition, NIV may avert iatrogenic complications associated with invasive ventilation (ie, complications associated with endotracheal intubation)[1] and may reduce the risk of infections (ie, ventilator-associated pneumonia).[2]

[a] Department of Anesthesia and Intensive Care, Azienda Ospedaliero Universitaria "Città della Salute e della Scienza", Corso Dogliotti 14, Turin 10126, Italy; [b] Department of Specialistic, Diagnostic and Experimental Medicine (DIMES), Respiratory and Critical Care, Sant'Orsola Malpighi Hospital, Alma Mater Studiorum, University of Bologna, Via Massarenti 9, Bologna 40126, Italy; [c] Department of Biopathology, Medical and Forensic Biotechnologies (DIBIMEF), Section of Anesthesiology, Analgesia, Emergency and Intensive Care, Policlinico "P. Giaccone," University of Palermo, Palermo, Italy
* Corresponding author. Department of Anesthesia and Intensive Care, Azienda Ospedaliero Universitaria "Città della Salute e della Scienza", Corso Dogliotti 14, Turin 10126, Italy.
E-mail address: C.gregoretti@gmail.com

Crit Care Clin 31 (2015) 435–457
http://dx.doi.org/10.1016/j.ccc.2015.03.002
0749-0704/15/$ – see front matter © 2015 Elsevier Inc. All rights reserved.

criticalcare.theclinics.com

The rationale behind its use can be divided in 2 distinct categories:

1. Patients with lung failure caused by alveolar perfusion mismatching (ie, the ratio of arterial oxygen partial pressure to fractional inspired oxygen (PaO_2FiO_2) <300] and hypoxemia but without hypercapnia). In these patients the rationale of using NIV is to open derecruited alveoli, maintain them open, and decrease the patient's dyspnea through a reduction of the work of breathing (WOB) and respiratory rate.
2. Patients with ventilatory pump failure with hypercapnia and respiratory acidosis ($Paco_2$ >45 mm Hg and pH <7.35). This subgroup should be further divided into:
   a. Hypercapnia caused by an acute exacerbation of chronic obstructive pulmonary disease (AECOPD) in which carbon dioxide (CO_2) increase is not homogeneous in the lung. The reduction of CO_2 level is obtained with an amelioration of alveolar ventilation and an amelioration of ventilation-perfusion mismatching. In these patients WOB may be reduced by resting the respiratory muscles (patients are fatigued but not weak) and also counterbalancing intrinsic positive end-expiratory pressure (PEEPi).[3–5]
   b. Hypercapnia caused by genuine alveolar hypoventilation (ie, neuromuscular patients or other restrictive chest/lung disorders). In these patients, in contrast with patients with AECOPD, the reduction of WOB is achieved mainly by resting the respiratory muscles. Some patients with neuromuscular disorders have weak respiratory muscles and are thus incapable of regaining muscle strength[6] after resting on NPPV. Some patients in this subgroup need to counterbalance with PEEPi (ie, patients with severe obesity or quadriplegic patients in supine position).[7,8]
   c. Hypercapnia in end-stage interstitial lung diseases. These patients show impaired oxygen diffusion and Ventilation-Perfusion ratio (VA/Q) inequalities; the level of hypoxemia depends critically on the interplay between mixed venous Po_2 and the degree of VA/Q mismatching. Thus patients with a high cardiac output can have little hypoxemia if there are severe VA/Q mismatching, whereas patients with inadequate cardiac output can have moderately severe hypoxemia with little VA/Q mismatching; in contrast with patients with acute de novo hypoxemia, in whom pulmonary shunt is often present, the arterial Po_2 alone cannot indicate the severity of VA/Q mismatch in any given situation. However although these patients are often normocapnic/hypocapnic in the early stage of the disease, persistent hypercapnic respiratory failure is a feature of advancing end-stage interstitial pulmonary disease caused by both severe alteration in pulmonary diffusion and pump failure.[9,10]

As a consequence, although hypoxia and/or hypercapnia and muscle fatigue are always the basis of NIV treatment, the NIV settings and the clinical response may be different for different causes of acute respiratory failure (ARF).

This article provides physicians and respiratory therapists with a comprehensive, practical guideline for using NIV in critical care.

EPIDEMIOLOGY OF NONINVASIVE VENTILATION

Since its first application in the late 1980s,[11] NIV has become a first-line intervention for certain forms of ARF.[12–14] However, NIV is still underused in certain parts of the world because of lack of experience and inadequate training and economic resources.[15,16] In Europe, NIV use ranges from 35% of ventilated patients in intensive care units (ICUs) to about (60%) in respiratory ICUs (RICUs) or emergency departments (EDs).[16] In North America, where NIV is most often begun in the ED, data are similar to those from Europe.[15,17,18] Nevertheless, several studies have found that the use of NIV varies widely between hospitals and countries. It has also been changing over time.[12,19,20] Demoule and colleagues[20] found that, in France, overall NIV use increased from 16% to 23% of ventilated patients. The study also found that, between 1997 and 2002, its use increased from 35% to 52% of patients not intubated before ICU admission.

TYPES OF VENTILATORS

As mentioned earlier, NIV may be delivered for ARF as NPPV or as CPAP. NPPV may be delivered by traditional highly compressed gas-driven ICU ventilators, or dedicated turbine-driven or micropiston-driven NIV ventilator.[21–23]

Basic knowledge of the principles of ventilator functioning may be helpful when choosing a ventilator for NIV.[24] This knowledge enables physicians/respiratory therapists to consider the ventilator's technical performance in relation to the patient's clinical characteristics, underlying disease, the setting, and the available financial resources.[25] Although new highly compressed gas-driven ICU ventilators have embedded NIV algorithms to manage leaks and to promote improved patient-ventilator synchrony[23,26] by adjusting triggering, flow, and cycling mechanisms, turbine-driven ventilators in their intentional-leak circuit configuration may outperform compressed-driven ventilators in ICUs.[21,23,27–30]

All ventilators, except for portable transport ventilators that may be driven pneumatically, require electricity (alternating current external power or a direct current internal battery). The gas source can be (1) external high-pressure gas (centralized gas system or tanks), (2) an internal compressor, (3) a turbine or piston; (4) a combination of (1) and (3) or (1) and (2). Based on the gas source, mechanical ventilators for NIV in critical care can in practice be divided into 2 categories: those that work with oxygen and air at high pressure (4 atmospheres, 400 kPa), and those that work with oxygen at high pressure (4 atmospheres, 400 kPa) and atmospheric air driven by a turbine. Fast turbines (dynamic blower systems that change speed to reach the preset ventilator output) or turbines rotating at constant speed (constant-revolution blower systems) driven by a proportional valve make the latest generation of turbine-driven ventilators as efficient as ICU ventilators, driven by high-pressure gas.[24,25,31] A recent study showed that, on average, turbine-based ventilators performed better than conventional ventilators.[31] From the standpoint of high responsiveness to patients' flow demands, constant-revolution blower systems with proportional valves perform well. However, although in the past these systems had a clear responsiveness advantage compared with dynamic blower systems, recent developments show that dynamic blowers with a small turbine size and a high revolution rate per minute are also extremely responsive to patient demand.[21] In contrast, CPAP is usually provided by a CPAP flow generator that delivers constant positive pressure or by mechanical ventilators.[32,33]

Ventilators can deliver noninvasive positive pressure to the patient's airway by the respiratory circuit (RC) connected to the interface. RCs are of 2 types[21]:

1. Double-limb RCs, composed of an inspiratory and an expiratory limb whose proximal ends are connected to the interface. This is the typical RC used in high-pressure ventilators but it is also found in turbine-drive ventilators.
2. Single-limb circuit.
   a. A single RC with a true nonrebreathing expiratory valve (eg, a mushroom valve driven by ventilator pressure) usually labeled as nonvented RC. This valve has an on-off function and often works as a positive end-expiratory pressure (PEEP) valve.

b. A single RC without a true nonrebreathing valve, usually labeled as vented RC or intentional-leak RC. This type is a feature, so far, only of turbine-driven ventilators. CO_2 is vented out through a vented system embedded in the interface (some slots or holes on the frame or on the swivel elbow) or through a vented system placed into the RC proximal to the interface.[34–38]

NONINVASIVE VENTILATION MODES
Continuous Positive Airway Pressure

Unlike NPPV, during CPAP the pressure applied to the respiratory system is only generated by the patient's respiratory muscles. CPAP is aimed at improving oxygenation by increasing functional residual capacity, promoting alveolar recruitment (and maintaining open alveoli), and by reducing shunting. Theoretically CPAP should switch the patient's tidal volume to a flatter portion of the pressure-volume curve.[39] It is also designed to reduce WOB by counteracting PEEPi.[3,4] CPAP is commonly used for mild hypoxemic ARF without clear signs of respiratory muscle fatigue. It may also be effective to counterbalance PEEPi in patients with AECOPD associated with NPPV.[3–5]

However, the level of evidence of CPAP support in manifested ARF without cardiopulmonary edema (CPE) is still low,[40] whereas preemptive post-extubation CPAP in abdominal surgery has been found to reduce the need for re-intubation compared to usual post-extubation.[41,42] CPAP may be considered as a first-line therapy in CPE.[43–46]

Noninvasive Positive Pressure Ventilation

During NPPV the pressure applied to the respiratory system may be generated only by the ventilator (so-called controlled modes) or in a different degree by patient's respiratory muscles and by the ventilator (so-called assisted modes).

NPPV is usually applied both in time-cycled (assisted pressure controlled ventilation [APCV]) and flow-cycled (pressure support ventilation [PSV]) pressure targeted mode. The setup level of positive inspiratory pressure can be "above" or "below" the EPAP/PEEP level according to the manufacturer's algorithm. The former is usually labeled as PSV while the latter as inspiratory positive airway pressure [IPAP]. Inspiratory pressure can be combined with positive expiratory end positive pressure (EPAP or PEEP; an equal level of IPAP and EPAP/PEEP generates CPAP). In assisted pressure targeted flow-cycled mode, in which the pressure applied to the respiratory system is generated both by the patient's respiratory muscles and by the ventilator, the ventilator detects the patient's inspiratory effort and delivers inspiratory pressure. Expiration starts when the patient's inspiratory flow decreases to a preset percentage of inspiratory flow decay[47] (this threshold, also called the expiratory trigger, is usually set at 25% of inspiratory flow decay, but may be adjustable in most ventilators). The rationale behind expiratory trigger adjustability is to cope with different respiratory mechanics. The higher the value (eg, 50%), the lower the inspiratory time, and vice versa. Usually patients with chronic obstructive pulmonary disease (COPD) benefit from a threshold value around 40%, whereas restrictive conditions benefit from lower values (ie, 5%–25%). PSV have been found to increase tidal volume and unload the inspiratory muscles. Furthermore, the combined use of PSV/IPAP and PEEP/EPAP may counteract the effects of PEEPi in patients with COPD, further improving dyspnea, gas exchange, and inspiratory muscle effort.[5]

In PSV mode, the operator sets a given level of inspiratory and (whenever needed) expiratory pressure, an inspiratory and expiratory trigger threshold (whenever allowed), and a pressure ramp. Pressure ramp, namely the time that the ventilator takes to reach the set pressure, can interfere in the mechanical inspiratory time.[48] Some turbine-driven ventilators allow a backup rate to be set (so-called spontaneous timed [ST] mode). Turbine-driven ventilators in intentional-leak configuration always have a given amount of default EPAP/PEEP that may vary, according to the manufacturer, from 2 to 4 cm H_2O.[21]

APCV is an assisted pressure targeted time-cycled mode in which the operator sets a preset pressure (and an expiratory pressure whenever needed), a respiratory rate, an inspiratory time, and an inspiratory trigger sensitivity (whenever allowed). Its use during NIV may be appropriate in the presence of several leaks hindering expiratory cycling in pressure targeted flow-cycled mode[49,50] or when a back rate is needed. Although pressure targeted modes are able to compensate for nonintentional leaks better than volume-targeted ventilation,[51] a constant tidal volume [V_T] may not be guaranteed to the patient when respiratory impedance changes.[21] To maintain V_T during pressure-targeted ventilation, a guaranteed volume (V_{TG}) can be set in most ICUs and bilevel turbine-driven ventilators can be used in the so-called dual modes of ventilation.[24,52–55] In the presence of modifications to respiratory impedance, a dual mode is able to guarantee a preset volume independently of circuit configuration. However, there are differences between V_{TG} delivered by vented versus nonvented RCs in the presence of nonintentional leaks.[54,55] Recent studies[54,55] found that the ability of the V_{TG} mode to compensate for nonintentional leaks depends strictly on whether a vented or nonvented circuit configuration is used. In simple terms, in the absence of nonintentional leaks in vented or nonvented RC configuration, all ventilators in vented configuration increased the inspiratory pressure to guarantee the V_{TG}. In contrast, in nonvented RC configuration, all tested ventilators showed a reduction in inspiratory pressure in the presence of leaks, resulting in a concomitant reduction in V_{Texp}. This difference must be taken into account as a possible risk when a V_{TG} mode is used in the presence of nonintentional linear or nonlinear leaks. Operators must be aware of the advantages and drawbacks of dual modes of ventilation and understand that patients are no longer supported when their ventilatory demand produces a V_T higher than the preset V_T. For this reason, the minimum value of the preset pressure should be carefully set by the operator.

NEW MODES

Manufacturers often propose new modes, but scientific evidence proving their effectiveness and clinical benefit is often lacking.[56]

Neurally adjusted ventilator assist (NAVA) is designed to enhance patient-ventilator synchrony. NAVA uses an esophageal catheter to detect diaphragmatic activity and thus the patient's effort regulating the amount of delivered pressure. Triggering and cycling of the ventilator are activated by NAVA. It decreases ineffective efforts (trigger asynchrony) and premature and delayed cycling (cycle asynchrony) compared with pressure-controlled flow-cycled ventilation (ie, PSV), thereby improving patient-ventilator synchrony.[57–59] Its role seems promising during helmet ventilation.[60,61]

WHICH INTERFACE FOR WHICH PATIENTS IN THE ACUTE SETTING?

The perfect NIV interface does not exist, but the choice of an adequate interface should be tailored to the patient's characteristics and influenced by ventilator setting and the patient's underlying type of respiratory failure. A good seal to prevent leaks, and patient comfort with the prevention of drawbacks and complications should be the major goals for clinicians. Fitting the mask to the patient rather than trying to make the patient fit the mask is mandatory, but this is only possible with a large range of interfaces and sizes. The larger the availability of interfaces and sizes, the higher the probability of success in fitting the interface to the patient. In the acute setting, the oronasal interface (covering the surface around the nose and the mouth) is the most commonly used. Total full-face mask (TFMs; covering the entire anterior surface of the face, including the mouth, eyes, and nose) and helmet (a transparent hood and soft polyvinyl chloride or silicon collar that includes the neck and whole head) may also be used in the critical care setting. Nasal masks, oronasal masks, and TFMs are available in vented and nonvented versions. Vented mask have some holes or slots in the frame or on the swivel elbow that allow CO_2 diffusion. CO_2 levels may increase in vented masks because of CO_2 rebreathing.[34] However, as recently underlined,[35,36] a proper setting and larger leaks from the new vented system embedded in the interface reduce the likelihood of CO_2 rebreathing.[35,36] The vented configuration of oronasal masks and TFMs is always equipped with an antiasphyxia valve with automatic opening to prevent rebreathing in case of a pressure failure or when airway pressure decreases to less than 2 to 3 cm H_2O.[62] Nonvented masks are completely closed and require the use of a double-limb or single-limb circuit with an expiratory valve.[62] A recent study[63] found that effective dead space in nonvented interfaces with large volumes is not related to the internal gas volume of the interface, suggesting that this internal volume should not be considered as a limiting factor for their efficacy during noninvasive ventilation. Compared with nasal masks, oronasal interfaces have the potential advantage of fewer air leaks and greater stability in the delivered mean airway pressure, especially in the acute setting or during sleep. In the acute setting, less patient cooperation is required during NIV. For these reasons its use should be preferred to nasal interfaces during the acute phase of respiratory failure; when patients are intensively dyspneic and, generally, in open-mouth breathers. The TFM avoids the nasal bridge, creating an effective seal around the less pressure-sensitive perimeter of the face, limiting the risk of deleterious cutaneous side effects.[62,64] The TFM mask also has the advantage of rapid and easy application, and it is a valid alternative for patients who are unable to obtain a good seal with other masks. It can also be used in the case of nasal bridge skin breakdown and facial irregularities. Its use has some limitations in claustrophobic patients.[65,66] There is no clear evidence yet on the advantages in terms of effectiveness and compliance of TFM compared with other conventional oronasal masks.[66–69] However, in patients with hypercapnic ARF, for whom escalation to intubation is deemed inappropriate, switching to a total face mask has been proposed as a last-resort therapy when face mask–delivered NIV has already failed to reverse ARF.[70] This strategy has been found to provide prolonged periods of continuous NIV while preventing facial pressure sores.[71] Moreover, it allows a clear and unrestricted view, as with the helmet. Helmet interfaces were originally used to deliver a precise oxygen concentration during hyperbaric oxygen therapy. The United States Food and Drug Administration has not approved any of the available helmets, but helmets have been approved in some other countries.[41,64,72–87] When using a helmet with a CPAP generator, a minimum flow of 40 L/min is mandatory to avoid CO_2 rebreathing.[88,89] For the same reason, CPAP alone should not be used with ICU ventilators in the nonvented configuration because the flow that is generated is too low to wash CO_2.[90,91]

Recent engineering improvements gave helmets more comfortable seals, better seal against leaks, and better patient-ventilator interaction.[92,93]

A new type of full-face mask, provided with nasal and oral ports that can be used in ongoing endoscopic procedures in case of respiratory failure without interrupting the procedure, has recently been introduced as a prototype. This mask is able to support ventilation in a few seconds because it is made of 2 symmetric parts that can be divided in order to place it in on the patient during the procedure, even if an endoscopic probe is already inserted.[94,95]

AIR HUMIDIFICATION

There are no current standards regarding the humidification system during NIV. Theoretically the passive heat and moisture exchangers are not suggested for NIV because it can increase dead space ventilation, resistance to gas flow, and WOB compared with heated humidifiers.[96,97]

However, Lellouche and colleagues[98] recently assessed the impact of different types of humidification system on the success rate of NIV delivered for ARF with ICU ventilators. The intubation rate was not influenced by the humidification system used.[99]

Indication and Contraindication for the Use of Noninvasive Ventilation

NIV should be considered in all patients with increased dyspnea (moderate to severe), tachypnea (with respiratory rate >24 breaths/min), and the use of accessory muscles or paradoxic abdominal movements. General inclusion criteria include the presence of ventilatory pump failure with hypercapnia and respiratory acidosis ($Paco_2$ >45 mm Hg and pH <7.35) and/or hypoxemia Pao_2/Fio_2 ratio less than 200.[13]

Inability to fit the mask and respiratory arrest are considered the absolute contraindications to NIV.

Relative contraindications include[13]:

- Medically unstable: hypotensive shock, uncontrolled cardiac ischemia or arrhythmia, uncontrolled copious upper gastrointestinal bleeding
- Agitated, uncooperative
- Unable to protect airway
- Swallowing impairment
- Excessive secretions not managed by secretion clearance techniques
- Multiple (ie, 2 or more) organ failure
- Recent upper airway or upper gastrointestinal surgery

WHERE TO APPLY NONINVASIVE VENTILATION

When applied appropriately, NIV may reduce morbidity and mortality, and may allow more efficient use of scarce medical resources compared with the previously standard medical therapy. Other important criteria that to be considered before starting NIV with the aim of producing a successful outcome is choosing the best location, matching the patient's clinical status, and the severity of ARF.

The question of where to start NIV has generated much debate because there are only a few studies that have clearly addressed this question. In addition, the model of hospital care varies between different countries, and the units' capabilities to deliver NIV differ substantially, even in the same hospital. A patient who requires ICU admission in one institution may therefore be appropriately treated in the RICU or even in the ward in another.[14]

Emergency Room

Many studies have produced uncertain results about the effectiveness of NIV in the ED.[100–102] The choice of starting NIV in the ED may be convenient, especially because

NIV initiation should not be delayed until the patient can be transferred to another ward and because most EDs have special high-intensity areas, a nurse/patient ratio of up to 1:1, and have proper monitoring.

Although fast-responding diseases, such as acute cardiogenic pulmonary edema, may be appropriately ventilated in the ED, unstable patients with slowly resolving disorders (eg, COPD exacerbations, pneumonia, acute respiratory distress syndrome [ARDS]) should be rapidly moved to specialized departments.[100]

Recently, an approach (the so-called NIV trial strategy) in which NIV was started in the ED and then continued in the intermediate care unit showed a decrease in in-hospital mortality and length of stay for patients admitted with ARF.[103] This finding means that early initiation for NIV should be strongly encouraged in order to avoid delays that could contribute to NIV failure.

Intensive Care Unit

The ICU represents the ideal location for critical ill patients with ARF secondary to respiratory disorders in which the role of NIV is uncertain (eg, pneumonia, ARDS). These patients should be observed closely in order to prevent a worsening of the situation, managing an immediate intervention like endotracheal intubation. Most of the randomized controlled trials on NIV for ARF have been performed in ICUs.[100] Despite important benefits (eg, a decrease in the need for endotracheal intubation and length of both ICU and hospital stay) the higher costs and the limited beds availability should be taken into account.

Therefore, significant cost reductions should be possible through the careful selection of patients admitted to ICUs, according to the underlying diseases and the severity of ARF.

Respiratory Intensive Care Units

RICUs, also known as intermediate care units, are specialized settings that represent a step-up service from the general wards and a step down for patients coming from ICUs in terms of level of care and intensity of monitoring. Although the European Respiratory Society has proposed specific recommendations[104] for the standard of care of these services, the model of step-down units differs from country to country and even between institutions in the same country. These units usually include staff with training and expertise in NIV, a better nurse/patient ratio than the general ward, facilities for close observation, and respiratory therapy equipment.[105] In addition, in most of these units the staff are able to manage endotracheal intubation for IMV. Although a recent Italian survey showed that the number of RICUs increased from 26 to 44 over a period of 10 years,[106] in several countries the number of these units is still small.

General Ward

The success of NIV outside a high-dependency setting depends on staff skills, severity of ARF, and underlying conditions.[107,108]

Standard wards typically have low ratios of staff to patients and are usually not able to manage unstable patients. In a randomized controlled trial performed on general respiratory wards of hospitals in the United Kingdom, Plant and colleagues,[109] showed that NIV delivered by trained nurses reduced the overall intubation rate and mortality compared with their control group. However, in the subgroup of patients with pH less than 7.30, the intubation rate and mortality were not significantly different. Care must therefore be taken, especially when starting NIV in borderline patients. One exception is when NIV is applied in do-not-intubate or do-not-resuscitate patients, when the goal is palliation of symptoms, as shown in a recent American survey.[110] The investigators found that the inclination to use NIV in end-of-life patients was greater for pulmonologists than for intensivists.

NONINVASIVE VENTILATION IN MAJOR DISEASES
Hypercapnic Chronic Obstructive Pulmonary Disease

NIV is currently considered the gold standard in the management of patients with exacerbation of COPD and acute hypercapnic respiratory failure. These patients are the group most likely to be successfully treated with NIV. The addition of NIV to standard medical therapy reduces mortality, intubation rate, and hospital length of stay.[109,111,112] More recently, a large retrospective cohort study of more than 25,000 patients with COPD confirmed these findings.[113] Among patients hospitalized for exacerbation of COPD those who were treated with NIV on the first or second hospital day had lower inpatient mortality, shorter length of stay, and lower costs compared with those treated with IMV.[113] Despite NIV providing positive results with success rates of 70% to 75%,[114] NIV is not suitable for all patients and, in particular, for those who have refractory respiratory acidosis and altered mentation. Confalonieri and colleagues[115] found that a pH less than 7.25 after 1 hour of NIV use was associated with an increased risk of failure and that the risk of failure was even greater than when the pH levels were less than 7.25 at admission. Alternatively, as a last resort, in selected patients not responding to NIV, respiratory acidosis and hypercapnia may be managed by an extracorporeal circuit with a venovenous bypass designed to remove CO_2 by extracorporeal CO_2 removal ($ECCO_2R$). Recently, data from a matched cohort study with historical control indicated a reduction of intubation rate by adding $ECCO_2R$ to NIV compared with NIV-only in patients with COPD with acute hypercapnic respiratory failure who were at risk of NIV failure. However, $ECCO_2R$-related complications were observed in half of the patients.[116]

Hypercapnic Nonchronic Obstructive Pulmonary Disease

As highlighted earlier, the rationale for the use of NIV in neuromuscular diseases (NMDs) or in patients with other chest disorders is to improve alveolar ventilation that is ineffective as a result of the respiratory muscles weakness. These patients typical have a restrictive lung function disorder with a decrease of vital capacity, total lung capacity, and functional residual capacity. The hypercapnic respiratory failure usually develops when the vital capacity decreases to less than 55% of predicted.[117] In addition, most patients with NMD are also hypoxemic. The expiratory and bulbar muscle weakness leads to coughing and swallowing impairment, causing, respectively, the development of atelectasis and aspiration pneumonia.[118–122]

Based on the clinical onset of ARF, 2 classes of NMD can be distinguished[123]:

1. Slowly progressive NMDs (ie, amyotrophic lateral sclerosis, spinal muscular atrophy, and Duchenne muscular dystrophy) with acute exacerbations of chronic respiratory failure.
2. Rapidly progressive NMDs (ie, Guillain-Barré syndrome, myasthenia gravis, and inflammatory myopathies) that usually present with ARF as a first sign and in which the fast deterioration of gas exchange often requires immediate intubation.

NIV plays a role in the management of the first group of patients both in the acute and chronic settings. In particular, the combined approach of secretion clearance techniques and of NIV is strongly recommended and is considered an effective tool to avoid intubation, especially in patients without significant bulbar impairment.[121,124,125] Therefore, clinicians have to identify the appropriate patients in order to optimize the success of the ventilatory strategy.

The outcome of patients with idiopathic pulmonary fibrosis referred to the ICU for ARF is poor and is not improved by mechanical ventilation. Without a clearly identified reversible cause of ARF, these patients do not benefit from admission to the ICU.[126,127]

Hypoxemia

There is a clear rationale for using NIV in hypoxemic ARF because it addresses the hypoxemia keeping underventilated alveoli open and improves WOB.[128] However, the beneficial effects of NIV remain unclear and robust randomized controlled trials conducted in patients with de novo acute hypercapnic respiratory failure (AHRF) are scarce[40,129–131] except in immunosuppressed patients.[81,132,133] It is also true that hypoxemic ARF represents a heterogeneous group of diseases with different prognoses and treatments. This large heterogeneity explains some of the literature's contradictory results, depending on the study population.[128] Some of the most challenging patients are those with ARDS.[134] In general, NIV is more likely to fail in patients with ARDS,[135,136] particularly in the presence of shock, metabolic acidosis, and high severity scores of illness (simplified acute physiology score [SAPS] II).[137] Antonelli and collegues[138] showed that a SAPS II score greater than 34 and a Pao_2/Fio_2 ratio less than 175 mm Hg after 1 hour of NIV were strong predictors of NIV failure, with an intubation rate of 78% when both were present. In the new Berlin definition of ARDS, the term acute lung injury has been abandoned and patients are now categorized into 3 different classes, based on the severity of hypoxemia.[134] According to this definition, Thille and colleagues[139] showed in a recent observational cohort study that intubation rate in patients without ARDS was lower than in those with ARDS (35% vs 61%; $P = .015$) and that the ICU mortality was significantly different among separate categories (31% in mild, 62% in moderate, and 84% in severe ARDS). In a small, randomized controlled trial, NPPV was compared with high-concentration oxygen therapy in 40 selected patients with acute lung injury (200 mm Hg <Pao_2/Fio_2 ratio ≤300 mm Hg).[140] Twenty-one patients were assigned to the NIV group and 19 to the control group. Patients receiving NIV had a more significant improvement in oxygenation and a lower intubation rate (4.8% vs 36.8%). However, NIV was again compared with a therapy that has a purely cosmetic effect, namely oxygen therapy. All this evidence suggests that NIV should not be used in moderate to severe ARDS, but additional studies are necessary before more precise recommendations can be provided about the role of NIV in this patient population.

Acute Pulmonary Edema

Acute cardiogenic pulmonary edema (ACPE) is a common medical emergency. ACPE is characterized by the rapid accumulation of fluid within the lung's interstitial and/or alveolar spaces, commonly caused by left ventricular systolic dysfunction and an acute increase in systemic vascular resistance.[141] Consequently, the lungs become less compliant and the WOB increases.[45,142] Both NPPV and CPAP rapidly improve patients' symptoms, gas exchange, respiratory mechanics, and hemodynamics by rearranging intra-alveolar fluid and reducing left ventricular afterload and preload.[43,44,143] By contrast, the beneficial effects of NIV on mortality in patients with ACPE still remain unclear.[144] A recent update of a systematic review previously published in 2008 showed that both NPPV and CPAP significantly reduced hospital mortality (relative risk [RR], 0.66; 95% confidence interval [CI], 0.48–0.89) and endotracheal intubation (RR, 0.52; 95% CI, 0.36–0.75) compared with standard medical treatment alone in patients with ACPE.[45] According to robust evidence, CPAP and NPPV are also equivalent in terms of efficacy in hypercapnic patients with ACPE.[145] For this reason CPAP is often the first treatment choice in the ED or in a prehospital setting because is considered cheaper and easier than NPPV.[146]

Tables 1 and **2** summarize the possibility of using NIV in different clinical settings.

WEANING AND DISCONTINUATION OF NONINVASIVE VENTILATION

No validated protocols are defined for weaning NIV in ARF, compared with weaning protocols for invasive ventilation. After resolution of the acute episode that was the cause for initiating ventilation, the decision to stop NIV should be based on an integrated analysis of clinical signs and functional parameters. In general, different strategies are possible as methods of withdrawing NIV: direct discontinuation, partial nocturnal ventilation or gradual discontinuation (especially in patients with COPD), neuromuscular disease, or sleep disordered breathing (obstructive sleep apnea and obesity-hypoventilation syndrome).[147,148] In addition, Cuvelier and colleagues[149] showed that long-term dependency (LTD) on noninvasive ventilation after ARF is a common situation in respiratory intermediate care units, usually in patients with non-COPD causes of respiratory failure. Future randomized clinical trials are required to determine the best NIV discontinuation method and to individualize care in patients with LTD-NIV as soon as possible.

Table 1	
Noninvasive ventilation for hypercapnic ARF	
Cause of Hypercapnic ARF	**Suggestions**
Obstructive Conditions	
Status Asthmaticus	There are no clear indication for using NIV in status asthmaticus even in critical care[150] although NIV has been found to improve ABG and WOB[151]
COPD: acute exacerbation	In severely ill ICU patients, compared with IMV, it showed similar improvements in ABG, duration of ventilatory support, ICU LOS, and mortality.[112,152,153] Its use even in sicker patients expected to be intubated did not show increase in mortality[153]
COPD: weaning, early extubation, and postextubation prophylactic NIV	During weaning it reduced mortality, duration of IMV, postextubation ARF, ICU and hospital LOS, and rates of complications.[154,155] After extubation, in patients with risk factors for extubation failure, it reduced the need for reintubation[156–159]
Restrictive Conditions	
NMD	There is no clear evidence for using NIV in the acute setting. However NIV may prevent intubation in patients with intact upper airway patency[121–124]
OHS	Patients with OHS can be treated with NIV during an episode of AHRF with similar efficacy and better outcomes than in patients with COPD[160]

Abbreviations: ABG, arterial blood gases; LOS, length of stay; OHS, obesity-hypoventilation syndrome.

Table 2
Noninvasive ventilation for hypoxemic ARF

Cause of Hypoxemic ARF	Suggestions
Immunocompromised patients	There is evidence to use NIV vs IMV given the possible lower associated risk for complications, including VAP[81,132,133,161,162]
ACPE	Strong supporting evidence has been found both with NPPV and CPAP in reducing intubation compared with standard medical therapy.[43,44,143] However the evidence to date on the potential benefit of CPAP and NPPV in reducing mortality is derived from small-trials and further large-scale trials are needed[45]
Pneumonia	Although NIV in patients with CAP both CPAP and NPPV have been found to improve oxygenation and outcomes,[129,131,132,163,164] NIV failure rate is still high[136,138,165,166]
ARDS	Use of NIV in moderate to severe ARDS (PaO_2/FiO_2 <150 mm Hg) is generally discouraged because of high failure risk (50%–70%).[144,145,167] When NPPV is used, patients with mild ARDS had reduced intubation rates and mortality compared with unsupported patients with standard oxygen therapy[147]
Postextubation in surgical patients and weaning	When appropriately applied in selected surgical patients, NPPV and CPAP can be considered both as prophylactic and therapeutic tools to improve gas exchange.[42] In patients having risk factors for extubation failure it reduced the need for reintubation.[156] In a pilot study, the feasibility of early extubation followed by immediate NIV was shown to be comparable with conventional weaning in 20 patients resolving hypoxemic ARF[169]
Trauma	Early NIV use reduced mortality, intubation rate, and ICU LOS, and improved oxygenation by promoting recruitment of collapsed lung regions[168]

Abbreviations: CAP, community-acquired pneumonia; LOS, length of stay; VAP, ventilator-associated pneumonia.

SLEEP AND NONINVASIVE VENTILATION

Patients receiving IMV may show severe sleep disturbances, even after withdrawal of sedation.[170,171] Sleep disturbance may also promote delirium, which has been found to be an independent risk factor for death in mechanically ventilated critically ill patients.[172] Poor sleep quality has also been reported during NIV in chronically ventilated patients[173] and a lower activities-of-daily-living score (indicating greater functional impairment) was found in the patients who subsequently failed NIV.[174]

Some of the effects of NIV on sleep may be linked to a reduction in CO_2 leading to[175,176]:

- A decrease in respiratory drive that may cause central apneas, possibly associated with obstructive hypopnea
- A lower apnea threshold causing central apnea, possibly associated with airway obstruction
- Induced active progressive vocal cord closure, causing central apnea or obstructive hypopnea/apnea

Campo and colleagues[177] assessed whether sleep quality helps to predict noninvasive ventilation outcome in patients with acute hypercapnic respiratory failure. They prospectively studied 27 hypercapnic patients in a medical ICU who required NIV for greater than 48 hours and underwent 17-hour polysomnography (3 PM–8 AM) from 2 to 4 days after NIV initiation. Late NIV failure was defined as death, endotracheal intubation, or persistent need for NIV on day 6. An abnormal electroencephalographic pattern was noted in 7 (50%) of the 14 patients with late NIV failure compared with 1 (8%) of the 13 patients successfully treated with NIV. Patients failing noninvasive ventilation had poorer sleep quality with greater circadian sleep cycle disruption and less significant nocturnal rapid eye movement (REM) sleep compared with patients successfully treated with noninvasive ventilation. NIV failure was associated with delirium during the ICUs stay (64% vs 0%). Abnormal electroencephalogram (EEG) patterns in NIV-treated patients without clinical encephalopathy may reflect subclinical acute brain dysfunction, because no typical features of electrical activity could be detected. This notion is supported by another study that evaluated EEG in delirious ICU patients and found EEG patterns that resembled the pattern of abnormal wakefulness described in their study,[178] These abnormal polysomnographic patterns of wakefulness and sleep were similar to polysomnography features of wakefulness, quiet sleep (non-REM), and active sleep (REM) used to classify sleep stages in newborns and may correspond with the reappearance of primary sleep in their patients.[177]

Cordoba-Izquierdo and colleagues[179] compared sleep quality between conventional mechanical ventilators and dedicated noninvasive ventilators to evaluate sleep during and between noninvasive ventilation sessions in critically ill patients. Patients were randomly assigned to receive noninvasive ventilation with either an ICU ventilator (n = 12) or a dedicated noninvasive ventilator (n = 12), and their sleep and respiratory parameters were recorded by polysomnography from 4 PM to 9 AM on the second, third, or fourth day after noninvasive ventilation initiation. Sleep architecture was similar between ventilator groups, including sleep fragmentation (number of arousals and awakenings per hour), but the dedicated noninvasive ventilator group showed a significantly higher patient-ventilator asynchrony–related fragmentation, whereas the ICU ventilator group showed a higher noise-related fragmentation. More sleep time occurred and sleep quality was better during noninvasive ventilation sessions than during spontaneous breathing periods as a result of greater slow wave and REM sleep and lower fragmentation. The investigators concluded that there were no observed differences in sleep quality associated with the type of ventilator used despite slight differences in patient-ventilator asynchrony. Noninvasive ventilation sessions did not prevent patients from sleeping; on the contrary, they seem to aid sleep compared with unassisted breathing.

SUMMARY

NIV has a clear role in selected critically ill patients as an initial therapy in addition to standard medical therapy. NIV requires an experienced team, a tailored approach in terms of monitoring and equipment availability, taking into account all the possible drawbacks and contraindications because starting and maintaining NIV means initiating and maintaining optimal mechanical ventilation. Signs of impending NIV failure must be promptly recognized to avoid intubation delay, especially in de novo hypoxemic respiratory failure.[20]

Discontinuation of NPPV in case of failure often means removing high levels of support and therefore great caution is needed in patients with severe acute hypoxemic failure, in which NPPV discontinuation to intubate the patient may lead to acute decompensation and cardiac arrest.

REFERENCES

1. Stauffer JL, Olson DE, Petty TL. Complications and consequences of endotracheal intubation and tracheotomy. A prospective study of 150 critically ill adult patients. Am J Med 1981;70:65–76.
2. Sinuff T, Muscedere J, Cook DJ, et al. Implementation of clinical practice guidelines for ventilator-associated pneumonia: a multicenter prospective study. Crit Care Med 2013;41:15–23.
3. Coussa ML, Guerin C, Eissa NT, et al. Partitioning of work of breathing in mechanically ventilated COPD patients. J Appl Physiol (1985) 1993;75:1711–9.
4. Goldberg P, Reissmann H, Maltais F, et al. Efficacy of noninvasive CPAP in COPD with acute respiratory failure. Eur Respir J 1995;8:1894–900.
5. Appendini L, Patessio A, Zanaboni S, et al. Physiologic effects of positive end-expiratory pressure and mask pressure support during exacerbations of chronic obstructive pulmonary disease. Am J Respir Crit Care Med 1994;149:1069–76.
6. Grassino AE, Clanton T. Mechanisms of muscle fatigue. Monaldi Arch Chest Dis 1993;48:94–8.
7. Chergui K, Choukroun G, Meyer P, et al. Prone positioning for a morbidly obese patient with acute respiratory distress syndrome: an opportunity to explore intrinsic positive end-expiratory pressure-lower inflexion point interdependence. Anesthesiology 2007;106:1237–9.
8. Alvisi V, Marangoni E, Zannoli S, et al. Pulmonary function and expiratory flow limitation in acute cervical spinal cord injury. Arch Phys Med Rehabil 2012;93:1950–6.
9. Wagner PL. Gas exchange in chronic pulmonary disease. Clin Physiol 1985;3:9–17.
10. Young IH, Bye PT. Gas exchange in disease: asthma, chronic obstructive pulmonary disease, cystic fibrosis, and interstitial lung disease. Compr Physiol 2011;1:663–97.
11. Brochard L, Isabey D, Piquet J, et al. Reversal of acute exacerbations of chronic obstructive lung disease by inspiratory assistance with a face mask. N Engl J Med 1990;323:1523–30.
12. Boldrini R, Fasano L, Nava S. Noninvasive mechanical ventilation. Curr Opin Crit Care 2012;18:48–53.
13. Nava S, Hill N. Noninvasive ventilation in acute respiratory failure. Lancet 2009;374:250–9.
14. Olivieri C, Carenzo L, Vignazia GL, et al. Does noninvasive ventilation delivery in the ward provide early effective ventilation? Respir Care 2014;60(1):6–11.
15. Maheshwari V, Paioli D, Rothaar R, et al. Utilization of noninvasive ventilation in acute care hospitals. A regional survey. Chest 2006;129:1226–33.
16. Crimi C, Noto A, Princi P, et al. A European survey of noninvasive ventilation practices. Eur Respir J 2010;36:362–9.
17. Templier F, Labastire L, Pes P, et al. Noninvasive ventilation use in French out-of-hospital settings: a preliminary national survey. Am J Emerg Med 2012;30:765–9.
18. Crimi C, Noto A, Princi P, et al. Survey of noninvasive ventilation practices: a snapshot of Italian practice. Minerva Anestesiol 2011;77:971–8.

19. Esteban A, Ferguson ND, Meade MO, et al. Evolution of mechanical ventilation in response to clinical research. Am J Respir Crit Care Med 2008;177:170–7.
20. Demoule A, Girou E, Richard JC, et al. Increased use of noninvasive ventilation in French intensive care units. Intensive Care Med 2006;32:1747–55.
21. Gregoretti C, Navalesi P, Ghannadian S, et al. Choosing a ventilator for home mechanical ventilation. Breathe 2013;10:395–408.
22. Scala R, Naldi M. Ventilators for noninvasive ventilation to treat acute respiratory failure. Respir Care 2008;53:1054–80.
23. Carteaux G, Lyazidi A, Cordoba-Izquierdo A, et al. Patient-ventilator asynchrony during noninvasive ventilation: a bench and clinical study. Chest 2012;142:367–76.
24. Kacmarek RM, Chipman D. Basic principles of ventilator machinery. In: Tobin MJ, editor. Principles and practice of mechanical ventilation. 2nd edition. New York: McGraw-Hill; 2006. p. 53–95.
25. Make BJ, Hill NS, Goldberg AI, et al. Mechanical ventilation beyond the intensive care unit. Report of a consensus conference of the American College of Chest Physicians. Chest 1998;113(Suppl):289S–344S.
26. Vignaux L, Vargas F, Roeseler J, et al. Patient-ventilator asynchrony during noninvasive ventilation for acute respiratory failure: a multicenter study. Intensive Care Med 2009;35:840–6.
27. Oto J, Chenelle CT, Marchese AD, et al. A comparison of leak compensation in acute care ventilators during non-invasive and invasive ventilation; a lung model study. Respir Care 2013;58:2027–37.
28. Ferreira JC, Chipman DW, Hill NS, et al. Bilevel vs ICU ventilators providing noninvasive ventilation: effect of system leaks: a COPD lung model comparison. Chest 2009;136:448–56.
29. Vignaux L, Tassaux D, Jolliet P. Performance of noninvasive ventilation modes on ICU ventilators during pressure support: a bench model study. Intensive Care Med 2007;33:1444–51.
30. Vignaux L, Tassaux D, Carteaux G, et al. Performance of noninvasive ventilation algorithms on ICU ventilators during pressure support: a clinical study. Intensive Care Med 2010 Dec;36:2053–9.
31. Thille AW, Lyazidi A, Richard JC, et al. A bench study of intensive-care-unit ventilators: new versus old and turbine-based versus compressed gas-based ventilators. Intensive Care Med 2009;35:1368–76.
32. Fu C, Caruso P, Lucatto JJ, et al. Comparison of two flow generators with a noninvasive ventilator to deliver continuous positive airway pressure: a test lung study. Intensive Care Med 2005;31:1587–91.
33. Takeuchi M, Williams P, Hess D, et al. Continuous positive airway pressure in new-generation mechanical ventilators: a lung model study. Anesthesiology 2002;96:162–72.
34. Ferguson GT, Gilmartin M. CO_2 rebreathing during BiPAP ventilatory assistance. Am J Respir Crit Care Med 1995;151:1126–35.
35. Saatci E, Miller DM, Stell IM, et al. Dynamic dead space in face masks used with non-invasive ventilators: a lung model study. Eur Respir J 2004;23:129–35.
36. Schettino GP, Chatmongkolchart S, Hess DR, et al. Position of exhalation port and mask design affect CO_2 rebreathing during non-invasive positive pressure ventilation. Crit Care Med 2003;31:2178–82.
37. Szkulmowski Z, Belkhouja K, Le QH, et al. Bilevel positive airway pressure ventilation: factors influencing carbon dioxide rebreathing. Intensive Care Med 2010;36:688–91.

38. Chatburn RL. Classification of mechanical ventilators. In: Tobin MJ, editor. Principles and practice of mechanical ventilation. 2nd Edition. New York: McGraw-Hill; 2006. p. 37–52.

39. L'Her E, Deye N, Lellouche F, et al. Physiologic effects of noninvasive ventilation during acute lung injury. Am J Respir Crit Care Med 2005;172:1112–8.

40. Delclaux C, L'Her E, Alberti C, et al. Treatment of acute hypoxemic nonhypercapnic respiratory insufficiency with continuous positive airway pressure delivered by a face mask: a randomized controlled trial. JAMA 2000;284:2352–60.

41. Squadrone V, Coha M, Cerutti E, et al. Continuous positive airway pressure for treatment of postoperative hypoxemia: a randomized controlled trial. JAMA 2005;293:589–95.

42. Chiumello D, Chevallard G, Gregoretti C. Non-invasive ventilation in postoperative patients: a systematic review. Intensive Care Med 2011;37:918–29.

43. Masip J, Roque M, Sanchez B, et al. Noninvasive ventilation in acute cardiogenic pulmonary edema: systematic review and meta-analysis. JAMA 2005; 294:3124–30.

44. Winck JC, Azevedo LF, Costa-Pereira A, et al. Efficacy and safety of noninvasive ventilation in the treatment of acute cardiogenic pulmonary edema–a systematic review and meta-analysis. Crit Care 2006;10:R69.

45. Vital FM, Ladeira MT, Atallah AN. Non-invasive positive pressure ventilation (CPAP or bilevel NPPV) for cardiogenic pulmonary oedema. Cochrane Database Syst Rev 2013;(5):CD005351.

46. Collins SP, Mielniczuk LM, Whittingham HA, et al. The use of noninvasive ventilation in emergency department patients with acute cardiogenic pulmonary edema: a systematic review. Ann Emerg Med 2006;48:260–9, 269.e1–4.

47. Hess DR. Ventilator waveforms and the physiology of pressure support ventilation. Respir Care 2005;50:166–86 [discussion: 183–6].

48. Aliverti A, Carlesso E, Dellacà R, et al. Chest wall mechanics during pressure support ventilation. Crit Care 2006;10(2):R54.

49. Calderini E, Confalonieri M, Puccio PG, et al. Patient-ventilator asynchrony during noninvasive ventilation: the role of expiratory trigger. Intensive Care Med 1999;25:662–7.

50. Gregoretti C, Foti G, Beltrame F, et al. Pressure control ventilation and minitracheotomy in treating severe flail chest trauma. Intensive Care Med 1995;21:1054–6.

51. Highcock MP, Shneerson JM, Smith IE. Functional differences in bi-level pressure preset ventilators. Eur Respir J 2001;17:268–73.

52. Amato MB, Barbas CS, Bonassa J, et al. Volume-assured pressure support ventilation (VAPSV). A new approach for reducing muscle workload during acute respiratory failure. Chest 1992;102:1225–34.

53. Fauroux B, Leroux K, Pépin JL, et al. Are home ventilators able to guarantee a minimal tidal volume? Intensive Care Med 2010;36:1008–14.

54. Carlucci A, Schreiber A, Mattei A, et al. The configuration of bi-level ventilator circuits may affect compensation for non-intentional leaks during volume-targeted ventilation. Intensive Care Med 2013;39:59–65.

55. Khirani S, Louis B, Leroux K, et al. Harms of unintentional leaks during volume targeted pressure support ventilation. Respir Med 2013;107:1021–9.

56. Branson RD, Johannigman JA. What is the evidence base for the newer ventilation modes? Respir Care 2004;49:742–60.

57. Piquilloud L, Tassaux D, Bialais E, et al. Neurally adjusted ventilatory assist (NAVA) improves patient-ventilator interaction during non-invasive ventilation delivered by face mask. Intensive Care Med 2012;38:1624–31.

58. Schmidt M, Dres M, Raux M, et al. Neurally adjusted ventilatory assist improves patient-ventilator interaction during postextubation prophylactic noninvasive ventilation. Crit Care Med 2012;40:1738–44.

59. Bertrand PM, Futier E, Coisel Y, et al. Neurally adjusted ventilatory assist vs pressure support ventilation for noninvasive ventilation during acute respiratory failure: a crossover physiologic study. Chest 2013;143:30–6.

60. Racca F, Appendini L, Gregoretti C, et al. Effectiveness of mask and helmet interfaces to deliver noninvasive ventilation in a human model of resistive breathing. J Appl Physiol (1985) 2005;99:1262–71.

61. Cammarota G, Olivieri C, Costa R, et al. Noninvasive ventilation through a helmet in postextubation hypoxemic patients: physiologic comparison between neurally adjusted ventilatory assist and pressure support ventilation. Intensive Care Med 2011;37:1943–50.

62. Nava S, Navalesi P, Gregoretti C. Interfaces and humidification for noninvasive mechanic ventilation. Respir Care 2009;54:71–84.

63. Fodil R, Lellouche F, Mancebo J, et al. Comparison of patient-ventilator interfaces based on their computerized effective dead space. Intensive Care Med 2011;37:257–62.

64. Gregoretti C, Confalonieri M, Navalesi P, et al. Evaluation of patient skin breakdown and comfort with a new face mask for non-invasive ventilation: a multicenter study. Intensive Care Med 2002;28:278–84.

65. Fraticelli AT, Lellouche F, L'her E, et al. Physiological effects of different interfaces during noninvasive ventilation for acute respiratory failure. Crit Care Med 2009;37:939–45.

66. Cuvelier A, Pujol W, Pramil S, et al. Cephalic versus oronasal mask for noninvasive ventilation in acute hypercapnic respiratory failure. Intensive Care Med 2009;35:519–26.

67. Girault C, Briel A, Benichou J, et al. Interface strategy during noninvasive positive pressure ventilation for hypercapnic acute respiratory failure. Crit Care Med 2009;37:124–31.

68. Chacur FH, Vilella Felipe LM, Fernandes CG, et al. The total face mask is more comfortable than the oronasal mask in noninvasive ventilation but is not associated with improved outcome. Respiration 2011;82:426–30.

69. Ozsancak A, Sidhom SS, Liesching TN, et al. Evaluation of the total face mask for noninvasive ventilation to treat acute respiratory failure. Chest 2011;139:1034–41.

70. Roy B, Cordova FC, Travaline JM, et al. Full face mask for noninvasive positive-pressure ventilation in patients with acute respiratory failure. J Am Osteopath Assoc 2007;107:148–56.

71. Lemyze M, Mallat J, Nigeon O, et al. Rescue therapy by switching to total face mask after failure of face mask-delivered noninvasive ventilation in do-not-intubate patients in acute respiratory failure. Crit Care Med 2013;41:481–8.

72. Antonelli M, Conti G, Pelosi P, et al. New treatment of acute hypoxemic respiratory failure: noninvasive pressure support ventilation delivered by helmet–a pilot controlled trial. Crit Care Med 2002;30:602–8.

73. Tonnelier JM, Prat G, Nowak E, et al. Noninvasive continuous positive airway pressure ventilation using a new helmet interface: a case-control prospective pilot study. Intensive Care Med 2003;29:2077–80.

74. Chiumello D, Pelosi P, Carlesso E, et al. Noninvasive positive pressure ventilation delivered by helmet vs standard face mask. Intensive Care Med 2003;29:1671–9.

75. Antonelli M, Pennisi MA, Pelosi P, et al. Noninvasive positive pressure ventilation using a helmet in patients with acute exacerbation of chronic obstructive pulmonary disease: a feasibility study. Anesthesiology 2004;100:16–24.
76. Costa R, Navalesi P, Antonelli M, et al. Physiologic evaluation of different levels of assistance during noninvasive ventilation delivered through a helmet. Chest 2005;128:2984–90.
77. Moerer O, Fischer S, Hartelt M, et al. Influence of two different interfaces for noninvasive ventilation compared to invasive ventilation on the mechanical properties and performance of a respiratory system: a lung model study. Chest 2006;129:1424–31.
78. Navalesi P, Costa R, Ceriana P, et al. Non-invasive ventilation in chronic obstructive pulmonary disease patients: helmet versus facial mask. Intensive Care Med 2007;33:74–81.
79. Foti G, Sangalli F, Berra L, et al. Is helmet CPAP first line pre-hospital treatment of presumed severe acute pulmonary edema? Intensive Care Med 2009;35(4):656–62.
80. Principi T, Pantanetti S, Catani F, et al. Noninvasive continuous positive airway pressure delivered by helmet in hematological malignancy patients with hypoxemic acute respiratory failure. Intensive Care Med 2004;30:147–50.
81. Rocco M, Dell'Utri D, Morelli A, et al. Noninvasive ventilation by helmet or face mask in immunocompromised patients: a case-control study. Chest 2004;126:1508–15.
82. Antonelli M, Pennisi MA, Conti G, et al. Fiberoptic bronchoscopy during noninvasive positive pressure ventilation delivered by helmet. Intensive Care Med 2003;29:126–9.
83. Pelosi P, Severgnini P, Aspesi M, et al. Non-invasive ventilation delivered by conventional interfaces and helmet in the emergency department. Eur J Emerg Med 2003;10(2):79–86.
84. Piastra M, Antonelli M, Chiaretti A, et al. Treatment of acute respiratory failure by helmet-delivered non-invasive pressure support ventilation in children with acute leukemia: a pilot study. Intensive Care Med 2004;30:472–6.
85. Piastra M, Conti G, Caresta E, et al. Noninvasive ventilation options in pediatric myasthenia gravis. Paediatr Anaesth 2005;15:699–702.
86. Piastra M, Antonelli M, Caresta E, et al. Noninvasive ventilation in childhood acute neuromuscular respiratory failure: a pilot study. Respiration 2006;73:791–8.
87. Cavaliere F, Conti G, Costa R, et al. Exposure to noise during continuous positive airway pressure: influence of interfaces and delivery systems. Acta Anaesthesiol Scand 2008;52:52–6.
88. Patroniti N, Foti G, Manfio A, et al. Head helmet versus face mask for non-invasive continuous positive airway pressure: a physiological study. Intensive Care Med 2003;29(10):1680–7.
89. Patroniti N, Saini M, Zanella A, et al. Danger of helmet continuous positive airway pressure during failure of fresh gas source supply. Intensive Care Med 2007;33(1):153–7.
90. Taccone P, Hess D, Caironi P, et al. Continuous positive airway pressure delivered with a "helmet": effects on carbon dioxide rebreathing. Crit Care Med 2004;32(10):2090–6.
91. Racca F, Appendini L, Gregoretti C, et al. Helmet ventilation and carbon dioxide rebreathing: effects of adding a leak at the helmet ports. Intensive Care Med 2008;34:1461–8.

92. Vaschetto R, De Jong A, Conseil M, et al. Comparative evaluation of three interfaces for non-invasive ventilation: a randomized cross-over design physiologic study on healthy volunteers. Crit Care 2014;18:R2.
93. Olivieri C, Costa R, Spinazzola G, et al. Bench comparative evaluation of a new generation and standard helmet for delivering non-invasive ventilation. Intensive Care Med 2013;39:734–8.
94. Antonelli M, Conti G, Rocco M, et al. Noninvasive positive-pressure ventilation vs conventional oxygen supplementation in hypoxemic patients undergoing diagnostic bronchoscopy. Chest 2002;121:1149–54.
95. Scala R, Naldi M, Maccari U. Early fiberoptic bronchoscopy during non-invasive ventilation in patients with decompensated chronic obstructive pulmonary disease due to community-acquired-pneumonia. Crit Care 2010;14:R80.
96. Lellouche F, Pignataro C, Maggiore SM, et al. Short-term effects of humidification devices on respiratory pattern and arterial blood gases during noninvasive ventilation. Respir Care 2012;57:1879–86.
97. Jaber S, Chanques G, Matecki S, et al. Comparison of the effects of heat and moisture exchangers and heated humidifiers on ventilation and gas exchange during non-invasive ventilation. Intensive Care Med 2002;28:1590–4.
98. Lellouche F, L'Her E, Abroug F, et al. Impact of the humidification device on intubation rate during noninvasive ventilation with ICU ventilators: results of a multicenter randomized controlled trial. Intensive Care Med 2014;40:211–9.
99. Restrepo RD, Walsh BK, American Association for Respiratory Care. Humidification during invasive and noninvasive mechanical ventilation: 2012. Respir Care 2012;57:782–8.
100. Scala R, Latham M. How to start a patient on non-invasive ventilation. In: Elliott M, Nava S, Schonhofer B, editors. Non-invasive ventilation and weaning: principles and practice. London: Hodder Arnold Publication; 2010. p. 70–83.
101. Wood KA, Lewis L, Von Harz B, et al. The use of noninvasive positive pressure ventilation in the emergency department: results of a randomized clinical trial. Chest 1998;113:1339–46.
102. Barbé F, Togores B, Rubí M, et al. Noninvasive ventilator support does not facilitate recovery from acute respiratory failure in chronic obstructive disease. Eur Respir J 1996;9:1240–5.
103. Tomii K, Seo R, Tachikawa R, et al. Impact of noninvasive ventilation trial for various types of acute respiratory failure in the emergency department: decreased mortality and use of the ICU. Respir Med 2009;103:67–73.
104. Evans T, Elliott MW, Ranieri M, et al. Pulmonary medicine and (adult) critical care medicine in Europe. Eur Respir J 2002;19:1202–6.
105. Torres A, Ferrer M, Blanquer JB, et al. Intermediate respiratory intensive care units: definitions and characteristics. Arch Bronconeumol 2005;41(9):505–12.
106. Scala R, Corrado A, Confalonieri M, et al. Increased number and expertise of Italian respiratory high-dependency care units: the second national survey. Respir Care 2011;56:1100–7.
107. Landoni G, Zangrillo A, Cabrini L. Non invasive ventilation outside the ICU. In: Vincent JL, editor. Annual update of intensive care and emergency medicine. Berlin, Heidelberg: Springer-Verlag; 2012. p. 207–18.
108. Cabrini L, Antonelli M, Savoia G, et al. Noninvasive ventilation outside the intensive care unit: an Italian survey. Minerva Anestesiol 2011;77:313–22.
109. Plant PK, Owen JL, Elliott MW. Early use of non-invasive ventilation for acute exacerbations of chronic obstructive pulmonary disease on general respiratory wards: a multicentre randomised controlled trial. Lancet 2000;355:1931–5.

110. Sinuff T, Cook DJ, Keenan SP, et al. Noninvasive ventilation for acute respiratory failure near the end of life. Crit Care Med 2008;36:789–94.

111. Kramer N, Meyer TJ, Meharg J, et al. Randomized, prospective trial of noninvasive positive pressure ventilation in acute respiratory failure. Am J Respir Crit Care Med 1995;151:1799–806.

112. Keenan SP, Sinuff T, Cook DJ, et al. Which patients with acute exacerbation of chronic obstructive pulmonary disease benefit from noninvasive positive-pressure ventilation? A systematic review of the literature. Ann Intern Med 2003;138:861–70.

113. Lindenauer PK, Stefan MS, Shieh Meng-Shiou, et al. Outcomes associated with invasive and noninvasive ventilation among patients hospitalized with exacerbations of chronic obstructive pulmonary disease. JAMA Intern Med 2014;174: 1982–93.

114. Carlucci A, Delmastro M, Rubini F, et al. Changes in the practice of noninvasive ventilation in treating COPD patients over eight years. Intensive Care Med 2003; 29:419–25.

115. Confalonieri M, Garuti G, Cattaruzza MS, et al. A chart of failure risk for noninvasive ventilation in patients with COPD exacerbation. Eur Respir J 2005;25: 348–55.

116. Del Sorbo L, Pisani L, Filippini C, et al. Extracorporeal CO_2 removal in hypercapnic patients at risk of noninvasive ventilation failure: a matched cohort study with historical control. Crit Care Med 2015;43:120–7.

117. Ragette R, Mellies U, Schwake C, et al. Patterns and predictors of sleep disordered breathing in primary myopathies. Thorax 2002;57:724–8.

118. Poponick JM, Jacobs I, Supinski G, et al. Effect of upper respiratory tract infection in patients with neuromuscular disease. Am J Respir Crit Care Med 1997; 156:659–64.

119. Tzeng AC, Bach JR. Prevention of pulmonary morbidity for patients with neuromuscular disease. Chest 2000;118:1390–6.

120. Bach JR, Rajaraman R, Ballanger F, et al. Neuromuscular ventilatory insufficiency: effect of home mechanical ventilator use vs oxygen therapy on pneumonia and hospitalization rates. Am J Phys Med Rehabil 1998;77:8–19.

121. Mehta S. Neuromuscular disease causing acute respiratory failure. Respir Care 2006;51:1016–21.

122. Hill NS. Neuromuscular disease in respiratory and critical care medicine. Respir Care 2006;51:1065–71.

123. Racca F, Del Sorbo L, Mongini T, et al. Respiratory management of acute respiratory failure in neuromuscular diseases. Minerva Anestesiol 2010;76:51–62.

124. Racca F, Appendini L, Berta G, et al. Helmet ventilation for acute respiratory failure and nasal skin breakdown in neuromuscular disorders. Anesth Analg 2009;109:164–7.

125. Shneerson JM, Simonds AK. Noninvasive ventilation for chest wall and neuromuscular disorders. Eur Respir J 2002;20:480–7.

126. Blivet S, Philit F, Sab JM, et al. Outcome of patients with idiopathic pulmonary fibrosis admitted to the ICU for respiratory failure. Chest 2001;120:209–12.

127. Vianello A, Arcaro G, Battistella L, et al. Noninvasive ventilation in the event of acute respiratory failure in patients with idiopathic pulmonary fibrosis. J Crit Care 2014;29:562–7.

128. Brochard L, Lefebvre JC, Cordioli RL, et al. Noninvasive ventilation for patients with hypoxemic acute respiratory failure. Semin Respir Crit Care Med 2014;35: 492–500.

129. Confalonieri M, Potena A, Carbone G, et al. Acute respiratory failure in patients with severe community-acquired pneumonia. A prospective randomized evaluation of noninvasive ventilation. Am J Respir Crit Care Med 1999;160:1585–91.
130. Martin TJ, Hovis JD, Costantino JP, et al. A randomized, prospective evaluation of noninvasive ventilation for acute respiratory failure. Am J Respir Crit Care Med 2000;161:807–13.
131. Ferrer M, Esquinas A, Leon M, et al. Noninvasive ventilation in severe hypoxemic respiratory failure: a randomized clinical trial. Am J Respir Crit Care Med 2003; 168:1438–44.
132. Hilbert G, Gruson D, Vargas F, et al. Noninvasive ventilation in immunosuppressed patients with pulmonary infiltrates, fever, and acute respiratory failure. N Engl J Med 2001;344:481–7.
133. Antonelli M, Conti G, Bufi M, et al. Noninvasive ventilation for treatment of acute respiratory failure in patients undergoing solid organ transplantation: a randomized trial. JAMA 2000;283:235–41.
134. Ferguson ND, Fan E, Camporota L, et al. The Berlin definition of ARDS: an expanded rationale, justification, and supplementary material. Intensive Care Med 2012;38:1573–82.
135. Antonelli M, Conti G, Rocco M, et al. A comparison of noninvasive positive-pressure ventilation and conventional mechanical ventilation in patients with acute respiratory failure. N Engl J Med 1998;339:429–35.
136. Honrubia T, García López FJ, Franco N, et al. Noninvasive vs conventional mechanical ventilation in acute respiratory failure: a multicenter, randomized controlled trial. Chest 2005;1286:3916–24.
137. Rana S, Jenad H, Gay PC, et al. Failure of non-invasive ventilation in patients with acute lung injury: observational cohort study. Crit Care 2006;10:R79–1619.
138. Antonelli M, Conti G, Moro ML, et al. Predictors of failure of noninvasive positive pressure ventilation in patients with acute hypoxemic respiratory failure: a multicenter study. Intensive Care Med 2001;27:1718–28.
139. Thille AW, Contou D, Fragnoli C, et al. Non-invasive ventilation for acute hypoxemic respiratory failure: intubation rate and risk factors. Crit Care 2013;17:R269.
140. Zhan Q, Sun B, Liang L, et al. Early use of noninvasive positive pressure ventilation for acute lung injury: a multicenter randomized controlled trial. Crit Care Med 2012;40:455–60.
141. Poppas A, Rounds S. Congestive heart failure. Am J Respir Crit Care Med 2002; 165:4–8.
142. Chadda K, Annane D, Hart N, et al. Cardiac and respiratory effects of continuous positive airway pressure and noninvasive ventilation in acute cardiac pulmonary edema. Crit Care Med 2002;30:2457–61.
143. Ho KM, Wong K. A comparison of continuous and bi-level positive airway pressure non-invasive ventilation in patients with acute cardiogenic pulmonary oedema: a meta-analysis. Crit Care 2006;10:R49.
144. Gray A, Goodacre S, Newby DE, et al. Noninvasive ventilation in acute cardiogenic pulmonary edema. N Engl J Med 2008;359:142–51.
145. Bellone A, Vettorello M, Monari A, et al. Noninvasive pressure support ventilation vs continuous positive airway pressure in acute hypercapnic pulmonary edema. Intensive Care Med 2005;31:807–11.
146. Bakke SA, Botker MT, Riddervold IS, et al. Continuous positive airway pressure and noninvasive ventilation in prehospital treatment of patients with acute respiratory failure: a systematic review of controlled studies. Scand J Trauma Resusc Emerg Med 2014;22:69.

147. Damas C, Andrade C, Araujo JP, et al. Weaning from non-invasive positive pressure ventilation: experience with progressive periods of withdraw. Rev Port Pneumol 2008;14:49–53.
148. Duan J, Tang X, Huang SS, et al. Protocol-directed versus physician-directed weaning from noninvasive ventilation: the impact in chronic obstructive pulmonary disease patients. J Trauma Acute Care Surg 2012;72:1271–5.
149. Cuvelier A, Viacroze C, Benichou J, et al. Dependency on mask ventilation after acute respiratory failure in the intermediate care unit. Eur Respir J 2005;26:289–97.
150. Lim WJ, Mohammed Akram R, Carson KV, et al. Non-invasive positive pressure ventilation for treatment of respiratory failure due to severe acute exacerbations of asthma. Cochrane Database Syst Rev 2012;(12):CD004360.
151. Meduri GU, Cook TR, Turner RE, et al. Noninvasive positive pressure ventilation in status asthmaticus. Chest 1996;110:767–74.
152. Conti G, Antonelli M, Navalesi P, et al. Noninvasive vs conventional mechanical ventilation in patients with chronic obstructive pulmonary disease after failure of medical treatment in the ward: a randomized trial. Intensive Care Med 2002;28:1701–7.
153. Squadrone E, Frigerio P, Fogliati C, et al. Noninvasive vs invasive ventilation in COPD patients with severe acute respiratory failure deemed to require ventilatory assistance. Intensive Care Med 2004;30:1303–10.
154. Girault C, Bubenheim M, Abroug F, et al. Noninvasive ventilation and weaning in patients with chronic hypercapnic respiratory failure: a randomized multicenter trial. Am J Respir Crit Care Med 2011;184:672–9.
155. Burns KE, Meade MO, Premji A, et al. Noninvasive ventilation as a weaning strategy for mechanical ventilation in adults with respiratory failure: a Cochrane systematic review. CMAJ 2014;186:E112–22.
156. Nava S, Gregoretti C, Fanfulla F, et al. Noninvasive ventilation to prevent respiratory failure after extubation in high-risk patients. Crit Care Med 2005;33:2465–70.
157. Ferrer M, Valencia M, Nicolas JM, et al. Early noninvasive ventilation averts extubation failure in patients at risk: a randomized trial. Am J Respir Crit Care Med 2006;173:164–70.
158. Ferrer M, Sellares J, Valencia M, et al. Non-invasive ventilation after extubation in hypercapnic patients with chronic respiratory disorders: randomised controlled trial. Lancet 2009;374:1082–8.
159. Ornico SR, Lobo SM, Sanches HS, et al. Noninvasive ventilation immediately after extubation improves weaning outcome after acute respiratory failure: a randomized controlled trial. Crit Care 2013;17:R39.
160. Carrillo A, Ferrer M, Gonzalez-Diaz G, et al. Noninvasive ventilation in acute hypercapnic respiratory failure caused by obesity hypoventilation syndrome and chronic obstructive pulmonary disease. Am J Respir Crit Care Med 2012;186:1279–85.
161. Squadrone V, Massaia M, Bruno B, et al. Early CPAP prevents evolution of acute lung injury in patients with hematologic malignancy. Intensive Care Med 2010;36:1666–74.
162. Confalonieri M, Calderini E, Terraciano S, et al. Noninvasive ventilation for treating acute respiratory failure in AIDS patients with *Pneumocystis carinii* pneumonia. Intensive Care Med 2002;28:1233–8.
163. Cosentini R, Brambilla AM, Aliberti S, et al. Helmet continuous positive airway pressure vs oxygen therapy to improve oxygenation in community-acquired pneumonia: a randomized, controlled trial. Chest 2010;138:114–20.

164. Brambilla AM, Aliberti S, Prina E, et al. Helmet CPAP vs oxygen therapy in severe hypoxemic respiratory failure due to pneumonia. Intensive Care Med 2014;40:942–9.

165. Jolliet P, Abajo B, Pasquina P, et al. Non-invasive pressure support ventilation in severe community-acquired pneumonia. Intensive Care Med 2001;27:812–21.

166. Domenighetti G, Gayer R, Gentilini R. Noninvasive pressure support ventilation in non-COPD patients with acute cardiogenic pulmonary edema and severe community-acquired pneumonia: acute effects and outcome. Intensive Care Med 2002;28:1226–32.

167. Antonelli M, Conti G, Esquinas A, et al. A multiple-center survey on the use in clinical practice of noninvasive ventilation as a first-line intervention for acute respiratory distress syndrome. Crit Care Med 2007;35:18–25.

168. Chiumello D, Coppola S, Froio S, et al. Noninvasive ventilation in chest trauma: systematic review and meta-analysis. Intensive Care Med 2013;39:1171–80.

169. Vaschetto R, Turucz E, Dellapiazza F, et al. Noninvasive ventilation after early extubation in patients recovering from hypoxemic acute respiratory failure: a single-centre feasibility study. Intensive Care Med 2012;38:1599–606.

170. Cabello B, Thille AW, Drouot X, et al. Sleep quality in mechanically ventilated patients: Comparison of three ventilatory modes. Crit Care Med 2008;36: 1749–55.

171. Parthasarathy S, Tobin MJ. Effect of ventilator mode on sleep quality in critically ill patients. Am J Respir Crit Care Med 2002;166:1423–9.

172. Ely EW, Shintani A, Truman B, et al. Delirium as a predictor of mortality in mechanically ventilated patients in the intensive care unit. JAMA 2004;291: 1753–62.

173. Fanfulla F, Delmastro M, Berardinelli A, et al. Effects of different ventilator settings on sleep and inspiratory effort in patients with neuromuscular disease. Am J Respir Crit Care Med 2005;172:619–24.

174. Moretti M, Cilione C, Tampieri A, et al. Incidence and causes of non-invasive mechanical ventilation failure after initial success. Thorax 2000;55:819–25.

175. Parreira VF, Jounieaux V, Aubert G, et al. Nasal two-level positive-pressure ventilation in normal subjects. Effects of the glottis and ventilation. Am J Respir Crit Care Med 1996;153:1616–23.

176. Moreau-Bussière F, Samson N, St-Hilaire M, et al. Laryngeal response to nasal ventilation in non sedated newborn lambs. J Appl Physiol (1985) 2007;102: 2149–57.

177. Campo FR, Drouot X, Thille AW, et al. Poor sleep quality is associated with late noninvasive ventilation failure in patients with acute hypercapnic respiratory failure. Crit Care Med 2010;38:477–85.

178. Plaschke K, Hill H, Engelhardt R, et al. EEG changes and serum anticholinergic activity measured in patients with delirium in the intensive care unit. Anaesthesia 2007;62:1217–23.

179. Cordoba-Izquierdo A, Drouot X, Thille AW, et al. Sleep in hypercapnic critical care patients under noninvasive ventilation: conventional versus dedicated ventilators. Crit Care Med 2013;41:60–8.

Restless Legs Syndrome

Saiprakash B. Venkateshiah, MD,
Octavian C. Ioachimescu, MD, PhD*

KEYWORDS

- Restless legs syndrome • Periodic leg movements of sleep • Iron deficiency
- Dopaminergic agents • Alpha-2-delta calcium channel ligands • Opioid agents

KEY POINTS

- Restless legs syndrome is characterized by an urge to move and associated with an uncomfortable sensation in the legs.
- Restless legs syndrome can lead to sleep-onset or sleep-maintenance insomnia, and excessive daytime sleepiness leading to significant morbidity.
- Brain iron deficiency and dopaminergic neurotransmission abnormalities play a central role in the pathogenesis of this disorder.
- Dopaminergic agents, alpha-2-delta calcium channel ligands, opioids, and benzodiazepines are commonly used agents to treat restless legs syndrome with variable efficacy.

INTRODUCTION

Restless legs syndrome/Willis-Ekbom disease (RLS/WED) is a neurologic sensorimotor disorder that is mainly characterized by an urge to move, which is often associated with paresthesias. The urge to move is usually worse during rest and at night. RLS/WED is commonly associated with periodic leg movements of sleep (PLMS), which are involuntary jerking leg movements. RLS/WED was first described in 1672 by the English physician Thomas Willis.[1] The term "restless legs syndrome" was coined by Professor Karl-Axel Ekbom in 1944.[2,3] RLS/WED is a common disorder, but often underdiagnosed in the general population.

PREVALENCE

There is a wide variation of the age of onset; as such, RLS could present from childhood to older than 80 years of age.[4] Prevalence estimates of RLS/WED vary significantly, depending on the criteria used to define this condition in surveys. Approximately 5% to 10% of adults are estimated to have RLS/WED in North America

Disclosures: None.
Division of Pulmonary, Critical Care and Sleep Medicine, Department of Medicine, Emory University School of Medicine, Atlanta, GA, USA
* Corresponding author. 1670 Clairmont Road (Sleep 111), Decatur, GA 30033.
E-mail address: oioac@yahoo.com

Crit Care Clin 31 (2015) 459–472
http://dx.doi.org/10.1016/j.ccc.2015.03.003
0749-0704/15/$ – see front matter Published by Elsevier Inc.

criticalcare.theclinics.com

and Europe. The prevalence estimates are lower when the frequency and severity of symptoms are included in the definition.[5] Prevalence of clinically significant RLS is estimated to be around 2% to 3%.[6–9] Increasing prevalence of RLS has been described in women and also with increasing age.[10] Nearly one-third of pregnant women experience RLS in the third trimester and the risk of RLS increases with the number of live births.[11] Prevalence also varies by ethnicity, with lower prevalence in Asian populations.[5] RLS has been described in 2% of school-age children.[12]

ETIOLOGY

The cause of most cases of RLS/WED is unknown, and hence is called primary RLS. A positive family history is present in approximately 40% of patients, with autosomal-dominant inheritance patterns.[13] Familial aggregation of RLS is well described and the proportion of phenotypic variation attributable to genes is 54% to 83%.[14,15] Genetic linkage studies have identified several potential regions of interest. The gene RLS1 on chromosome 12 is common in Icelandic, German, and French-Canadian families, implicating a role for neuronal nitric oxide synthase (NOS1).[16] Multiple single-nucleotide polymorphisms have been identified by genome-wide association studies, suggesting involvement of at least six different gene products: BTBD9, Meis1, PTPRD, MAP2K5, LBXCOR1, and TOX3.[17–21] The implicated genes are widely expressed in the central nervous system and other organs, and at-risk single-nucleotide polymorphisms in each instance are common and present within non-coding, intronic, or intergenic regions. A single single-nucleotide polymorphism (rs3923809) in an intron of BTBD9 is associated with increased risk of RLS and PLMS by 70% to 80%. Nearly one-half of subjects of northern European ancestry were found to carry two copies of this common at-risk variant, which accounts for at least 50% of the population-attributable risk for RLS/PLMS.[22] A dose-dependency between the BTBD9 variant and decrements in iron stores has been observed.[17] The Meis1 variant was found to influence iron homeostasis causing functional decrements.[23] Other genetic factors are also possibly involved, suggesting that RLS expressivity is influenced by a substantial inheritable component.

RLS occurs in association with several disorders (called secondary RLS). The conditions where the frequency of RLS occurs higher than expected than in the general population include iron deficiency; end-stage renal disease; diabetes mellitus; rheumatologic disorders, such as rheumatoid arthritis, Sjögren syndrome, and systemic lupus erythematosus; pulmonary disorders, such as chronic obstructive pulmonary disease and pulmonary hypertension; neurologic conditions, such as Parkinson disease, multiple sclerosis, and migraine; and gastrointestinal conditions, such as gastric surgery, celiac, and Crohn disease.[24–42]

PATHOGENESIS

There is increasing evidence for the role of brain iron insufficiency and dopamine neurotransmission abnormalities in the development of RLS/WED. The remarkable treatment response seen with levodopa and dopaminergic agonists in alleviating RLS symptoms, and the symptomatic worsening observed with dopamine antagonists, has led to the natural hypothesis of a possible role of dopaminergic abnormalities in RLS. The exact mechanisms by which abnormalities in dopaminergic neurotransmission or in dopamine metabolism result in the development of RLS remain unclear.[43–45]

Clinical investigations, neuroimaging modalities, autopsy tissue analysis, cerebrospinal fluid analysis, and experimental models of dietary iron deficiency suggest an intimate interplay between systemic and brain iron and central dopaminergic tone.[24,46–48]

RLS is observed in 30% to 40% of patients with iron deficiency anemia.[49,50] Clinical iron-deficient states and epidemiologic considerations show that systemic iron deficiency is neither sufficient, nor necessary to produce RLS. In a community-based sample, no relationship was observed between the degree of anemia or iron deficiency and RLS.[49] In contrast, smaller studies evaluating serum or cerebrospinal fluid iron and MRI of the substantia nigra have found an association between RLS and low iron stores.[25,51–53] Normal iron transport from plasma into the brain occurs at the level of the choroid plexus of the cerebral ventricles, and by binding to the transferrin receptor expressed by the endothelial cells of the brain microvasculature.[54,55] Autopsy studies suggest that the expression and activity of iron management proteins, including transferrin and its receptor in the choroid plexus and the brain microvasculature, differ in patients with RLS versus healthy control subjects.[56,57] This can possibly explain the existence of a brain-specific iron deficit in the absence of a systemic iron deficiency.

Another pathophysiologic hypothesis focused on observed hypodopaminergic states in the nigrostriatal circuits. This is congruent with levodopa and dopamine agonists' efficacy in relieving RLS/PLMS and that basal ganglia are involved in hypokinetic and hyperkinetic movement disorders. As such, it is not surprising that the peak time for RLS symptoms coincides with the natural nadirs in the synthesis, release, and signaling of dopamine.[58] The rate-limiting enzyme in the synthesis of dopamine is tyrosine hydroxylase, for which iron is an important cofactor.[59,60] Furthermore, recycling and signaling of synaptic dopamine in the basal ganglia is impaired by dietary iron deficiency. Indeed, an excess in extracellular dopamine in the basal ganglia caused by altered presynaptic dopamine-releasing mechanisms, as opposed to reduced synthesis, has been observed in dietary models of iron deficiency.[61,62]

Several clinical and biologic observations suggest that other neurotransmitter systems may also be involved in the pathogenesis of RLS. For example, diminished opiate function may be part of the pathology of RLS.[63,64] This may explain why opiates are successful in the treatment of RLS. The central nervous system opiate systems have significant interactions with dopaminergic systems.[65] Magnetic resonance spectroscopy data also show an increase in glutamate in the thalami of patients with RLS.[66] Alpha-2 delta drugs, such as gabapentin and pregabalin, which are also effective in treating RLS, act by modifying calcium channels and thus decrease the release of neurotransmitters, such as glutamate.[67,68] It is of interest that methadone, which is one of the most effective treatment agents for RLS, is both a mu-receptor agonist and an N-methyl-D-aspartate receptor antagonist, thus affecting both the opiate and the glutamatergic systems.[69] Hypocretin, which is one of the activating hypothalamic peptidergic neurotransmitters, has also been shown to interact with the dopaminergic system. Increased levels of hypocretin in the cerebrospinal fluid were associated in one study with a high incidence of RLS.[70,71] In summary, although the exact pathophysiologic mechanisms in RLS/WED are still unclear, there is a complex interplay between multiple neurotransmitters, dopaminergic and nondopaminergic.

CLINICAL FEATURES

RLS is characterized by complaints of a nearly irresistible urge to move the limbs. The urge to move is often accompanied by other uncomfortable sensations felt deep inside the limbs. The sensorial perception is generally difficult to describe by the patients, but such characterizations as creeping, crawling, aching, itching, twitching, stretching, or pulling have been published. Pain and tingling paresthesia are usually absent, unless an algic form of peripheral neuropathy exists. "Restless legs" is also a misnomer because, even though the legs are most prominently affected, one-quarter to one-half of individuals with RLS describe some upper extremity sensations. These symptoms usually begin or worsen during periods of rest or inactivity, such as sitting or lying down. Symptoms are partially or totally relieved by movement, such as stretching or walking, as long as the activity continues. Patients may fidget, kick, or massage their legs, or move in bed to obtain relief in mild cases. Patients may get out of bed and start pacing around when the symptoms are severe. These symptoms occur exclusively or predominantly in the evening or night rather than during the day. The symptoms usually become worse toward the end of the day and reach their peak at night when they occur within 30 minutes of lying in bed. In severe cases of RLS, patients may have symptoms earlier in the day while resting.

Onset of RLS symptoms may occur at all ages. The mean age of onset for familial RLS is in the third or fourth decade of life, with onset before age 21 years in about one-third of cases. The clinical course of RLS varies based on the age of onset. Slow progression of symptoms is found in about two-thirds of cases in early onset RLS (ie, before age 45 years). Stable symptoms over time have been reported in most of the remaining third. Rapid progression is more typical in late-onset RLS.

Patients with RLS may complain about difficulty falling asleep and frequent night awakenings with leg symptoms.[7,13] Approximately half of the patients may complain of excessive daytime sleepiness. About 80% to 90% of patients with RLS present with periodic limb movements. Periodic limb movements may be seen in sleep (PLMS) or wakefulness (PLMW). PLMS are jerking leg movements lasting between 0.5 and 10 seconds, and with time between onsets of consecutive PLMS ranging from 5 to 90 seconds.[72] PLMS are repetitive stereotyped movements involving flexion of the hip and knee, dorsiflexion of the ankle, and extension of the great toe, which resemble the spinal reflex mechanism designed to withdraw the limb from noxious stimuli. PLMS are frequently associated with arousal from sleep. PLMS with arousals may (rarely) lead to sleep fragmentation and subsequent excessive daytime sleepiness. PLMW occur during quiet rest and frequently at the transition between waking and sleep. A few observational studies have reported an association of cardiovascular disease with RLS and/or PLMS, but there is no definitive evidence for a causal relationship.[73–79]

DIAGNOSIS

International Restless Legs Syndrome Study Group consensus diagnostic criteria for RLS are noted next.[80] RLS is diagnosed by ascertaining symptom patterns that meet the following five essential criteria (all must be met):

1. An urge to move the legs usually but not always accompanied by, or felt to be caused by, uncomfortable and unpleasant sensations in the legs.
2. The urge to move the legs and any accompanying unpleasant sensations begin or worsen during periods of rest or inactivity, such as lying down or sitting.
3. The urge to move the legs and any accompanying unpleasant sensations are partially or totally relieved by movement, such as walking or stretching, at least as long as the activity continues.
4. The urge to move the legs and any accompanying unpleasant sensations during rest or inactivity only occur or are worse in the evening or night than during the day.
5. The occurrence of the previously mentioned features is not solely accounted for as symptoms primary to another medical or a behavioral condition (eg, myalgia,

venous stasis, leg edema, arthritis, leg cramps, positional discomfort, habitual foot tapping).

The clinical features supporting the diagnosis of RLS (although nonessential) for diagnosis are (1) periodic limb movements (presence of PLMS or PLMW at rates or intensity greater than expected for age or medical/medication status), (2) dopaminergic treatment response (reduction in symptoms at least initially with dopaminergic treatment), (3) family history of RLS/WED among first-degree relatives, and (4) lack of profound daytime sleepiness.

More recently, International Classification of Sleep Disorders, 3rd edition lists roughly similar diagnostic criteria for RLS (ICD-9-CM code: 333.94; ICD-10-CM code: G25.81) (**Table 1**).[81]

RESTLESS LEGS SYNDROME IN THE INTENSIVE CARE UNIT

There is a paucity of literature on the subject of RLS in the intensive care unit (ICU) setting. In a small study of 30 patients admitted to critical care unit, 36.3% showed signs of RLS based on questionnaires. In groups with and without sleep disturbance, 52.7% and 20% of participants, respectively, were suffering from RLS.[82] There is a small case series reporting on RLS exacerbation in the perioperative recovery room setting in patients with known RLS, but does not address any ICU presentation.[83] Sleep deprivation is common in hospitalized patients. Environmental noise is the most often cited cause of sleep disturbance in the hospital and the ICU. Multiple factors in the ICU environment can potentially exacerbate RLS. Some of these factors commonly seen in the ICU patient population are rest and immobilization; irregular sleep-wake schedule and sleep restriction; and metabolic factors, such as uremia and iron and folate deficiency. Commonly used medications that could worsen RLS symptoms are antipsychotics (eg, haloperidol, perphenazine), antiemetics (eg, metoclopramide, prochlorperazine), antihistamines (eg, diphenhydramine, cimetidine, ranitidine), calcium channel blockers (eg, verapamil, nifedipine, diltiazem), anticonvulsants (eg, phenytoin), and antidepressants (eg, amitriptyline, lithium, mirtazapine, fluoxetine).[22,84] However, the use of opiates and benzodiazepine in the ICU may be protective against RLS exacerbations.

Table 1
New diagnostic criteria for RLS

Criteria	Specifications
A. An urge to move the legs, usually accompanied by uncomfortable and unpleasant sensations in the legs.	These symptoms must 1. Begin or worsen during rest or inactivity (eg, lying down or sitting); 2. Be partially or totally relieved by movement, such as walking or stretching; and 3. Occur exclusively or predominantly in the evening or night rather than during the day.
B. These features are not solely accounted for as symptoms of another medical or a behavioral condition.	Examples: habitual foot tapping, leg cramps or positional discomfort, myalgia, venous stasis, leg edema, arthritis.
C. The symptoms of RLS cause dysfunction.	Levels of dysfunction: concern; distress; sleep disturbance; or impairment in mental, physical, social, occupational, educational, behavioral, or other important functional areas.

All three criteria (A, B, and C) must be present for the RLS/WED diagnosis.[81]

Circadian rhythm abnormalities are also common in the ICU patient population. In a study of ICU patients whose urinary 6-sulfa-oxymelatonin (a metabolite of melatonin measured as a marker for circadian rhythm) levels were analyzed, the nocturnal peak of melatonin secretion was absent, and the concentration/time curve was flat.[85] Circadian rhythm disturbances have also been described in postoperative patients. A delay was found in the endogenous rhythm of plasma melatonin and excretion of the 6-sulfa-oxymelatonin in urine the first night after either minimally invasive or major surgery. The amplitude in 6-sulfa-oxymelatonin was reduced the first night after minimally invasive surgery.[86] RLS has a strong circadian rhythmicity, with worsening during the evening or night. It is plausible that these circadian rhythm abnormalities noted in the ICU subjects might potentially lead to atypical presentations of RLS, but unfortunately there is no literature on this topic.

Unmasking or worsening of RLS should be a consideration if an ICU patient manifests restlessness or agitation that cannot be otherwise explained. All of the factors that can incite RLS can also provoke periodic limb movements. The periodic limb movements can potentially mimic more serious conditions seen in the ICU, such as myoclonus caused by metabolic derangements or anoxic encephalopathy.[87] There is also a theoretic possibility that the periodic limb movements, if severe, can cause dislodgement of monitoring or life support devices.

TREATMENT OF RESTLESS LEGS SYNDROME

There is a paucity of data on the management of RLS in the ICU setting. The following discussion extrapolates to the ICU the treatment principles of outpatient RLS management (**Table 2**).

Nonpharmacologic Strategies

Nonpharmacologic measures

Some of the nonpharmacologic measures include mental alerting activities, sleep hygiene, and circadian re-entrainment. Lower extremity compression devices may be considered based on anecdotal clinical experience, but there is no sufficient evidence to support their regular use. A randomized controlled trial that involved wearing pneumatic compression devices for a minimum of 1 hour per day, found the devices to be significantly superior to sham treatment, and one-third of patients experienced complete resolution of symptoms.[88] As such, this strategy could be a consideration

Table 2
Main therapeutic modalities for RLS

Modality/Strategy	Measures	Examples/Agents
Nonpharmacologic strategies	Nonpharmacologic measures	Sleep hygiene, circadian re-entrainment, and so forth
	Iron replacement	Oral or intravenous preparations
Pharmacologic strategies	Dopaminergic agents	Ropinirole, pramipexole, rotigotine, levodopa/carbidopa
	Apha-2-delta calcium channel ligands	Gabapentin, gabapentin enacarbil (prodrug of gabapentin), pregabalin
	Opioid agents	Tramadol, oxycodone, hydrocodone, or methadone
	Benzodiazepines	Temazepam, zolpidem, zaleplon, eszopiclone
	Others	Carnitine, and so forth

for application in an ICU setting. Similarly, discontinuing drugs that may be provoking RLS (if feasible), and trial of abstinence from caffeine should be considered.[89,90]

Iron replacement

A variety of causes may lead to iron deficiency in ICU patients (eg, gastrointestinal or other sources of blood loss, repeated laboratory blood draws). We recommend that the iron status of the ICU patient should be determined (iron, serum ferritin, total iron-binding capacity, transferrin saturation, and soluble transferrin receptors, if available). If iron stores are low, iron replacement should be administered, unless fulminant sepsis exists and concerns related to the availability of this important cofactor for the microbial metabolism. If the serum ferritin concentration is less than 20 μg/L or percentage of transferrin saturation is low (<18%), a cause of iron deficiency should be sought and iron replacement instituted, if possible. In general, an increased severity of RLS has been associated with a serum ferritin concentration lower than 45 to 50 μg/L.[51,91] Ferrous sulfate, 325 mg (65 mg of elemental iron), combined with 100 to 200 mg of vitamin C with each dose to enhance absorption two to three times a day is usually administered.[89] Parenteral iron therapy is administered if oral iron therapy is not tolerated or if there are issues with gut absorption of iron. The practice parameters for the treatment of RLS issued by the American Academy of Sleep Medicine have recommended iron supplementation in patients with refractory RLS or with iron deficiency, but this recommendation is based on low level of evidence.[90]

Pharmacologic Strategies

Dopaminergic agents

Dopaminergic agents are very effective in the treatment of RLS. They are represented by carbidopa/levodopa; non–ergot-derived dopamine agonists, such as pramipexole, ropinirole, and rotigotine; and ergot-derived dopamine agonists, such as pergolide and cabergoline. Ergot agonists are not recommended because of their association with cardiac valvular fibrosis and other fibrotic reactions.[90,92] Carbidopa/levodopa, 25 mg/100 mg, has been used for RLS and controlled trials have shown good efficacy.[90] Carbidopa/levodopa combination has a relatively short duration of action and may lead to rebound phenomenon (recurrence of RLS in early morning) in 20% to 35% of patients.[93] Augmentation may occur in up to 70% of patients taking levodopa daily, and hence levodopa should be considered for intermittent use only.[94] Augmentation is the phenomenon of worsening of RLS symptoms earlier in the day after an evening dose of medication, including earlier symptom onset, increased symptom intensity, or symptom spread to the arms.[95] Nonergot dopamine agonists, such as pramipexole, ropinirole, and rotigotine patch, are approved by the Food and Drug Administration for treatment of RLS. Dopamine agonists are preferred for severe RLS, patients with comorbid depression or dysthymia, obesity, or metabolic syndrome.[89] Pramipexole is usually started at 0.125 mg once daily taken 2 hours before onset of major RLS symptoms and increased by 0.125 mg every 2 to 3 days until symptom relief. Most patients require 0.5 mg or less. Ropinirole is started at 0.25 to 0.5 mg, taken 1.5 hours before onset of major symptoms and increased by 0.25 to 0.5 mg every 2 to 3 days to a maximum of 4 mg daily. Rotigotine patch is applied once daily starting at 1 mg and increased as required, to a maximum of 3 mg.[89] Minor adverse effects, such as nausea, light headedness, nasal stuffiness, constipation, insomnia, leg edema, hypersomnia, and sleep attacks (with higher doses), can occur with dopamine agonists. Major adverse effects are augmentation (40%–70%) with pramipexole and probably similar frequency with ropinirole (36% with rotigotine patch).[89,96,97] Impulse control disorders, such as pathologic gambling, compulsive shopping or eating, and hypersexuality, may be seen in 6% to 17% of patients.[89,90,98–100] Rotigotine transdermal patch may be a consideration for use in ICU patients who are unable to take any oral medications.

Apha-2-delta calcium channel ligands

Apha-2-delta calcium channel ligands, such as gabapentin, gabapentin enacarbil (prodrug of gabapentin), and pregabalin, are also used in the treatment of RLS. These agents are preferred as the initial agents of choice for patients with algic RLS (ie, with comorbid pain), anxiety, or insomnia, and also those with a history of addiction or impulse control disorder. Gabapentin is started at 300 mg and increased every few days as required. Many patients require 900 to 1800 mg of gabapentin daily. Maximum dose of 3600 mg/day has been tried. Pregabalin is started at 100 mg daily and effective doses are between 150 and 450 mg. Gabapentin enacarbil is administered as a single daily dose of 600 mg at 5 PM. Class-specific adverse effects of these agents include dizziness, drowsiness, unsteadiness, weight gain, and depression.[89,90,92]

Opioid agents

Opioid agents are another class of agents that are effective in treating RLS. Intermittent use of low-potency opioids, such as 30 to 60 mg of codeine, or opioid receptor agonists, such as 50 to 100 mg of tramadol, can be used at bedtime. Tramadol is the only nondopaminergic drug occasionally associated with augmentation phenomenon. Low-potency opioids are useful for treatment of intermittent RLS. High-potency opioids, such as oxycodone, hydrocodone, or methadone, are highly effective and can be particularly helpful in refractory RLS. Daily effective doses of these agents are 5 to 20 mg, in single or divided doses. The risk of dependence is rarely seen when used for RLS, and hence they should not be withheld for fear of developing opioid dependence. Opioids can cause daytime somnolence, constipation, nausea, and may worsen obstructive sleep apnea or induce central sleep apnea. Opioids are particularly appealing for use in an ICU because they can be used in injectable forms and they are used routinely as part of pain management in the ICU.[89,90]

Benzodiazepines

Another class of agents used to treat RLS is benzodiazepines or benzodiazepine receptor agonists. Zolpidem, 5 to 10 mg, zaleplon, 5 to 10 mg, temazepam, 15 to 30 mg, and eszopiclone, 1 to 3 mg, have been used. They are helpful in treating insomnia symptoms, and that is probably how they help patients with RLS rather than treating the sensorimotor symptoms. There are no good controlled trials of benzodiazepines and there is insufficient information on the effect of benzodiazepines for treatment of RLS. Adverse effects include drowsiness, unsteadiness, and daytime cognitive impairment.[89,90] These agents are commonly used in the ICU as part of sedation armamentarium and are available in intravenous form, making them appealing for consideration for treatment of RLS unless delirium is a confounder, as a significant and frequent ICU complication.

SUMMARY

RLS is a common sensorimotor disorder characterized by an urge to move and associated with an uncomfortable sensation in the lower extremities. PLMS are seen in 80% to 90% of patients with RLS. RLS may lead to sleep initiation or sleep maintenance insomnia, and/or excessive daytime sleepiness, all leading to significant morbidity. Brain iron deficiency and dopaminergic neurotransmission abnormalities play a central role in the pathogenesis of this disorder, along with other nondopaminergic systems, although the exact mechanisms are still unclear. Dopaminergic agents, alpha-2-delta calcium channel ligands, opioids, and benzodiazepines are commonly used agents to treat RLS, with variable efficacy. ICU patients are especially vulnerable to have unmasking or frank exacerbation of RLS caused by sleep deprivation, circadian rhythm disturbances, immobilization, iron deficiency, and/or use of medications that can antagonize dopamine. There is a paucity of literature on RLS in ICU patients. Future research is warranted in the area of RLS in ICU patients.

REFERENCES

1. Willis T. De anima brutorum. London: Wells and Scott; 1672.
2. Ekbom KA. Restless legs: a clinical study. Acta Med Scand 1945;158(Suppl): 1–122.
3. Ekbom KA. Asthenia crurum paraesthetica (irritable legs). Acta Med Scand 1944;118:197–209.
4. Winkelmann J, Wetter TC, Collado-Seidel V, et al. Clinical characteristics and frequency of the hereditary restless legs syndrome in a population of 300 patients. Sleep 2000;23(5):597–602.
5. Ohayon MM, O'Hara R, Vitiello MV. Epidemiology of restless legs syndrome: a synthesis of the literature. Sleep Med Rev 2012;16(4):283–95.
6. Allen RP, Bharmal M, Calloway M. Prevalence and disease burden of primary restless legs syndrome: results of a general population survey in the United States. Mov Disord 2011;26(1):114–20.
7. Allen RP, Walters AS, Montplaisir J, et al. Restless legs syndrome prevalence and impact: REST general population study. Arch Intern Med 2005;165(11): 1286–92.
8. Allen RP, Stillman P, Myers AJ. Physician-diagnosed restless legs syndrome in a large sample of primary medical care patients in western Europe: prevalence and characteristics. Sleep Med 2010;11(1):31–7.
9. Phillips B, Young T, Finn L, et al. Epidemiology of restless legs symptoms in adults. Arch Intern Med 2000;160(14):2137–41.
10. Berger K, Luedemann J, Trenkwalder C, et al. Sex and the risk of restless legs syndrome in the general population. Arch Intern Med 2004;164(2):196–202.
11. Manconi M, Govoni V, De Vito A, et al. Restless legs syndrome and pregnancy. Neurology 2004;63(6):1065–9.
12. Picchietti D, Allen RP, Walters AS, et al. Restless legs syndrome: prevalence and impact in children and adolescents–the Peds Rest study. Pediatrics 2007; 120(2):253–66.
13. Montplaisir J, Boucher S, Poirier G, et al. Clinical, polysomnographic, and genetic characteristics of restless legs syndrome: a study of 133 patients diagnosed with new standard criteria. Mov Disord 1997;12(1):61–5.
14. Desai AV, Cherkas LF, Spector TD, et al. Genetic influences in self-reported symptoms of obstructive sleep apnoea and restless legs: a twin study. Twin Res 2004;7(6):589–95.
15. Ondo WG, Vuong KD, Wang Q. Restless legs syndrome in monozygotic twins: clinical correlates. Neurology 2000;55(9):1404–6.
16. Winkelmann J, Lichtner P, Schormair B, et al. Variants in the neuronal nitric oxide synthase (nNOS, NOS1) gene are associated with restless legs syndrome. Mov Disord 2008;23(3):350–8.
17. Stefansson H, Rye DB, Hicks A, et al. A genetic risk factor for periodic limb movements in sleep. N Engl J Med 2007;357(7):639–47.

18. Winkelmann J, Schormair B, Lichtner P, et al. Genome-wide association study of restless legs syndrome identifies common variants in three genomic regions. Nat Genet 2007;39(8):1000–6.
19. Vilarino-Guell C, Farrer MJ, Lin SC. A genetic risk factor for periodic limb movements in sleep. N Engl J Med 2008;358(4):425–7.
20. Schormair B, Kemlink D, Roeske D, et al. PTPRD (protein tyrosine phosphatase receptor type delta) is associated with restless legs syndrome. Nat Genet 2008; 40(8):946–8.
21. Winkelmann J, Czamara D, Schormair B, et al. Genome-wide association study identifies novel restless legs syndrome susceptibility loci on 2p14 and 16q12.1. PLoS Genet 2011;7(7):e1002171.
22. Rye DB, Trotti LM. Restless legs syndrome and periodic leg movements of sleep. Neurol Clin 2012;30(4):1137–66.
23. Catoire H, Dion PA, Xiong L, et al. Restless legs syndrome-associated MEIS1 risk variant influences iron homeostasis. Ann Neurol 2011;70(1):170–5.
24. Earley CJ, Allen RP, Beard JL, et al. Insight into the pathophysiology of restless legs syndrome. J Neurosci Res 2000;62(5):623–8.
25. Silber MH, Richardson JW. Multiple blood donations associated with iron deficiency in patients with restless legs syndrome. Mayo Clin Proc 2003;78(1):52–4.
26. Winkelman JW, Chertow GM, Lazarus JM. Restless legs syndrome in end-stage renal disease. Am J Kidney Dis 1996;28(3):372–8.
27. Merlino G, Fratticci L, Valente M, et al. Association of restless legs syndrome in type 2 diabetes: a case-control study. Sleep 2007;30(7):866–71.
28. Salih AM, Gray RE, Mills KR, et al. A clinical, serological and neurophysiological study of restless legs syndrome in rheumatoid arthritis. Br J Rheumatol 1994; 33(1):60–3.
29. Gudbjornsson B, Broman JE, Hetta J, et al. Sleep disturbances in patients with primary Sjogren's syndrome. Br J Rheumatol 1993;32(12):1072–6.
30. Hassan N, Pineau CA, Clarke AE, et al. Systemic lupus and risk of restless legs syndrome. J Rheumatol 2011;38(5):874–6.
31. Kaplan Y, Inonu H, Yilmaz A, et al. Restless legs syndrome in patients with chronic obstructive pulmonary disease. Can J Neurol Sci 2008;35(3):352–7.
32. Lo Coco D, Mattaliano A, Lo Coco A, et al. Increased frequency of restless legs syndrome in chronic obstructive pulmonary disease patients. Sleep Med 2009; 10(5):572–6.
33. Minai OA, Malik N, Foldvary N, et al. Prevalence and characteristics of restless legs syndrome in patients with pulmonary hypertension. J Heart Lung Transplant 2008;27(3):335–40.
34. Poewe W, Hogl B. Akathisia, restless legs and periodic limb movements in sleep in Parkinson's disease. Neurology 2004;63(8 Suppl 3):S12–6.
35. Nomura T, Inoue Y, Miyake M, et al. Prevalence and clinical characteristics of restless legs syndrome in Japanese patients with Parkinson's disease. Mov Disord 2006;21(3):380–4.
36. Gomez-Esteban JC, Zarranz JJ, Tijero B, et al. Restless legs syndrome in Parkinson's disease. Mov Disord 2007;22(13):1912–6.
37. Manconi M, Fabbrini M, Bonanni E, et al. High prevalence of restless legs syndrome in multiple sclerosis. Eur J Neurol 2007;14(5):534–9.
38. Rhode AM, Hosing VG, Happe S, et al. Comorbidity of migraine and restless legs syndrome: a case-control study. Cephalalgia 2007;27(11):1255–60.
39. Banerji NK, Hurwitz LJ. Restless legs syndrome, with particular reference to its occurrence after gastric surgery. Br Med J 1970;4(5738):774–5.

40. Manchanda S, Davies CR, Picchietti D. Celiac disease as a possible cause for low serum ferritin in patients with restless legs syndrome. Sleep Med 2009; 10(7):763–5.
41. Weinstock LB, Walters AS, Mullin GE, et al. Celiac disease is associated with restless legs syndrome. Dig Dis Sci 2010;55(6):1667–73.
42. Weinstock LB, Bosworth BP, Scherl EJ, et al. Crohn's disease is associated with restless legs syndrome. Inflamm Bowel Dis 2010;16(2):275–9.
43. Trenkwalder C, Hening WA, Montagna P, et al. Treatment of restless legs syndrome: an evidence-based review and implications for clinical practice. Mov Disord 2008;23(16):2267–302.
44. Trenkwalder C, Paulus W. Restless legs syndrome: pathophysiology, clinical presentation and management. Nat Rev Neurol 2010;6(6):337–46.
45. Winkelman JW, Allen RP, Tenzer P, et al. Restless legs syndrome: nonpharmacologic and pharmacologic treatments. Geriatrics 2007;62(10):13–6.
46. Allen R. Dopamine and iron in the pathophysiology of restless legs syndrome (RLS). Sleep Med 2004;5(4):385–91.
47. Allen RP, Earley CJ. The role of iron in restless legs syndrome. Mov Disord 2007; 22(Suppl 18):S440–8.
48. Connor JR. Pathophysiology of restless legs syndrome: evidence for iron involvement. Curr Neurol Neurosci Rep 2008;8(2):162–6.
49. Allen RP, Auerbach S, Bahrain H, et al. The prevalence and impact of restless legs syndrome on patients with iron deficiency anemia. Am J Hematol 2013; 88(4):261–4.
50. Akyol A, Kiylioglu N, Kadikoylu G, et al. Iron deficiency anemia and restless legs syndrome: is there an electrophysiological abnormality? Clin Neurol Neurosurg 2003;106(1):23–7.
51. O'Keeffe ST, Gavin K, Lavan JN. Iron status and restless legs syndrome in the elderly. Age Ageing 1994;23(3):200–3.
52. Earley CJ, Connor JR, Beard JL, et al. Abnormalities in CSF concentrations of ferritin and transferrin in restless legs syndrome. Neurology 2000;54(8): 1698–700.
53. Allen RP, Barker PB, Wehrl F, et al. MRI measurement of brain iron in patients with restless legs syndrome. Neurology 2001;56(2):263–5.
54. Beard JL, Connor JR, Jones BC. Iron in the brain. Nutr Rev 1993;51(6):157–70.
55. Fishman JB, Rubin JB, Handrahan JV, et al. Receptor-mediated transcytosis of transferrin across the blood-brain barrier. J Neurosci Res 1987;18(2):299–304.
56. Connor JR, Ponnuru P, Wang XS, et al. Profile of altered brain iron acquisition in restless legs syndrome. Brain 2011;134(Pt 4):959–68.
57. Connor JR, Boyer PJ, Menzies SL, et al. Neuropathological examination suggests impaired brain iron acquisition in restless legs syndrome. Neurology 2003;61(3):304–9.
58. Freeman A, Rye D. Dopamine in behavioral state control. In: Sinton C, Perumal P, Monti J, editors. Cambridge (United Kingdom): Cambridge University Press; 2008. p. 179–223.
59. Ramsey AJ, Hillas PJ, Fitzpatrick PF. Characterization of the active site iron in tyrosine hydroxylase. Redox states of the iron. J Biol Chem 1996;271(40): 24395–400.
60. Nagatsu T. Tyrosine hydroxylase: human isoforms, structure and regulation in physiology and pathology. Essays Biochem 1995;30:15–35.
61. Nelson C, Erikson K, Pinero DJ, et al. In vivo dopamine metabolism is altered in iron-deficient anemic rats. J Nutr 1997;127(12):2282–8.

62. Bianco LE, Wiesinger J, Earley CJ, et al. Iron deficiency alters dopamine uptake and response to L-DOPA injection in Sprague-Dawley rats. J Neurochem 2008; 106(1):205–15.

63. Walters AS, Ondo WG, Zhu W, et al. Does the endogenous opiate system play a role in the restless legs syndrome? a pilot post-mortem study. J Neurol Sci 2009; 279(1–2):62–5.

64. Walters AS. Review of receptor agonist and antagonist studies relevant to the opiate system in restless legs syndrome. Sleep Med 2002;3(4):301–4.

65. Pert A, DeWald L, Gallager D. Effects of opiates on nigrostriatal dopaminergic activity: electrophysiological and behavioral analysis. In: Usdin E, Kopin I, Barchas J, editors. New York: Pergamon; 1979. p. 1041–3.

66. Allen RP, Barker PB, Horska A, et al. Thalamic glutamate/glutamine in restless legs syndrome: increased and related to disturbed sleep. Neurology 2013; 80(22):2028–34.

67. Hoppa MB, Lana B, Margas W, et al. Alpha2delta expression sets presynaptic calcium channel abundance and release probability. Nature 2012;486(7401):122–5.

68. Coderre TJ, Kumar N, Lefebvre CD, et al. A comparison of the glutamate release inhibition and anti-allodynic effects of gabapentin, lamotrigine, and riluzole in a model of neuropathic pain. J Neurochem 2007;100(5):1289–99.

69. Inturrisi CE. Pharmacology of methadone and its isomers. Minerva Anestesiol 2005;71(7–8):435–7.

70. Taheri S, Zeitzer JM, Mignot E. The role of hypocretins (orexins) in sleep regulation and narcolepsy. Annu Rev Neurosci 2002;25:283–313.

71. Allen RP, Mignot E, Ripley B, et al. Increased CSF hypocretin-1 (orexin-A) in restless legs syndrome. Neurology 2002;59(4):639–41.

72. Berry RB, Brooks R, Gamaldo CE, et al. The AASM manual for the scoring of sleep and associated events: rules, terminology and technical specifications. Darien (IL): American Academy of Sleep Medicine; 2014.

73. Winter AC, Berger K, Glynn RJ, et al. Vascular risk factors, cardiovascular disease, and restless legs syndrome in men. Am J Med 2013;126(3):228–35, 235.e1–2.

74. Winter AC, Schurks M, Glynn RJ, et al. Vascular risk factors, cardiovascular disease, and restless legs syndrome in women. The Am J Med 2013;126(3):220–7, 227.e1–2.

75. Walters AS, Rye DB. Review of the relationship of restless legs syndrome and periodic limb movements in sleep to hypertension, heart disease, and stroke. Sleep 2009;32(5):589–97.

76. Coelho FM, Georgsson H, Narayansingh M, et al. Higher prevalence of periodic limb movements of sleep in patients with history of stroke. J Clin Sleep Med 2010;6(5):428–30.

77. Koo BB, Blackwell T, Ancoli-Israel S, et al. Association of incident cardiovascular disease with periodic limb movements during sleep in older men: outcomes of sleep disorders in older men (MrOS) study. Circulation 2011;124(11):1223–31.

78. Winkelman JW, Shahar E, Sharief I, et al. Association of restless legs syndrome and cardiovascular disease in the sleep heart health study. Neurology 2008; 70(1):35–42.

79. Szentkiralyi A, Volzke H, Hoffmann W, et al. A time sequence analysis of the relationship between cardiovascular risk factors, vascular diseases and restless legs syndrome in the general population. J Sleep Res 2013;22(4):434–42.

80. Allen RP, Picchietti DL, Garcia-Borreguero D, et al. Restless legs syndrome/ Willis-Ekbom disease diagnostic criteria: updated International Restless Legs

Syndrome Study Group (IRLSSG) consensus criteria–history, rationale, description, and significance. Sleep Med 2014;15(8):860–73.

81. Sateia M. International classification of sleep disorders third edition (ICSD-3). Darien (IL): American Academy of Sleep Medicine; 2014.

82. Habibzade H, Khalkhali H, Ghaneii R. Study of the relationship between restless legs syndrome and sleep disturbance among patients in critical care units. Iran J Crit Care Nurs 2011;4(3):153.

83. Karroum EG, Raux M, Riou B, et al. Acute exacerbation of restless legs syndrome during perioperative procedures: case reports and suggested management. Ann Fr Anesth Reanim 2010;29(12):920–4 [in French].

84. Ahmed QA. Effects of common medications used for sleep disorders. Crit Care Clin 2008;24(3):493–515, vi.

85. Shilo L, Dagan Y, Smorjik Y, et al. Patients in the intensive care unit suffer from severe lack of sleep associated with loss of normal melatonin secretion pattern. Am J Med Sci 1999;317(5):278–81.

86. Gogenur I. Postoperative circadian disturbances. Dan Med Bull 2010;57(12): B4205.

87. Brown LK, Arora M. Nonrespiratory sleep disorders found in ICU patients. Crit Care Clin 2008;24(3):589–611, viii.

88. Lettieri CJ, Eliasson AH. Pneumatic compression devices are an effective therapy for restless legs syndrome: a prospective, randomized, double-blinded, sham-controlled trial. Chest 2009;135(1):74–80.

89. Silber MH, Becker PM, Earley C, et al. Medical advisory board of the Willis-Ekbom disease. F. Willis-Ekbom Disease Foundation revised consensus statement on the management of restless legs syndrome. Mayo Clin Proc 2013; 88(9):977–86.

90. Aurora RN, Kristo DA, Bista SR, et al. The treatment of restless legs syndrome and periodic limb movement disorder in adults–an update for 2012: practice parameters with an evidence-based systematic review and meta-analyses: an American Academy of Sleep Medicine clinical practice guideline. Sleep 2012; 35(8):1039–62.

91. Sun ER, Chen CA, Ho G, et al. Iron and the restless legs syndrome. Sleep 1998; 21(4):371–7.

92. Garcia-Borreguero D, Ferini-Strambi L, Kohnen R, et al. European guidelines on management of restless legs syndrome: report of a joint task force by the European Federation of Neurological Societies, the European Neurological Society and the European Sleep Research Society. Eur J Neurol 2012;19(11):1385–96.

93. Guilleminault C, Cetel M, Philip P. Dopaminergic treatment of restless legs and rebound phenomenon. Neurology 1993;43(2):445.

94. Earley CJ, Allen RP. Pergolide and carbidopa/levodopa treatment of the restless legs syndrome and periodic leg movements in sleep in a consecutive series of patients. Sleep 1996;19(10):801–10.

95. Garcia-Borreguero D, Allen RP, Kohnen R, et al. Diagnostic standards for dopaminergic augmentation of restless legs syndrome: report from a world association of sleep medicine-international restless legs syndrome study group consensus conference at the Max Planck Institute. Sleep Med 2007;8(5): 520–30.

96. Oertel W, Trenkwalder C, Benes H, et al. Long-term safety and efficacy of rotigotine transdermal patch for moderate-to-severe idiopathic restless legs syndrome: a 5-year open-label extension study. Lancet Neurol 2011;10(8): 710–20.

97. Silver N, Allen RP, Senerth J, et al. A 10-year, longitudinal assessment of dopamine agonists and methadone in the treatment of restless legs syndrome. Sleep Med 2011;12(5):440–4.

98. Moore TJ, Glenmullen J, Mattison DR. Reports of pathological gambling, hypersexuality, and compulsive shopping associated with dopamine receptor agonist drugs. JAMA Intern Med 2014;174(12):1930–3.

99. Cornelius JR, Tippmann-Peikert M, Slocumb NL, et al. Impulse control disorders with the use of dopaminergic agents in restless legs syndrome: a case-control study. Sleep 2010;33(1):81–7.

100. Garcia-Borreguero D, Kohnen R, Silber MH, et al. The long-term treatment of restless legs syndrome/Willis-ekbom disease: evidence-based guidelines and clinical consensus best practice guidance: a report from The International Restless Legs Syndrome Study Group. Sleep Med 2013;14(7):675–84.

Congestive Heart Failure and Central Sleep Apnea

 CrossMark

Scott A. Sands, PhD[a,b], Robert L. Owens, MD[c],*

KEYWORDS

- Congestive heart failure • Central sleep apnea • Cheyne stokes respiration
- Loop gain

KEY POINTS

- Congestive heart failure (CHF) is a common clinical syndrome among patients in the intensive care unit (ICU), who frequently require noninvasive or mechanical ventilation.
- CHF affects breathing control by increasing chemosensitivity and circulatory delay, predisposing to central sleep apnea, classically in a crescendo–decrescendo pattern of respiration known as Cheyne–Stokes respiration (CSR).
- Few data are available to determine prevalence of CSR in the ICU, or how CSR might affect clinical management and weaning from mechanical ventilation.

CLINICAL CONSIDERATIONS
Historical Perspective

An abnormal respiratory pattern has long been recognized as an ominous sign of congestive heart failure (CHF). The observations of 3 physicians who have lent their names to the pattern remain informative:

> His breathing was very particular: he would cease breathing for twenty or thirty seconds, and then begin to breathe softly, which increased until he breathed extremely strong, or rather with violent strength, which gradually died away till we could not observe that he breathed at all. He could not lie down without running the risk of being suffocated, therefore he was obliged to sit up in his chair.
> —John Hunter, 1781[1]

Disclosure Statement: Dr S.A. Sands is supported by a National Health and Medical Research Council of Australia Early Career Fellowship and R.G. Menzies award (1053201). Dr R.L. Owens is supported by the National Institutes of Health K23 HL105542. He has previously consulted for Philips Respironics.
a Division of Sleep Medicine, Brigham and Women's Hospital and Harvard Medical School, 221 Longwood Avenue, Boston, MA 02115, USA; b Department of Allergy, Immunology and Respiratory Medicine and Central Clinical School, Alfred Hospital and Monash University, 55 Commercial Rd, Melbourne, VIC 3004, Australia; c Division of Pulmonary and Critical Care Medicine, University of California San Diego, 9300 Campus Point Drive, #7381, La Jolla, CA 92037, USA
* Corresponding author.
E-mail address: rowens@ucsd.edu

Crit Care Clin 31 (2015) 473–495
http://dx.doi.org/10.1016/j.ccc.2015.03.005
0749-0704/15/$ – see front matter © 2015 Elsevier Inc. All rights reserved.
criticalcare.theclinics.com

The patient suddenly developed palpitations and displayed signs of severe congestive heart failure. The only particularity in the last period of his illness, which lasted eight or nine days, was in the state of respiration. For several days his breathing was irregular; it would entirely cease for a quarter of a minute, then it would become perceptible, though very low, then by degrees it became heaving and quick, and then it would gradually cease again. This revolution in the state of his breathing occupied about a minute, during which there were about thirty acts of respiration.

—John Cheyne, 1818

This symptom [periodic breathing], as occurring in its highest degree, I have only seen during a few weeks previous to the death of the patient.

—William Stokes, 1854

The initial observations by Hunter, Cheyne, and Stokes were made in patients close to death. They were the first to note the characteristic waxing and waning respiratory pattern of "Cheyne–Stokes respiration" (CSR), a common pattern of central sleep apnea in patients with CHF. CSR is characterized by complete cessation of respiratory effort and airflow (apnea phase) alternating with profound hyperventilation (hyperventilation phase). Such patterns occur during wakefulness, but are typically more prominent during sleep (**Fig. 1**). The apnea phase of CSR causes arterial hypoxemia, and the hyperventilation phase produces surges in blood pressure, arousal from sleep, and dyspnea (**Fig. 2**).[2–5] Typically, CSR has a periodicity of 45 to 90 seconds, and occurs during non–rapid eye movement (REM) sleep stages 1 and 2. CSR severity is typically measured by quantifying the percent of total sleep time in CSR, and by the number of apneas and central hypopneas per hour of sleep (apnea–hypopnea index).[6] Despite advances in the treatment of CHF (eg, β-blockade, spironolactone), untreated CSR remains highly prevalent during sleep and retains its association with

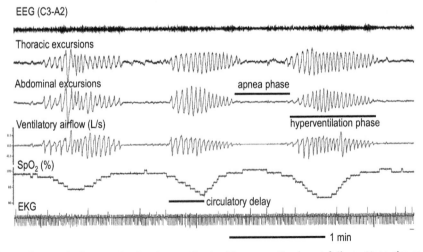

Fig. 1. Cheyne–Stokes respiration in a patient with congestive heart failure. Note the crescendo–decrescendo pattern of respiratory effort and airflow. The lung-to-ear circulatory delay can be approximated by the time from resumption of airflow to the start of the increase in oxygen saturation. EEG, electroencephalogram; EKG, electrocardiogram; SpO_2, oxygen saturation.

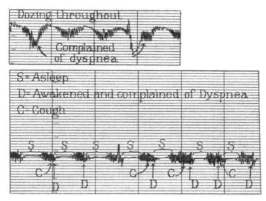

Fig. 2. Increased ventilatory drive during the hyperventilation phase of Cheyne–Stokes respiration results in dyspnea in a patient with heart failure. (*Adapted from* Harrison TR, King CE, Calhoun JA, et al. Congestive heart failure: Xx. Cheyne-Stokes respiration as the cause of paroxysmal dyspnea at the onset of sleep. Arch Intern Med 1934;53(6):897; with permission.)

increased morbidity and mortality independent of the severity of heart failure (**Boxes 1–4**).[7–10]

Box 1
Features of Cheyne–Stokes respiration

- Waxing and waning respiratory pattern
- Baseline hyperventilation and hypocapnia is typical
- Periodicity of 45–90 seconds
- Improved in REM and slow-wave sleep

Abbreviation: REM, rapid eye movement.

Epidemiology in Stable Congestive Heart Failure

One of the first rigorous studies to use polysomnography by Javaheri and colleagues[11] found a high prevalence (40%) of CSR in patients with systolic heart failure. This prevalence has been a relatively consistent finding depending on the population studied (with increased prevalence with worsening heart failure) and the threshold and technology used to diagnosis sleep disordered breathing.[12–15] Although early epidemiologic studies predated the widespread use of advanced heart failure therapies, even the most recent studies continue to show a consistently high prevalence of CSR.[14,16] CSR is not limited to systolic heart failure; CSR is common in patients with symptomatic heart failure with preserved ejection fraction[17] (diastolic dysfunction), and is also common in patients with asymptomatic systolic dysfunction.[18] Additional risk factors for CSR include male gender, older age, the presence of atrial fibrillation, nocturnal ventricular arrhythmias, low arterial partial pressure of CO_2 (Pa_{CO_2}), dyspnea with minimal exertion (New York Heart Association class $\geq$II), nocturnal dyspnea, very low ejection fraction (<20%), left atrial enlargement, and high N-terminal of the prohormone brain natriuretic peptide (NT-proBNP).[5,10,12,14,15,19,20]

Box 2
Types/causes of central sleep apnea in the intensive care unit

- Cheyne–Stokes respiration
- Stroke/neurologic disease
- Narcotic induced

Congestive Heart Failure in the Intensive Care Unit

CHF is among the most common causes of admission to hospitals in the United States, especially in those over 65 years of age, with more than 1 million hospital admissions per year.[21] Approximately 10% of these patients will require admission to the intensive care unit (ICU).[22] Despite the high number of hospital/ICU admissions, there are few data regarding the prevalence of CSR among hospitalized patients. Hoffman and colleagues[23] noted CSR in 44% of CHF patients after weaning from mechanical ventilation for cardiogenic pulmonary edema. More recently, Padeletti and colleagues[24] found moderate to severe CSR (apnea–hypopnea index of >15) in 75% of patients admitted for an acute exacerbation of systolic CHF, with an average of 51% of total sleep time spent exhibiting CSR. Thus, CSR seems to be more prevalent (~75%) in decompensated CHF in inpatients than in stable CHF outpatients (~40%).

Unfortunately, data on the prevalence of CSR in the ICU and effects on outcomes are lacking. Given the pathophysiologic changes that occur in severe heart failure (that requires ICU admission for management), we might expect a very high rate of CSR. However, the most acutely ill patients may be on mechanical ventilation and sedated, often with narcotics. Mechanical ventilation also provides ventilatory and cardiac support for the patient in heart failure, because both cardiac preload and afterload are reduced while on positive end-expiratory pressure (PEEP).[25,26] Thus, CSR is likely to be most relevant during the process of ventilator weaning[23] when such support is removed. It is during the process of moving toward liberation from mechanical ventilation that sedatives are decreased, PEEP and supplemental oxygen levels are lowered, and patients are placed on spontaneous modes (ie, patient triggered) of ventilation.

PATHOPHYSIOLOGIC CONSIDERATIONS
Control of Breathing

The physiologic control of breathing is maintained by a negative feedback system that acts to regulate acid–base status and the partial pressure of arterial carbon dioxide ($Paco_2$), and ensure adequate oxygenation. The primary components of the ventilatory control system are chemoreceptor inputs located in the medulla that respond to changes in acid–base status and the peripheral chemoreceptors in the carotid bodies that are sensitive to both changes in Pao_2 and $Paco_2$. Central and peripheral chemoreceptor inputs are integrated in the medulla and act to modulate breath amplitude (and timing to a lesser extent), ultimately resulting in a level of ventilation conducive to survival. Importantly, there are other sensors in the lungs and circulation whose inputs modify the behavior of the respiratory control system, including pulmonary stretch receptors, irritant receptors, and the "J" (juxtacapillary) receptors, which may become important in disease states and are discussed elsewhere in this article.[27–31]

Box 3
Pathophysiology/mechanisms of Cheyne–Stokes respiration in congestive heart failure

- Increased chemosensitivity owing to
  - Increased left atrial pressure
  - Hypoxemia
- Increased circulatory delay
- Low lung volumes

The Concept of Loop Gain

The stability of the respiratory feedback loop has been quantified using the engineering criterion, loop gain. Briefly, loop gain is the magnitude of the ventilatory response of the respiratory control system to a sinusoidal respiratory disturbance (at the frequency of CSR). Feedback loops with a value of loop gain that exceeds 1.0 (response is greater than the disturbance) are intrinsically unstable and periodic oscillations in breathing inevitably occur (**Fig. 3**). When loop gain is less than 1 (response < disturbance), transient oscillations are attenuated and thereby temporary. Detailed descriptions of loop gain have been given previously.[32–34] Consider a period of hyperventilation (disturbance) that causes a reduction in $Paco_2$. This reduction in $Paco_2$ is sensed by chemoreceptors after a circulatory delay, which in turn elicit a later reduction in ventilatory drive (response). In an unstable system, the decrease in ventilatory drive causes a greater degree of hypoventilation than the original hyperventilatory disturbance. Oscillations re amplified and self-sustained with no specific initiating factor required. The concept of loop gain has been applied successfully to predict the occurrence of CSR (**Fig. 4**)[35] and the resistance to its suppression with treatment.[36,37]

Detailed analyses of the control system consistently reveal 4 primary factors that contribute to loop gain,[32,35,36,38–40] according to the relationship:

$$\text{Loop gain} = G\frac{Paco_2}{\text{Lung Volume}}T \qquad (1)$$

where G is the chemosensitivity, defined as the change in ventilation in response to a change in $Paco_2$; $Paco_2$ is the arterial partial pressure of CO_2 (with the assumption here that inspired $Pco_2 = 0$); lung volume is the end-expiratory lung volume (eg, functional residual capacity); and T is a timing factor that incorporates the lung–chemoreceptor circulatory delay. A similar equation can be written for the ventilatory feedback control of arterial Po_2.

How Congestive Heart Failure Predisposes to Cheyne–Stokes respiration

Equation 1 provides the framework for identifying the factors that predispose an individual to CSR. Indeed, there is evidence that each of these factors plays a role in the development or effective treatment of CSR.

Circulatory Delay

Classically, an increased lung-to-chemoreceptor circulatory delay (T) has been implicated as the cause of CSR. Patients with heart failure can have elevated circulatory delay as a result of decreased cardiac output. CHF patients with a lower left ventricular ejection fraction, lower cardiac output, and elongated circulatory delays are at elevated risk of CSR.[11,19,41,42] Further evidence includes the observation that the

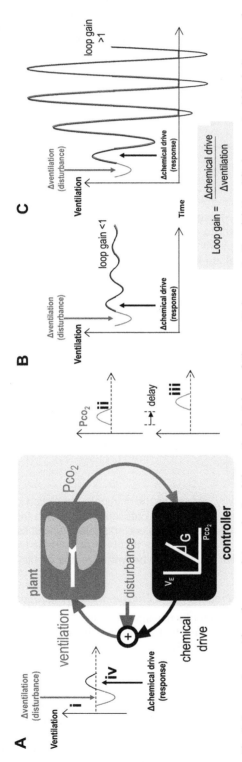

Fig. 3. Loop gain provides a framework to understand the pathophysiology of Cheyne–Stokes respiration. (A) Simplified conceptual block diagram of the respiratory control system. A disturbance to this system (*i*, hypoventilation) temporarily increases alveolar and arterial CO_2 (P_{CO_2}) at the lungs (*ii*) as determined by the "plant." After a circulatory delay (*iii*), the controller perceives the blood gas change and increases its output to oppose the original disturbance (*iv*). Whether or not this oscillation grows and manifests CSR depends on the loop gain of the system. (B) If loop gain is less than 1.0, each response is smaller than the prior disturbance and transient disturbances are damped away. (C) If loop gain exceeds 1.0, each response is greater than the prior disturbance, and oscillations grow until Cheyne–Stokes respiration is established. P_{CO_2}, partial pressure of CO_2; V_E, minute ventilation during exercise.

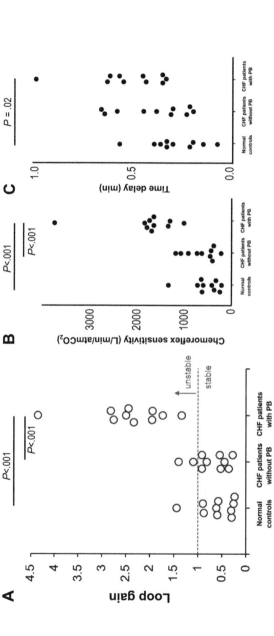

Fig. 4. Loop gain determines the presence or absence of Cheyne–Stokes respiration (periodic breathing [PBI]) during wakefulness. (A) Congestive heart failure (CHF) patients with PB had higher loop gain compared with CHF patients without PB and healthy controls. Increased loop gain in CHFPB was owing to elevated chemosensitivity (B) and increased circulatory delay (C). (*Data from* Francis DP, Willson K, Davies LC, et al. Quantitative general theory for periodic breathing in chronic heart failure and its clinical implications. Circulation 2000;102(18):2218; and Kee K, Sands SA, Edwards BA, et al. Positive airway pressure in congestive heart failure. Sleep Med Clin 2010;5:398.)

lung-to-ear circulation delay (approximating the lung-to-chemoreceptor delay) is equal to the delay between the nadir CO_2 level and apnea during CSR.[43] Raising cardiac output with exercise, pharmacologic intervention, or cardiac resynchronization can also reduce the ventilatory oscillations in CHF.[44–46] However, such interventions may also effect other factors (Equation 1) contributing to stabilization. Moreover, many CHF patients with low LVEF and increased circulatory delays do not have CSR.[35] Thus, the other factors identified in Equation 1 are likely important as well.

Chemosensitivity

Increased chemosensitivity (G) is the most powerful determinant of CSR.[35,47–49] Specifically, CHF–CSR severity is strongly associated with the dynamic ventilatory response to CO_2,[49] suggesting an essential role for elevated peripheral chemoreceptor (carotid bodies) activity in CSR. Increased chemosensitivity is thought to be owing to increased left atrial pressure (**Fig. 5**).[50] Additional evidence includes:

i. Increased pulmonary capillary wedge pressure (PCWP) is common in patients with CSR and is correlated with CSR severity.[42,46,50]
ii. CSR is associated with increased NT-proBNP levels,[10,51] a biomarker of left ventricular stretch and increased PCWP.[52–55]
iii. Left atrial size is associated with CSR and chemosensitivity.[56]
iv. PCWP is associated with hypocapnia,[57] a marker of increased chemosensitivity[58] and predictor of CSR.[12]
v. Raising left atrial pressure acutely increases chemosensitivity in dogs.[59]
vi. CSR is associated with cardiogenic pulmonary edema in the form of reduced pulmonary diffusing capacity,[60] presumably via increased pulmonary capillary pressure.
vii. CSR is linked with fluid status, including the degree of overnight rostral fluid shift.[61]
viii. The reduction in PCWP with vasodilator (nitroprusside) is linearly associated with the reduction in CSR.[46]

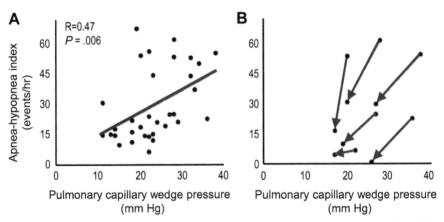

Fig. 5. Pulmonary capillary wedge pressure (PCWP) and Cheyne–Stokes respiration during sleep. (*A*) Correlation between the PCWP and Cheyne–Stokes respiration severity (apnea–hypopnea index). (*B*) Reducing PCWP with medical intervention for heart failure improves Cheyne–Stokes respiration. (*Adapted from* Solin P, Bergin P, Richardson M, et al. Influence of pulmonary capillary wedge pressure on central apnea in heart failure. Circulation 1999;99(12):1578; with permission.)

Increased left atrial pressure is believed to increase chemosensitivity directly via stretch receptors in the left atrium or pulmonary vein[31,62,63] and indirectly through pulmonary edema via juxtapulmonary capillary receptors (J receptors, pulmonary C fibers). It is important to note, however, that such vagal afferents may not explain entirely hypersensitive chemoreflexes in CHF–CSR, given that CSR has been seen to persist despite lung transplantation (and hence vagal denervation).[64] Other factors that may increase chemosensitivity include reduced cardiac output via reduced carotid arterial blood flow[65] and hypoxemia (via pulmonary congestion). Hypoxemia increases chemosensitivity both acutely and over time.[60,66] Indeed, recent evidence in rabbits suggests that afferent activity from carotid body glomus cells is increased in CHF, an effect which is unlikely to be related directly to cardiac pressures.[67]

Lung Volume

Reduced end-expiratory lung volume is another factor that can increase loop gain, destabilize breathing, and promote CSR.[35,36,68] End-expiratory lung volume is decreased in CHF as a result of lung edema and/or pleural effusions, cardiomegaly. Lowered lung volume acts to increase loop gain by lowering the lung gas volume for buffering ventilation-induced fluctuations in Pco_2 and Po_2.[36,68] Lowered end-expiratory lung volume, however, does not seem to differentiate between CHF patients and without CSR at baseline.[35] Nonetheless, manipulating lung volume can have an important effect on improving CSR.[36,68] Szollosi and colleagues[69] found that the lateral sleeping position attenuated the CSR severity (apnea–hypopnea index) by approximately 60% compared with the supine position. Importantly, the lateral position attenuates apnea-associated oxygen desaturation without affecting event duration. The decreased desaturation speed in lateral versus supine positions is consistent with the known increase in lung volume in the lateral position,[70] and provides indirect evidence that lung volume might be of major importance in the pathogenesis of CSR. Whether the lateral position affects other factors, including cardiac output or chemosensitivity in CHF patients, is currently unknown.

Behavioral State Effects

Behavioral state can also have a major effect on CSR severity. Although CSR can be observed during wakefulness, it is greatly exacerbated by the transition to sleep,[71] which may seem counterintuitive given the reduced chemosensitivity during sleep.[72–74] However, accompanying the transition from wake to sleep is an abrupt reduction in ventilatory drive (for any given $Paco_2$); likewise, accompanying the transition from sleep to wake (arousal) is an abrupt increase in ventilatory drive. Thus, any oscillation in ventilatory drive that is accompanied by transitions in state[75] is enhanced and hence ventilation is destabilized further.[76] CSR is most common in light non-REM sleep (stage 1) and is suppressed most powerfully in deep non-REM sleep (slow-wave sleep).[69,77] Deeper sleep presumably promotes stable breathing via increased arousal threshold (fewer arousals/awakenings) and reduced chemosensitivity compared with lighter sleep.[72–74] The observation that a sedative (zolpidem) can greatly improve CSR in patients without CHF[78] further highlights the importance of behavioral state on ventilatory instability. CSR is also reduced but not always absent in REM sleep,[36,69,77] whereas chemosensitivity is reduced in REM,[79] the arousal threshold is similar in REM to stage 1[80] and profound (non–CO_2-related) disturbances to ventilatory control are characteristic of this state. A final consideration is that sleep may promote CSR via the lowered end-expiratory lung volume that occurs with sleep onset.[81]

TREATMENT OF CHEYNE–STOKES RESPIRATION

In patients with CHF, untreated but not treated CSR is associated with increased mortality,[8,82,83] leading to the view that improving severe ventilatory oscillations of CSR may promote survival. Ongoing clinical trials are assessing whether CSR treatment improves mortality. In the meantime, clinicians treat symptomatic CSR to achieve improvements in quality of life, as well as nocturnal hypoxemia, sympathoexcitation, ventricular irritability, and for small improvements in cardiac function.[82,84–90] Although no such data exist for CSR in the ICU, we review the general treatment strategies in this article.

Treatment of Heart Failure

Based on the discussion so far, therapies for the treatment of CSR first focus on improving CHF. It is expected that treatments that improve cardiac output, decrease left atrial pressure, and improve lung volume should improve CSR. For example, intensive medical therapy that included diuretics and afterload reduction can successfully lower PCWP and improve CSR (see **Fig. 5**).[50] Similarly, β-blockers,[91–93] cardiac resynchronization therapy,[44,94] left ventricular assist devices[95] and transplantation[96–98] have been associated with improvements in CSR over time. Rapid changes in cardiac function, as might happen in the ICU, can quickly affect CSR severity. Kara and colleagues[99] have shown that there are acute improvements/worsening in the CSR with acute administration/withdrawal of cardiac resynchronization. Although CHF treatment can be effective at resolving CSR, in many patients CSR can persist despite the most aggressive therapies, including cardiac resynchronization therapy,[100] left ventricular assist devices,[101] and even heart transplantation.[96] Thus, additional treatments are needed for CSR.

Positive Airway Pressure

Positive airway pressure, whether applied as PEEP from a mechanical ventilator or in noninvasive form as continuous positive airway pressure (CPAP), has the potential to improve CSR acutely via multiple mechanisms:

i. Acutely increasing lung volume, which increases the gas volume for buffering ventilation-induced changes in P_{CO_2} and P_{O_2}.[36,68,102]
ii. Stabilization of the upper airway, which may play a covert role in CSR in some patients.[103]
iii. Improved hypoxemia that in turn reduces chemosensitivity, both acutely and further over time.[104,105] CPAP may improve oxygenation by improving microatelectasis in cardiogenic pulmonary edema.[106] CPAP also improves CSR-related desaturation independent of CSR resolution,[36] presumably via increased lung volume.
iv. Improved cardiac function by lowering cardiac preload and afterload. Such effects could theoretically increase cardiac output, decrease circulatory time, and lower PCWP (and chemosensitivity).[107] However, despite improvements in afterload, cardiac output and circulatory time do not typically change with CPAP.[26,84] Long-term CPAP can improve chemosensitivity over time.[84,89,104]

Although variability in the mechanism of action may help to explain the variable effect size of CPAP in CSR,[82,85] it is those with the most unstable breathing pattern (the greatest loop gain) that tend to respond insufficiently to CPAP.[36] The majority of CPAP-related suppression of CSR is immediate,[36,88] consistent with major effects of CPAP acting via increased lung volume[36,68,102] and relief of hypoxemia. Smaller additional suppression of CSR can be observed over time,[104] and are presumably via improvements in cardiac function. Such improvements in cardiac function are seen exclusively in those in whom CPAP improves CSR, and not in those in whom CPAP fails to resolve CSR nor in those with CHF but without CSR.[82,108] Given that CPAP is associated only with beneficial outcomes when CSR is suppressed, the early use of more aggressive therapy for CSR may be warranted.

Given the variable CSR response to CPAP, there has been increasing interested in bilevel positive airway pressure (PAP) and more advanced ventilation algorithms, such as adaptive-servo ventilation (ASV). Bilevel PAP offers the advantages of CPAP but, when used in a spontaneous/timed mode, can provide ventilation during periods of apnea. Importantly, bilevel PAP without any backup rate during periods of apnea may destabilize respiration further by augmenting hyperventilation (effectively raising chemosensitivity "G" in Equation 1), and can worsen central apneas during sleep.[109] When applied to patients with CSR, bilevel PAP (with a backup rate) can show small further improvements in the CSR severity over CPAP.[110] ASV also provides PEEP; however, the amount of inspiratory pressure varies dynamically to prevent hypopneas and maintain a constant minute ventilation. Inspiratory pressure increases as the patient's inspiratory effort decreases, but decreases as the patient augments their inspiratory effort. Preliminary data have been promising[83,100,111–119] and long-term outcome data are pending (NCT01128816 and NCT00733343).

Oxygen

Supplemental inspired oxygen therapy maintains arterial oxygenation during CSR, but can also resolve CSR effectively in many patients.[117,120–122] Relief of hypoxemia is expected to reduce chemosensitivity ("G" in Equation 1) and thereby reduce loop gain.[105] However, the effect of supplemental oxygen on CSR is heterogeneous (unlike the uniform resolution of CSR when oxygen is used for altitude-induced central sleep apnea), demonstrating that hypoxemia alone is not sufficient to explain CSR.

Medications

Ventilatory stimulants have also been used to improve CSR in CHF patients, including acetazolamide[71,87] and theophylline.[123] Stimulants act to lower $Paco_2$ (see Equation 1), which lowers plant gain and acts to stabilize breathing.[124] The administration of supplemental CO_2 has a similar effect on plant gain,[37] and can suppress CSR powerfully.[43,125] As yet, a long-term therapeutic benefit of stimulants for CHF–CSR has not yet been proven. Alternatively, the use of sedatives/hypnotics can improve CSR in patients without CHF[78]; the efficacy of this approach in heart failure patients is unknown. A mild dose of an opiate analgesic (eg, dihydrocodeine), as routinely administered in the ICU, can lower chemosensitivity and improve CSR and dyspnea during wakefulness[126,127]; however, improvements in CSR during sleep and long-term benefits have not been established. Judicious administration of medications on a case-by-case basis may be warranted to treat symptomatic CSR and associated sequelae in those who do not tolerate mask-pressure–based therapies.

Lung Volume Manipulation

One of the simplest yet underrecognized means to improve CSR is the manipulation of body position. Positional therapy via lateral positioning[69,77,128] and bed elevation[129] have potent effects on CSR severity. Given the low likelihood of "side effects," manipulating body position to treat CSR may yield improved outcomes (**Fig. 6**).

Novel and Future Therapies

Several new therapies are emerging for the treatment of CSR. Phrenic nerve stimulation, applied during the hypopnea phase of CSR, can resolve central events.[130,131] Dynamic CO_2 therapy, applied during the hyperventilation phase of CSR to prevent hypocapnia, can resolve CSR during wakefulness without considerably raising mean ventilation.[132,133] Finally, denervation of the carotid body chemoreceptors has been shown in animal studies to improve survival in CHF, and a case patient with CHF improved sleep disordered breathing, exercise capacity and quality of life.[134,135]

Box 4
Treatment of Cheyne–Stokes respiration

- Treat congestive heart failure
  - Improve cardiac function, left atrial pressure, and pulmonary congestion to decrease circulatory delay and decrease chemosensitivity
- Position patient to improve lung volumes
  - Lateral
  - Bed elevation
- PAP therapy
  - Continuous positive airway pressure
  - Bilevel positive airway pressure with backup rate
  - Adaptive servoventilation
- Supplemental oxygen therapy to reduce chemosensitivity
- Medication
  - Respiratory stimulants to lower CO_2
  - Sedatives to facilitate stable sleep
  - Low-dose opioids to reduce chemosensitivity

INTENSIVE CARE UNIT MANAGEMENT
General Considerations

Although data are not available, CSR is most likely to occur during the period of ventilator weaning. When sufficient clinical progress provides for reduced sedation, and a switch to a spontaneous mode of breathing, the underlying respiratory pattern will be revealed. Additionally, PEEP is frequently decreased as patients move toward liberation from mechanical ventilation. As PEEP is decreased, preload and afterload increase, which may tend to exacerbate CHF and CSR.

Recognition

The first step in the ICU management of CSR is recognition. Although apneas may be noted, especially by ventilator alarms, the initial management may be focused on (1) changing alarm settings to decrease alerts, or (2) changing ventilator modes from a spontaneous mode to an assist/control mode of ventilation. (An assist/control mode assists all spontaneous respiratory efforts, but in the absence of patient effort and apnea the ventilator controls minute ventilation by delivering a breath from the ventilator.) Alternatively, depending on the ventilator and alarm settings, some

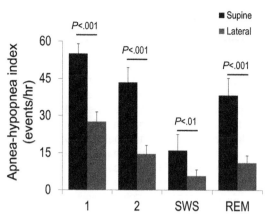

Fig. 6. Lateral position improves Cheyne–Stokes respiration in patients with heart failure in all sleep stages. Note also that Cheyne–Stokes respiration severity is mild in slow wave sleep (SWS) and most severe in stage 1 non-REM sleep. REM, rapid eye movement. (*Adapted from* Szollosi I, Roebuck T, Thompson B, et al. Lateral sleeping position reduces severity of central sleep apnea/Cheyne-Stokes respiration. Sleep 2006;29(8):1045–51; with permission.)

ventilators primarily alarm for a low minute ventilation (rather than apnea) when in a spontaneous mode of ventilation. The response may be to increase the amount of pressure support provided. As explained, this may paradoxically increase hyperventilation and further destabilize breathing.[136] Only with proper recognition can appropriate steps be taken to treat underlying heart failure, and manage the patient correctly. Respiratory therapists as well as physicians need to be familiar with the recognition of CSR.

Differential Diagnosis

For the patient not on mechanical ventilation, the differential for apnea includes obstructive sleep apnea. Although endotracheal intubation stents the upper airway open, patients on noninvasive positive pressure ventilation may still have upper airway obstruction if the airway pressure (expiratory positive airway pressure) is inadequate to hold open the upper airway. Obstructive sleep apnea is extremely common, and is likely as prevalent in patients with CHF as CSR. It too, may even more likely in the acutely decompensated patient as a result of excess edema fluid and narrowing of the pharyngeal airway.[137] Bedside evaluation of the sleeping patient should focus on signs of flow limitation, such as snoring, as well as evidence of ongoing respiratory effort during the apnea, such as paradoxic movement of the thorax and abdomen. CHF patients may have both obstructive and central sleep apnea, such that both upper airway and ventilator control require interventions.

Another important consideration is central sleep apnea owing to opioids, which are commonly used both for sedation while on mechanical ventilation, and for treatment of dyspnea in CHF.[138] Central sleep apnea owing to narcotics is generally believed to exhibit an ataxic, irregular pattern with reduced respiratory rate and occasional missed breaths.[139] However, many patients with narcotic-induced apneas exhibit a quasiperiodic or crescendo–decrescendo pattern similar to CSR (see **Fig. 6**).[140] The presence of CSR in the absence of hypocapnia may suggest opioid involvement.

Stroke (cerebral vascular accident) is another consideration. In fact, the patient described by Dr John Cheyne had both CHF and stroke.[141] CSR is seen in approximately 20% to 50% of patients recovering from recent stroke.[142-145] CSR is more common in patients with severe stroke, in those with concurrent CHF (low ejection fraction), and in those with longer hospital admissions.[143-145] The mechanisms of stroke-related CSR are not well-studied. Studies from more than 50 years ago illustrated that stroke, even in the absence of CHF, can cause an increase in chemosensitivity and CSR.[146,147] Likewise, more recent evidence suggests that CSR in stroke is caused by an increase in chemosensitivity (as indicated by observations of lower carbon dioxide) in stroke patients with CSR versus those without CSR.[143] The role of high chemosensitivity (and high loop gain) is confirmed further by the case observation that medical agents that stabilize breathing can ameliorate CSR.[148] Whether treating CSR has a beneficial effect on stroke outcomes remains unclear, but available observation data illustrate that stroke-related CSR and associated sleepiness can be managed effectively with ASV.[149] Thus, the new appearance of central sleep apnea in a patient with improving CHF should prompt a neurologic evaluation.

Treatment

As discussed, if possible, the best treatment includes further efforts at heart failure treatment, especially therapies designed to lower the left atrial/PCWP. Other medical therapies with respiratory stimulants may or may not be practical in critically ill patients.

Patient Positioning

Given the effects of lung volume on loop gain, proper patient positioning to maximize lung volumes may have an important clinical impact. Lung volumes are greater when sitting or lying lateral than when lying supine.[150] If possible, supine patients with CSR could be moved to a different position to improve lung volumes.

Ventilator Management

For patients with CSR manifest on a pressure support mode, it is worthwhile both diagnostically and therapeutically to decrease pressure support as much as possible to assess the underlying respiratory pattern. Again, a decrement in support may decrease apneic periods, which may be sufficiently brief (and without substantial oxygen desaturation) to consider moving toward liberation from the ventilator. The most robust stress test would be to monitor the patient in the absence of pressure support and PEEP, because this mimics the additional stress that the heart is under once liberated from mechanical ventilation. If prolonged apneas are noted, a spontaneous mode with a backup rate (eg, synchronized intermittent mandatory ventilation). Most modern ventilators can also provide ASV.

Noninvasive Positive Pressure Ventilation Management

Once extubated, the treatment algorithm may not be substantially different than the list in the discussion of Cheyne–Stokes respiration. Noninvasive positive pressure ventilation can be used to provide mechanical support to the left ventricle and limit CSR, especially during sleep. Again, CPAP, bilevel PAP with a backup rate, and ASV could all be tried. Such therapy may be necessary not only in the ICU but during the remainder of hospitalization and after discharge.

SUMMARY

There are few data about the prevalence of CSR owing to CHF in the ICU. Nevertheless, CSR is expected to be highly prevalent among those with CHF, and treatment should focus on the underlying mechanisms by which CHF increases loop gain and promotes unstable breathing. Several important questions await further study: Does earlier recognition of CSR facilitate ventilator management and ultimately hasten weaning from mechanical ventilation? Does treatment of CSR during acute illness facilitate faster recovery? The answers to these questions could substantially impact a large number of ICU patients.

REFERENCES

1. Ward M. Periodic respiration. A short historical note. Ann R Coll Surg Engl 1973; 52(5):330–4.
2. van de Borne P, Oren R, Abouassaly C, et al. Effect of Cheyne-Stokes respiration on muscle sympathetic nerve activity in severe congestive heart failure secondary to ischemic or idiopathic dilated cardiomyopathy. Am J Cardiol 1998;81(4): 432–6.
3. Trinder J, Merson R, Rosenberg JI, et al. Pathophysiological interactions of ventilation, arousals, and blood pressure oscillations during Cheyne-Stokes respiration in patients with heart failure. Am J Respir Crit Care Med 2000; 162(3 Pt 1):808–13.
4. Harrison TR, King CE, Calhoun JA, et al. Congestive heart failure: Xx. Cheyne-Stokes respiration as the cause of paroxysmal dyspnea at the onset of sleep. Arch Intern Med 1934;53(6):891–910.
5. Rees PJ, Clark TJ. Paroxysmal nocturnal dyspnoea and periodic respiration. Lancet 1979;2(8156–8157):1315–7.
6. Berry RB, Budhiraja R, Gottlieb DJ, et al. Rules for scoring respiratory events in sleep: update of the 2007 AASM manual for the scoring of sleep and associated events. Deliberations of the sleep apnea definitions task force of the American Academy of Sleep Medicine. J Clin Sleep Med 2012;8(5):597–619.
7. Lanfranchi PA, Braghiroli A, Bosimini E, et al. Prognostic value of nocturnal Cheyne-Stokes respiration in chronic heart failure. Circulation 1999;99(11): 1435–40.
8. Jilek C, Krenn M, Sebah D, et al. Prognostic impact of sleep disordered breathing and its treatment in heart failure: an observational study. Eur J Heart Fail 2010;13:68–75.
9. Yumino D, Wang H, Floras JS, et al. Relationship between sleep apnea and mortality in patients with ischemic heart failure. Heart 2009;95(10):819–24.
10. Amir O, Reisfeld D, Sberro H, et al. Implications of Cheyne-Stokes breathing in advanced systolic heart failure. Clin Cardiol 2010;33(3):E8–12.
11. Javaheri S, Parker TJ, Liming JD, et al. Sleep apnea in 81 ambulatory male patients with stable heart failure. Types and their prevalences, consequences, and presentations. Circulation 1998;97(21):2154–9.
12. Sin DD, Fitzgerald F, Parker JD, et al. Risk factors for central and obstructive sleep apnea in 450 men and women with congestive heart failure. Am J Respir Crit Care Med 1999;160(4):1101–6.
13. Tremel F, Pepin JL, Veale D, et al. High prevalence and persistence of sleep apnoea in patients referred for acute left ventricular failure and medically treated over 2 months. Eur Heart J 1999;20(16):1201–9.
14. Yumino D, Wang H, Floras JS, et al. Prevalence and physiological predictors of sleep apnea in patients with heart failure and systolic dysfunction. J Card Fail 2009;15(4):279–85.

15. Javaheri S. Sleep disorders in systolic heart failure: a prospective study of 100 male patients. The final report. Int J Cardiol 2006;106(1):21–8.
16. MacDonald M, Fang J, Pittman SD, et al. The current prevalence of sleep disordered breathing in congestive heart failure patients treated with beta-blockers. J Clin Sleep Med 2008;4(1):38–42.
17. Chan J, Sanderson J, Chan W, et al. Prevalence of sleep-disordered breathing in diastolic heart failure. Chest 1997;111(6):1488–93.
18. Lanfranchi PA, Somers VK, Braghiroli A, et al. Central sleep apnea in left ventricular dysfunction: prevalence and implications for arrhythmic risk. Circulation 2003;107(5):727–32.
19. Oldenburg O, Lamp B, Faber L, et al. Sleep-disordered breathing in patients with symptomatic heart failure: a contemporary study of prevalence in and characteristics of 700 patients. Eur J Heart Fail 2007;9(3):251–7.
20. Blackshear JL, Kaplan J, Thompson RC, et al. Nocturnal dyspnea and atrial fibrillation predict Cheyne-Stokes respirations in patients with congestive heart failure. Arch Intern Med 1995;155(12):1297–302.
21. Fang J, Mensah GA, Croft JB, et al. Heart failure-related hospitalization in the U.S., 1979 to 2004. J Am Coll Cardiol 2008;52(6):428–34.
22. Safavi KC, Dharmarajan K, Kim N, et al. Variation exists in rates of admission to intensive care units for heart failure patients across hospitals in the United States. Circulation 2013;127(8):923–9.
23. Hoffman R, Agatston A, Krieger B. Cheyne-Stokes respiration in patients recovering from acute cardiogenic pulmonary edema. Chest 1990;97(2):410–2.
24. Padeletti M, Green P, Mooney AM, et al. Sleep disordered breathing in patients with acutely decompensated heart failure. Sleep Med 2009;10(3):353–60.
25. Malhotra A, Owens RL. What is central sleep apnea? Respir Care 2010;55(9):1168–78.
26. Naughton MT, Rahman MA, Hara K, et al. Effect of continuous positive airway pressure on intrathoracic and left ventricular transmural pressures in patients with congestive heart failure. Circulation 1995;91(6):1725–31.
27. Adrian ED. Afferent impulses in the vagus and their effect on respiration. J Physiol 1933;79(3):332–58.
28. Hamilton RD, Winning AJ, Horner RL, et al. The effect of lung inflation on breathing in man during wakefulness and sleep. Respir Physiol 1988;73(2):145–54.
29. Hatridge J, Haji A, Perez-Padilla JR, et al. Rapid shallow breathing caused by pulmonary vascular congestion in cats. J Appl Physiol 1989;67(6):2257–64.
30. Lalani S, Remmers JE, MacKinnon Y, et al. Hypoxemia and low Crs in vagally denervated lambs result from reduced lung volume and not pulmonary edema. J Appl Physiol 2002;93(2):601–10.
31. Paintal AS. Mechanism of stimulation of type J pulmonary receptors. J Physiol 1969;203(3):511–32.
32. Khoo MC, Kronauer RE, Strohl KP, et al. Factors inducing periodic breathing in humans: a general model. J Appl Physiol 1982;53(3):644–59.
33. Edwards BA, Sands SA, Skuza EM, et al. Increased peripheral chemosensitivity via dopaminergic manipulation promotes respiratory instability in lambs. Respir Physiol Neurobiol 2008;164(3):419–28.
34. Wellman A, Jordan AS, Malhotra A, et al. Ventilatory control and airway anatomy in obstructive sleep apnea. Am J Respir Crit Care Med 2004;170(11):1225–32.
35. Francis DP, Willson K, Davies LC, et al. Quantitative general theory for periodic breathing in chronic heart failure and its clinical implications. Circulation 2000;102(18):2214–21.

36. Sands SA, Edwards BA, Kee K, et al. Loop gain as a means to predict a positive airway pressure suppression of Cheyne-Stokes respiration in patients with heart failure. Am J Respir Crit Care Med 2011;184(9):1067–75.
37. Sands SA, Edwards BA, Kee K, et al. Loop gain explains the resolution of Cheyne-Stokes respiration using inspired CO_2 in patients with heart failure [abstract]. Am J Respir Crit Care Med 2012;185:A6697.
38. Nugent ST, Finley JP. Periodic breathing in infants: a model study. IEEE Trans Biomed Eng 1987;34:482–5.
39. Wilkinson MH, Sia KL, Skuza EM, et al. Impact of changes in inspired oxygen and carbon dioxide on respiratory instability in the lamb. J Appl Physiol 2005; 98(2):437–46.
40. Carley DW, Shannon DC. A minimal mathematical model of human periodic breathing. J Appl Physiol 1988;65(3):1400–9.
41. Mortara A, Sleight P, Pinna GD, et al. Association between hemodynamic impairment and Cheyne-Stokes respiration and periodic breathing in chronic stable congestive heart failure secondary to ischemic or idiopathic dilated cardiomyopathy. Am J Cardiol 1999;84(8):900–4.
42. Oldenburg O, Bitter T, Wiemer M, et al. Pulmonary capillary wedge pressure and pulmonary arterial pressure in heart failure patients with sleep-disordered breathing. Sleep Med 2009;10(7):726–30.
43. Lorenzi-Filho G, Rankin F, Bies I, et al. Effects of inhaled carbon dioxide and oxygen on Cheyne-Stokes respiration in patients with heart failure. Am J Respir Crit Care Med 1999;159(5 Pt 1):1490–8.
44. Sinha AM, Skobel EC, Breithardt OA, et al. Cardiac resynchronization therapy improves central sleep apnea and Cheyne-Stokes respiration in patients with chronic heart failure. J Am Coll Cardiol 2004;44(1):68–71.
45. Murphy RM, Shah RV, Malhotra R, et al. Exercise oscillatory ventilation in systolic heart failure: an indicator of impaired hemodynamic response to exercise. Circulation 2011;124(13):1442–51.
46. Olson TP, Frantz RP, Snyder EM, et al. Effects of acute changes in pulmonary wedge pressure on periodic breathing at rest in heart failure patients. Am Heart J 2007;153(1):104.e1–7.
47. Topor ZL, Johannson L, Kasprzyk J, et al. Dynamic ventilatory response to CO(2) in congestive heart failure patients with and without central sleep apnea. J Appl Physiol 2001;91(1):408–16.
48. Javaheri S. A mechanism of central sleep apnea in patients with heart failure. N Engl J Med 1999;341(13):949–54.
49. Solin P, Roebuck T, Johns DP, et al. Peripheral and central ventilatory responses in central sleep apnea with and without congestive heart failure. Am J Respir Crit Care Med 2000;162(6):2194–200.
50. Solin P, Bergin P, Richardson M, et al. Influence of pulmonary capillary wedge pressure on central apnea in heart failure. Circulation 1999;99(12):1574–9.
51. Poletti R, Passino C, Giannoni A, et al. Risk factors and prognostic value of daytime Cheyne-Stokes respiration in chronic heart failure patients. Int J Cardiol 2009;137(1):47–53.
52. Speksnijder L, Rutten JH, van den Meiracker AH, et al. Amino-terminal pro-brain natriuretic peptide (NT-proBNP) is a biomarker of cardiac filling pressures in pre-eclampsia. Eur J Obstet Gynecol Reprod Biol 2010;153(1):12–5.
53. Tschope C, Kasner M, Westermann D, et al. Elevated NT-ProBNP levels in patients with increased left ventricular filling pressure during exercise despite preserved systolic function. J Card Fail 2005;11(5 Suppl):S28–33.

54. Knebel F, Schimke I, Pliet K, et al. NT-ProBNP in acute heart failure: correlation with invasively measured hemodynamic parameters during recompensation. J Card Fail 2005;11(5 Suppl):S38–41.

55. Pudil R, Tichy M, Praus R, et al. NT-proBNP and echocardiographic parameters in patients with acute heart failure. Acta Med 2007;50(1):51–6.

56. Calvin AD, Somers VK, Johnson BD, et al. Left atrial size, chemosensitivity, and central sleep apnea in heart failure. Chest 2014;146(1):96–103.

57. Lorenzi-Filho G, Azevedo ER, Parker JD, et al. Relationship of carbon dioxide tension in arterial blood to pulmonary wedge pressure in heart failure. Eur Respir J 2002;19(1):37–40.

58. Manisty CH, Willson K, Wensel R, et al. Development of respiratory control instability in heart failure: a novel approach to dissect the pathophysiological mechanisms. J Physiol 2006;577(Pt 1):387–401.

59. Chenuel BJ, Smith CA, Skatrud JB, et al. Increased propensity for apnea in response to acute elevations in left atrial pressure during sleep in the dog. J Appl Physiol 2006;101(1):76–83.

60. Szollosi I, Thompson BR, Krum H, et al. Impaired pulmonary diffusing capacity and hypoxia in heart failure correlates with central sleep apnea severity. Chest 2008;134(1):67–72.

61. Yumino D, Redolfi S, Ruttanaumpawan P, et al. Nocturnal rostral fluid shift: a unifying concept for the pathogenesis of obstructive and central sleep apnea in men with heart failure. Circulation 2010;121(14):1598–605.

62. Lloyd TC Jr. Breathing response to lung congestion with and without left heart distension. J Appl Physiol (1985) 1988;65(1):131–6.

63. Kappagoda CT, Ravi K. The rapidly adapting receptors in mammalian airways and their responses to changes in extravascular fluid volume. Exp Physiol 2006;91(4):647–54.

64. Solin P, Snell GI, Williams TJ, et al. Central sleep apnoea in congestive heart failure despite vagal denervation after bilateral lung transplantation. Eur Respir J 1998;12(2):495–8.

65. Ding Y, Li YL, Schultz HD. Role of blood flow in carotid body chemoreflex function in heart failure. J Physiol 2011;589(Pt 1):245–58.

66. Dempsey JA, Smith CA, Blain GM, et al. Role of central/peripheral chemoreceptors and their interdependence in the pathophysiology of sleep apnea. Adv Exp Med Biol 2012;758:343–9.

67. Schultz HD, Marcus NJ, Del Rio R. Mechanisms of carotid body chemoreflex dysfunction during heart failure. Exp Physiol 2015;100:124–9.

68. Edwards BA, Sands SA, Feeney C, et al. Continuous positive airway pressure reduces loop gain and resolves periodic central apneas in the lamb. Respir Physiol Neurobiol 2009;168(3):239–49.

69. Szollosi I, Roebuck T, Thompson B, et al. Lateral sleeping position reduces severity of central sleep apnea/Cheyne-Stokes respiration. Sleep 2006;29(8):1045–51.

70. Hurewitz AN, Susskind H, Harold WH. Obesity alters regional ventilation in lateral decubitus position. J Appl Physiol 1985;59(3):774–83.

71. Fontana M, Emdin M, Giannoni A, et al. Effect of acetazolamide on chemosensitivity, Cheyne-Stokes respiration, and response to effort in patients with heart failure. Am J Cardiol 2011;107(11):1675–80.

72. Douglas NJ, White DP, Weil JV, et al. Hypoxic ventilatory response decreases during sleep in normal men. Am Rev Respir Dis 1982;125(3):286–9.

73. Douglas NJ, White DP, Weil JV, et al. Hypercapnic ventilatory response in sleeping adults. Am Rev Respir Dis 1982;126(5):758–62.

74. White DP, Douglas NJ, Pickett CK, et al. Hypoxic ventilatory response during sleep in normal premenopausal women. Am Rev Respir Dis 1982;126(3): 530–3.

75. Domenico Pinna G, Robbi E, Pizza F, et al. Sleep-wake fluctuations and respiratory events during Cheyne-Stokes respiration in patients with heart failure. J Sleep Res 2014;23(3):347–57.

76. Khoo MC, Berry RB. Modeling the interaction between arousal and chemical drive in sleep-disordered breathing. Sleep 1996;19(10 Suppl):S167–9.

77. Sahlin C, Svanborg E, Stenlund H, et al. Cheyne-Stokes respiration and supine dependency. Eur Respir J 2005;25(5):829–33.

78. Quadri S, Drake C, Hudgel DW. Improvement of idiopathic central sleep apnea with zolpidem. J Clin Sleep Med 2009;5(2):122–9.

79. Hudgel DW, Martin RJ, Johnson B, et al. Mechanics of the respiratory system and breathing pattern during sleep in normal humans. J Appl Physiol 1984; 56(1):133–7.

80. Edwards BA, Eckert DJ, McSharry DG, et al. Clinical predictors of the respiratory arousal threshold in patients with obstructive sleep apnea. Am J Respir Crit Care Med 2014;190(11):1293–300.

81. Ballard RD, Irvin CG, Martin RJ, et al. Influence of sleep on lung volume in asthmatic patients and normal subjects. J Appl Physiol 1990;68(5):2034–41.

82. Arzt M, Floras JS, Logan AG, et al. Suppression of central sleep apnea by continuous positive airway pressure and transplant-free survival in heart failure: a post hoc analysis of the Canadian Continuous Positive Airway Pressure for Patients with Central Sleep Apnea and Heart Failure Trial (CANPAP). Circulation 2007;115(25):3173–80.

83. Oldenburg O, Bitter T, Wellmann B, et al. Reduced mortality in heart failure patients with nocturnal Cheyne-Stokes respiration receiving adaptive servoventilation therapy. J Am Coll Cardiol 2013;61(10_S).

84. Naughton MT, Benard DC, Rutherford R, et al. Effect of continuous positive airway pressure on central sleep apnea and nocturnal PCO2 in heart failure. Am J Respir Crit Care Med 1994;150(6 Pt 1):1598–604.

85. Naughton MT, Liu PP, Bernard DC, et al. Treatment of congestive heart failure and Cheyne-Stokes respiration during sleep by continuous positive airway pressure. Am J Respir Crit Care Med 1995;151(1):92–7.

86. Bradley TD, Logan AG, Kimoff RJ, et al. Continuous positive airway pressure for central sleep apnea and heart failure. N Engl J Med 2005;353(19): 2025–33.

87. Javaheri S. Acetazolamide improves central sleep apnea in heart failure: a double-blind, prospective study. Am J Respir Crit Care Med 2006;173(2):234–7.

88. Javaheri S. Effects of continuous positive airway pressure on sleep apnea and ventricular irritability in patients with heart failure. Circulation 2000;101(4): 392–7.

89. Arzt M, Schulz M, Wensel R, et al. Nocturnal continuous positive airway pressure improves ventilatory efficiency during exercise in patients with chronic heart failure. Chest 2005;127(3):794–802.

90. Sharma BK, Bakker JP, McSharry DG, et al. Adaptive servoventilation for treatment of sleep-disordered breathing in heart failure: a systematic review and meta-analysis. Chest 2012;142(5):1211–21.

91. Tamura A, Kawano Y, Naono S, et al. Relationship between beta-blocker treatment and the severity of central sleep apnea in chronic heart failure. Chest 2007;131(1):130–5.

92. Kohnlein T, Welte T. Does beta-blocker treatment influence central sleep apnoea? Respir Med 2007;101(4):850–3.
93. Silva CP, Lorenzi-Filho G, Marcondes B, et al. Reduction of central sleep apnea in heart failure patients with beta-blockers therapy. Arq Bras Cardiol 2010;94(2): 223–9, 39–45, 6–32. [in Portuguese, Spanish].
94. Skobel EC, Sinha AM, Norra C, et al. Effect of cardiac resynchronization therapy on sleep quality, quality of life, and symptomatic depression in patients with chronic heart failure and Cheyne-Stokes respiration. Sleep Breath 2005;9(4): 159–66.
95. Vazir A, Hastings PC, Morrell MJ, et al. Resolution of central sleep apnoea following implantation of a left ventricular assist device. Int J Cardiol 2010; 138(3):317–9.
96. Mansfield DR, Solin P, Roebuck T, et al. The effect of successful heart transplant treatment of heart failure on central sleep apnea. Chest 2003;124(5):1675–81.
97. Braver HM, Brandes WC, Kubiet MA, et al. Effect of cardiac transplantation on Cheyne-Stokes respiration occurring during sleep. Am J Cardiol 1995;76(8): 632–4.
98. Thalhofer SA, Kiwus U, Dorow P. Influence of orthotopic heart transplantation on breathing pattern disorders in patients with dilated cardiomyopathy. Sleep Breath 2000;4(3):121–6.
99. Kara T, Novak M, Nykodym J, et al. Short-term effects of cardiac resynchronization therapy on sleep-disordered breathing in patients with systolic heart failure. Chest 2008;134(1):87–93.
100. Miyata M, Yoshihisa A, Suzuki S, et al. Adaptive servo ventilation improves Cheyne-Stokes respiration, cardiac function, and prognosis in chronic heart failure patients with cardiac resynchronization therapy. J Cardiol 2012;60(3):222–7.
101. Padeletti M, Henriquez A, Mancini DM, et al. Persistence of Cheyne-Stokes breathing after left ventricular assist device implantation in patients with acutely decompensated end-stage heart failure. J Heart Lung Transpl 2007;26(7): 742–4.
102. Krachman SL, Crocetti J, Berger TJ, et al. Effects of nasal continuous positive airway pressure on oxygen body stores in patients with Cheyne-Stokes respiration and congestive heart failure. Chest 2003;123(1):59–66.
103. Jobin V, Rigau J, Beauregard J, et al. Evaluation of upper airway patency during Cheyne-Stokes breathing in heart failure patients. Eur Respir J 2012;40(6): 1523–30.
104. Arzt M, Schulz M, Schroll S, et al. Time course of continuous positive airway pressure effects on central sleep apnoea in patients with chronic heart failure. J Sleep Res 2009;18(1):20–5.
105. Lloyd BB, Jukes MG, Cunningham DJ. The relation between alveolar oxygen pressure and the respiratory response to carbon dioxide in man. Q J Exp Physiol Cogn Med Sci 1958;43(2):214–27.
106. Lenique F, Habis M, Lofaso F, et al. Ventilatory and hemodynamic effects of continuous positive airway pressure in left heart failure. Am J Respir Crit Care Med 1997;155(2):500–5.
107. Bradley TD, Holloway RM, McLaughlin PR, et al. Cardiac output response to continuous positive airway pressure in congestive heart failure. Am Rev Respir Dis 1992;145(2 Pt 1):377–82.
108. Sin DD, Logan AG, Fitzgerald FS, et al. Effects of continuous positive airway pressure on cardiovascular outcomes in heart failure patients with and without Cheyne-Stokes respiration. Circulation 2000;102(1):61–6.

109. Johnson KG, Johnson DC. Bilevel positive airway pressure worsens central apneas during sleep. Chest 2005;128(4):2141-50.
110. Kohnlein T, Welte T, Tan LB, et al. Assisted ventilation for heart failure patients with Cheyne-Stokes respiration. Eur Respir J 2002;20(4):934-41.
111. Oldenburg O, Schmidt A, Lamp B, et al. Adaptive servoventilation improves cardiac function in patients with chronic heart failure and Cheyne-Stokes respiration. Eur J Heart Fail 2008;10(6):581-6.
112. Pepperell JC, Maskell NA, Jones DR, et al. A randomized controlled trial of adaptive ventilation for Cheyne-Stokes breathing in heart failure. Am J Respir Crit Care Med 2003;168(9):1109-14.
113. Philippe C, Stoica-Herman M, Drouot X, et al. Compliance with and effectiveness of adaptive servoventilation versus continuous positive airway pressure in the treatment of Cheyne-Stokes respiration in heart failure over a six month period. Heart 2006;92(3):337-42.
114. Szollosi I, O'Driscoll DM, Dayer MJ, et al. Adaptive servo-ventilation and dead space: effects on central sleep apnoea. J Sleep Res 2006;15(2):199-205.
115. Teschler H, Dohring J, Wang YM, et al. Adaptive pressure support servo-ventilation: a novel treatment for Cheyne-Stokes respiration in heart failure. Am J Respir Crit Care Med 2001;164(4):614-9.
116. Owada T, Yoshihisa A, Yamauchi H, et al. Adaptive servoventilation improves cardiorenal function and prognosis in heart failure patients with chronic kidney disease and sleep-disordered breathing. J Card Fail 2013;19(4):225-32.
117. Yoshihisa A, Suzuki S, Miyata M, et al. A single night' beneficial effects of adaptive servo-ventilation on cardiac overload, sympathetic nervous activity, and myocardial damage in patients with chronic heart failure and sleep-disordered breathing. Circ J 2012;76(9):2153-8.
118. Haruki N, Takeuchi M, Kaku K, et al. Comparison of acute and chronic impact of adaptive servo-ventilation on left chamber geometry and function in patients with chronic heart failure. Eur J Heart Fail 2011;13(10):1140-6.
119. Kasai T, Usui Y, Yoshioka T, et al. Effect of flow-triggered adaptive servo-ventilation compared with continuous positive airway pressure in patients with chronic heart failure with coexisting obstructive sleep apnea and Cheyne-Stokes respiration. Circ Heart Fail 2010;3(1):140-8.
120. Javaheri S, Ahmed M, Parker TJ, et al. Effects of nasal O2 on sleep-related disordered breathing in ambulatory patients with stable heart failure. Sleep 1999;22(8):1101-6.
121. Hanly PJ, Millar TW, Steljes DG, et al. The effect of oxygen on respiration and sleep in patients with congestive heart failure. Ann Intern Med 1989;111(10):777-82.
122. Krachman SL, D'Alonzo GE, Berger TJ, et al. Comparison of oxygen therapy with nasal continuous positive airway pressure on Cheyne-Stokes respiration during sleep in congestive heart failure. Chest 1999;116(6):1550-7.
123. Javaheri S, Parker TJ, Wexler L, et al. Effect of theophylline on sleep-disordered breathing in heart failure. N Engl J Med 1996;335(8):562-7.
124. Edwards BA, Sands SA, Eckert DJ, et al. Acetazolamide improves loop gain but not the other physiological traits causing obstructive sleep apnoea. J Physiol 2012;590(Pt 5):1199-211.
125. Leung RS, Diep TM, Bowman ME, et al. Provocation of ventricular ectopy by Cheyne-Stokes respiration in patients with heart failure. Sleep 2004;27(7):1337-43.
126. Ponikowski P, Anker SD, Chua TP, et al. Oscillatory breathing patterns during wakefulness in patients with chronic heart failure: clinical implications and

role of augmented peripheral chemosensitivity. Circulation 1999;100(24): 2418–24.

127. Chua TP, Harrington D, Ponikowski P, et al. Effects of dihydrocodeine on chemosensitivity and exercise tolerance in patients with chronic heart failure. J Am Coll Cardiol 1997;29(1):147–52.

128. Zaharna M, Rama A, Chan R, et al. A case of positional central sleep apnea. J Clin Sleep Med 2013;9(3):265–8.

129. Soll BA, Yeo KK, Davis JW, et al. The effect of posture on Cheyne-Stokes respirations and hemodynamics in patients with heart failure. Sleep 2009;32(11):1499–506.

130. Zhang XL, Ding N, Wang H, et al. Transvenous phrenic nerve stimulation in patients with Cheyne-Stokes respiration and congestive heart failure: a safety and proof-of-concept study. Chest 2012;142(4):927–34.

131. Ponikowski P, Javaheri S, Michalkiewicz D, et al. Transvenous phrenic nerve stimulation for the treatment of central sleep apnoea in heart failure. Eur Heart J 2012;33(7):889–94.

132. Giannoni A, Baruah R, Willson K, et al. Real-time dynamic carbon dioxide administration: a novel treatment strategy for stabilization of periodic breathing with potential application to central sleep apnea. J Am Coll Cardiol 2010;56(22):1832–7.

133. Mebrate Y, Willson K, Manisty CH, et al. Dynamic CO2 therapy in periodic breathing: a modeling study to determine optimal timing and dosage regimes. J Appl Physiol 2009;107(3):696–706.

134. Marcus NJ, Del Rio R, Schultz EP, et al. Carotid body denervation improves autonomic and cardiac function and attenuates disordered breathing in congestive heart failure. J Physiol 2014;592(Pt 2):391–408.

135. Niewinski P, Janczak D, Rucinski A, et al. Carotid body removal for treatment of chronic systolic heart failure. Int J Cardiol 2013;168(3):2506–9.

136. Meza S, Mendez M, Ostrowski M, et al. Susceptibility to periodic breathing with assisted ventilation during sleep in normal subjects. J Appl Physiol 1998;85(5): 1929–40.

137. White LH, Bradley TD. Role of nocturnal rostral fluid shift in the pathogenesis of obstructive and central sleep apnoea. J Physiol 2013;591(Pt 5):1179–93.

138. Mogri M, Khan MI, Grant BJ, et al. Central sleep apnea induced by acute ingestion of opioids. Chest 2008;133(6):1484–8.

139. Walker JM, Farney RJ, Rhondeau SM, et al. Chronic opioid use is a risk factor for the development of central sleep apnea and ataxic breathing. J Clin Sleep Med 2007;3(5):455–61.

140. Wang D, Teichtahl H, Drummer O, et al. Central sleep apnea in stable methadone maintenance treatment patients. Chest 2005;128(3):1348–56.

141. Cheyne J. A case of apoplexy, in which the fleshy part of the heart was converted into fat. Dublin Hosp Rep 1818;12:216–22. Cardiac Classics 1941. p. 317–20 [reprint].

142. Nachtmann A, Siebler M, Rose G, et al. Cheyne-Stokes respiration in ischemic stroke. Neurology 1995;45(4):820–1.

143. Nopmaneejumruslers C, Kaneko Y, Hajek V, et al. Cheyne-Stokes respiration in stroke: relationship to hypocapnia and occult cardiac dysfunction. Am J Respir Crit Care Med 2005;171(9):1048–52.

144. Bonnin-Vilaplana M, Arboix A, Parra O, et al. Cheyne-Stokes respiration in patients with first-ever lacunar stroke. Sleep Disord 2012;2012:257890.

145. Siccoli MM, Valko PO, Hermann DM, et al. Central periodic breathing during sleep in 74 patients with acute ischemic stroke - neurogenic and cardiogenic factors. J Neurol 2008;255(11):1687–92.

146. Brown HW, Plum F. The neurologic basis of Cheyne-Stokes respiration. Am J Med 1961;30(6):849–60.
147. Heyman A, Birchfield RI, Sieker HO. Effects of bilateral cerebral infarction on respiratory center sensitivity. Neurology 1958;8(9):694–700.
148. Garcia-Pachon E. Severe Cheyne-Stokes respiration in an awake patient after stroke. Internet J Pulm Med 2006;7(1).
149. Brill AK, Rosti R, Hefti JP, et al. Adaptive servo-ventilation as treatment of persistent central sleep apnea in post-acute ischemic stroke patients. Sleep Med 2014;15(11):1309–13.
150. Watson RA, Pride NB. Postural changes in lung volumes and respiratory resistance in subjects with obesity. J Appl Physiol 2005;98(2):512–7.

Perioperative Issues and Sleep-Disordered Breathing

Karen L. Wood, MD*, Beth Y. Besecker, MD

KEYWORDS

- Obstructive sleep apnea • Perioperative • Anesthesia • Sleep-disordered breathing

KEY POINTS

- Patients undergoing surgery have higher rates of obstructive sleep apnea (OSA) than those in the general population.
- Many different preoperative screening questionnaires have been developed to assess patient risk for OSA but the STOP/STOP-Bang is typically the easiest to administer.
- In patients with known or suspected OSA, providers must weigh the risks and benefits of all medications given in the pre-, peri-, and postoperative settings. Sedative and opioid medications must be used cautiously in patients with known or suspected OSA.
- The guidelines for monitoring/management of surgical patients with known or suspected OSA are not well defined and more studies are needed to facilitate standard recommendations.
- The combination of a preoperative screening questionnaire for OSA in addition to assessment of postanesthesia care unit (PACU) events (eg, desaturations) may provide a reliable evaluation for those at risk of postoperative complications.

OSA is a condition of repetitive upper airway obstruction during sleep. The prevalence of OSA has been reported as low as 3% to 7% in men and 2% to 5% in women and as high as 28% in the general population.[1,2] Factors that increase the risk of OSA include age, male gender, obesity, family history, menopause, craniofacial abnormalities, cigarette smoking, and alcohol use.[1] In surgical patients and certain subsets of the population, the incidence has been estimated as higher.

Perioperative management of patients with OSA is an important aspect of critical care medicine. Complications that can develop postoperatively include respiratory failure, hypoxemia, and cardiac arrhythmias; these complications can lead to ICU

Disclosure Statement: All of the authors report no financial conflicts of interest in relation to the completion of this article.

Department of Internal Medicine, Division of Pulmonary, Allergy, Critical Care, and Sleep Medicine, The Wexner Medical Center at The Ohio State University, Columbus, OH, USA

* Corresponding author. 201 Davis Heart and Lung Institute, 473 West 12th Avenue, Columbus, OH 43210.

E-mail address: Karen.Wood@osumc.edu

Crit Care Clin 31 (2015) 497–510

http://dx.doi.org/10.1016/j.ccc.2015.03.008   criticalcare.theclinics.com admission. In addition, the question often arises as to which patients with known or suspected OSA should be routinely monitored in an ICU after surgery. Anesthesiologists have screening tools that may suggest OSA before surgery, but guidelines also address intraoperative and postoperative monitoring, analgesia, positioning, and use of continuous oximetry. Several studies have examined procedures, including endoscopy and sedation (eg, conscious sedation), in ambulatory settings. These issues are applicable to intensivists who frequently encounter procedural sedation in nonintubated patients with known or high risk of OSA. This review examines the preoperative screening and peri/postoperative management of patients with OSA or at high risk of OSA.

OBSTRUCTIVE SLEEP APNEA PREVALENCE IN SURGICAL PATIENTS

This variability is based on the overall prevalence of OSA in the general surgical population is estimated as higher than for the general population; however, there is a wide range in the literature. This is based on evaluation of different surgical populations as well as various screening techniques. In one retrospective, matched cohort study of 1255 patients undergoing total joint arthroplasty, 109 patients were found to have OSA, using 3 screening questionnaires, for a rate of OSA of 8.8%.[3] This study did not, however, validate the rate of OSA with a sleep study and 2 of the questions used were designed to pick up diagnosed OSA. Therefore, the incidence of OSA likely would have been higher using a more sensitive and validated screening questionnaire; most other studies have found the majority of OSA in this population is undiagnosed. Most other studies have shown much higher rates of OSA in the surgical population. One recent study looked at OSA in general surgery patients using the STOP-Bang and of 367 patients who did the STOP-Bang, 237 patients (64.6%) were classified as high risk of OSA on the questionnaire. Forty-nine of the patients had a polysomnogram (PSG) and, in those patients, 39 had OSA (10.6%).[4] Another study using a screening questionnaire found that 23.7% of participants screened as high risk for OSA in adult surgical patients in an academic medical center; using portable sleep studies, 82% of these patients had OSA.[5] Overall, these investigators estimated that approximately 33% of their population had OSA. Another study in Canada showed the rate of moderate to severe OSA in surgical populations as high as 38%.[6]

Furthermore, many surgical subgroups have a higher prevalence of OSA than the general surgical population. In patients with oropharyngeal cancer, the risk is likely higher than the general surgical population and is associated with an increased risk of postoperative complications.[7] In morbidly obese patients undergoing bariatric surgery, the prevalence may be as high as 44% to 78%.[8–10]

RISKS OF ELECTIVE SURGERY IN OBSTRUCTIVE SLEEP APNEA PATIENTS

Although not all studies have correlated OSA with risk for surgical complications, OSA has been found associated with an increased risk of postoperative respiratory complications (hypoxemia requiring prolonged oxygen therapy), cardiac complications (shock and cardiac arrest), neurologic complications (delirium, agitation, confusion, and drowsiness), unplanned ICU transfer, and longer hospital stay.[11,12] Reintubation rates, however, have not been shown to significantly increase in patients with OSA.[11]

Most practitioners believe OSA is a risk factor for complications. A recent survey of 783 United States practitioners in anesthesiology, general surgery, primary care, and sleep medicine revealed that 94% of those surveyed thought OSA was a risk factor for perioperative complications and the majority thought it was a moderate or major risk factor. Approximately half of the respondents had noticed a patient with an adverse outcome, but only approximately a quarter reported their hospital had a written policy for perioperative care of OSA patients.[13] One of the largest studies examined data from the National (Nationwide) Inpatient Sample database and reviewed more than 1 million elective surgeries between 2004 and 2008. In this cohort, sleep-disordered breathing (SDB) was independently associated with an increased odds ratio of post-operative complications, including emergent intubation and mechanical ventilation, noninvasive ventilation, and atrial fibrillation. Increased complications occurred in 4 subgroups of surgery: orthopedic, prostate, abdominal, and cardiovascular. There was not an increased risk of mortality and the association with length of stay (LOS) was mixed.[14] One study found that diagnosing OSA prior to surgery decreased the risk of cardiac complications (eg, shock and cardiac arrest) postoperatively but did not decrease the risk for respiratory complications.[15] There is discrepancy in results between studies that have tried to determine whether severity of OSA, defined by apnea-hypopnea index (AHI), correlates with postoperative complications and at this time there does not seem to be a consensus. Patient age, comorbidities, and type of surgery may contribute to postoperative risk and confound the evaluation.[15] There is also discrepancy as to whether use of PAP for diagnosed OSA prior to surgery reduces postoperative complication rates or LOS.[16,17] One group has shown, however, that diagnosing severe OSA and prescribing continuous positive airway pressure (CPAP) reduce postoperative cardiovascular complications.[15]

PREOPERATIVE ASSESSMENT
Screening

The American Society of Anesthesiologists (ASA) recommends screening prior to sur-gery to identify those patients who have sleep apnea. These guidelines recommend preoperative evaluation based on clinical criteria, including medical records review, patient symptoms, screening questionnaires, physical examination, and sleep study review. The 2006 ASA guidelines have an example of a screening questionnaire for OSA in adults, which is broken down into 3 sections. The first section assesses clinical signs, such as weight, neck circumference, craniofacial abnormalities, nasal obstruc-tion, and tonsils; the second section assesses symptoms, including snoring (loud or frequent), apneas, choking, and arousals; and the third section evaluates somnolence, including frequent somnolence or fatigue and falling asleep in a nonstimulating environment.[18]

Other commonly used screening tools include the STOP and STOP-Bang, and Berlin Questionnaire scores; the 4-Variable Screening tool; and the Epworth Sleepiness Scale (ESS).[18–23] The STOP and STOP-Bang were developed and validated in surgical pop-ulations.[21] These instruments consist of a 4-question assessment (STOP), which in-cludes history or symptoms of snoring, being tired, observed apneas, and history of high blood pressure, followed by a 4-question objective assessment that includes body mass index (BMI), age, neck circumference, and gender (**Box 1**). The Berlin Ques-tionnaire is an 11-question tool divided into 3 sections about snoring, fatigue, and high blood pressure. The 4-Variable tool gives points based on gender, BMI, blood pressure, and snoring. The ESS is an 8-question assessment of sleepiness. Of all of these ques-tionnaires, the easiest to administer and to score is the STOP/STOP-Bang.

In the Sleep Heart Health Study, investigators compared several of the tools and found the STOP-Bang to have the highest sensitivity for identifying moderate to severe and se-vere OSA.[24] The Berlin Questionnaire has also been shown to predict OSA in a preop-erative setting but the STOP-Bang may be easier to use.[25] On the STOP-Bang questionnaire, more than 3 positive questions are associated with high risk of OSA.

Box 1
Updated STOP-Bang questionnaire

Yes No Snoring?
○   ○   Do you **Snore Loudly** (loud enough to be heard through closed doors or your bed-partner elbows you for snoring at night)?

Yes No Tired?
○   ○   Do you often feel **Tired, Fatigued, or Sleepy** during the daytime (such as falling asleep during driving)?

Yes No Observed?
○   ○   Has anyone **Observed** you **Stop Breathing** or **Choking/Gasping** during your sleep?

Yes No Pressure?
○   ○   Do you have or are being treated for **High Blood Pressure**?

Yes No Body Mass Index more than 35 kg/m^2?
○   ○

Yes No Age older than 50 y old?
○   ○

Yes No Neck size large? (Measured around Adams apple)
○   ○   For male, is your shirt collar 17 inches/43 cm or larger?
         For female, is your shirt collar 16 inches/41 cm or larger?

Yes No Gender = Male?
○   ○

Scoring Criteria:

For general population

Low risk of OSA: Yes to 0–2 questions

Intermediate risk of OSA: Yes to 3–4 questions

High risk of OSA: Yes to 5–8 questions; or Yes to 2 or more of 4 STOP questions + male gender; or Yes to 2 or more of 4 STOP questions + BMI > 35 kg/m^2; or Yes to 2 or more of 4 STOP questions + neck circumference (17"/43 cm in male, 16"/41 cm in female)

Property of University Health Network. For personal use only, please contact for other uses. www.stopbang.ca. *Modified from* Chung F et al. Anesthesiology 2008;108:812–21, Chung F et al. Br J Anaesth 2012;108:768–75, Chung F et al. J Clin Sleep Med Sept 2014. Used with permission.

Recently, however, the investigators of the STOP-Bang re-evaluated outcomes using a higher score ($\geq$5) and found improved odds ratio and specificity.[26] They recommend using the lower cutoff in a patient population with a high probability of OSA (because a lower cutoff is good for ruling out OSA in that group) but increasing the scoring cutoff to greater than or equal to 5 for the general population. A recent study comparing the Berlin and STOP-Bang confirmed this finding of high sensitivity but low specificity of the STOP-Bang using the 3-question cutoff in a cardiac and abdominal surgery cohort.[27] A large Veteran's Affairs study using home sleep studies also found that with 3 positive questions on STOP-Bang there was a good sensitivity but poor specificity (almost all of their patients had 2 questions positive, however—age and male, so when they went up to 5 questions, they had similar results).[28] The investigators of the STOP-Bang have proposed another method of increasing the specificity of the screening tool, which is to combine the score with the serum bicarbonate level greater than 28.[29]

The STOP questionnaire has been shown to predict postoperative atelectasis.[30] The STOP-Bang has been shown to predict increased postoperative complications.[31,32] Higher preoperative STOP-Bang scores also predicted a higher odds ratio of ICU admission postoperatively. This study was in more than 5000 patients with an overall postoperative ICU admission rate of 6.2%. The odds ratio increased to greater than 5 when the STOP-Bang had greater than or equal to 5 positive responses.[33] This study did not, however, address how many of these were planned ICU admissions simply because of the higher STOP-Bang score.[34] The STOP-Bang has also been shown to predict difficult airway patients.[35] With the publication of more recent studies, separate ambulatory guidelines were written in 2012 that differ from the ASA guidelines by recommending the STOP-Bang as a screening tool.[36]

Besides screening questionnaires, overnight oximetry is often used as a screening test for OSA in clinical practice. A few studies have used this instead of screening questionnaires to determine risk of OSA. One study did screening overnight oximetry on 172 patients. Those with an oxygen desaturation index (ODI) (number of oxygen desaturation [>4%] events per hour of monitoring) of more than 5 (5 events of desaturation per hour) had a higher rate of postoperative complications, including respiratory and cardiac.[37] Another study compared overnight oximetry with home sleep testing in 68 bariatric surgery patients and found that an ODI greater than or equal to 3% had a negative predictive value of 95% to rule out OSA (using AHI of 10) and a positive predictive value of 73%.[9] There are several clinical prediction scores available, but recently a neural network prediction tool, the OSUNet, was developed, which outperformed the STOP-Bang as a prediction tool for moderate OSA. It includes age, history of hypertension, history of diabetes mellitus, BMT, neck circumference, and 4 questions that are asked of patients and graded on a 6-item Likert scale. Although its sensitivity was lower than the STOP-Bang or the modified neck circumference prediction tool, the specificity was higher and the positive predictive value and positive likelihood ratio made it a helpful test for predicting moderate OSA.[38]

Further Testing/Preoperative Continuous Positive Airway Pressure

One area of preoperative screening remains uncertain—If a patient is found at elevated risk of having moderate to severe OSA, should further testing be done prior to the surgery? This may include overnight oximetry, home sleep testing, and overnight in-laboratory PSG. The ASA guidelines recommend using a sleep study if available to stratify the risk based on AHI. If no sleep study is available, however, the guidelines recommend empiric treatment of those at high risk for OSA for purposes of perioperative and postoperative management. One recent study found a prevalence of 5.2% of surgical patients screened positive as "at risk" for OSA and most of this group was divided (463 patients) into those put on OSA protocol for the surgery and those who had formal PSG. There was no difference in postoperative complications or differences in LOS or ICU admissions based on having a PSG before surgery.[39]

In summary, there are many questionnaires available to screen for OSA, and at this time the STOP-Bang has the most evidence and recommendations supporting its use. It may be best to use different levels of cutoff depending on the risk of OSA in the population; however, further studies are needed. If patients screen positive for OSA, they can be cared for in the perioperative period with a presumptive diagnosis of OSA. They should then follow-up after surgery for a formal sleep study and diagnosis.

INTRAOPERATIVE/PERIOPERATIVE

Although morbid obesity and elevated Mallampati score (used to predict the ease of intubation) are risks for difficult intubation, OSA has been reported by some to be an independent risk factor for difficult intubation. At least 1 study of 180 morbidly obese patients, however, found that OSA was not a risk factor.[40] Whether it is the OSA, obesity, or difficult airway assessment that is the risk factor, patients with OSA or presumptive OSA should be intubated and monitored with extra caution before, during, and after anesthesia. Some techniques that reduce the pharyngeal closing pressure and improve intubation success in OSA patients include adequate preoxygenation (and denitrogenation), sniffing position, neck extension, mandibular advancement (with 2-handed mask ventilation), and sitting position. Capnography during mask ventilation may be a good marker for adequate ventilation.[41]

The finding of OSA affects intraoperative medication and anesthesia choice as well as recovery from sedation, position of extubation, and recovery.[18] Induction of anesthesia is thought possibly more difficult in patients with OSA. Eikermann and colleagues[42] did not find lower oxygen levels during induction, but theirs was a small study and the anesthesiologists may have treated the OSA patients differently. Using neuraxial anesthesia, intraoperative bilevel positive airway pressure (PAP), and pain control with epidural infusion of local anesthetic may all be options to help with difficult cases.[43]

One study in 73 bariatric surgery patients examined the effects of dexmedetomidine infusion started before the end of the case and discontinued in the PACU. These patients had fewer narcotic medications given during the hospital stay and were discharged sooner.[44] Although this study was not looking at OSA, there is a high prevalence (up to 78%) of OSA in the bariatric surgery population.[10]

After surgery, the recommended criteria for extubation include patients should be following commands, performing a sustained head lift greater than 5 seconds, a vital capacity greater than 15 mL/kg, a negative inspiratory force less than −25 cm H_2O, and a minimum spontaneous respiratory rate of 12 breaths per minute. After extubation, patients should be positioned in a 30° reverse Trendelenburg position to minimize compression of the abdomen against the diaphragm and facilitate effective ventilation mechanics.[45]

POSTOPERATIVE MANAGEMENT

There are many factors to consider in the postoperative period in patients diagnosed with or presumed to have OSA based on their preoperative screening assessment.

Medications

In the immediate postoperative period, the effects of sedative, analgesic (specifically opioids), and anesthetic agents can worsen OSA. Mechanisms associated with this worsening include reduced pharyngeal tone and arousal responses to hypoxia, hypercarbia, and obstruction and increased upper airway resistance.[46,47] Therefore, avoidance of systemic opioids and sedatives is preferred. Concerns regarding peri/postoperative narcotic use must be balanced, however, with the need for adequate pain control. Pain control is essential to allow patients to participate in deep breathing and coughing strategies postoperatively and prevent the development of atelectasis/pneumonia. If opioids are used, expert opinion regarding the risks of a basal opioid infusion is equivocal.[18]

In general, the strategy is to minimize agents that can worsen apnea and use alternatives where appropriate and available. For example, the risk-benefit of using neuraxial analgesia that includes an opioid medication compared with a local anesthetic agent alone must be weighed.[18] At least 2 studies have demonstrated, however, that epidural or intrathecal techniques using morphine can be safely used in OSA patients with appropriate monitoring—use was reported in obese surgical patients managed with thoracic, patient-controlled epidural analgesia[48] and intrathecal narcotics in patients with total joint arthroplasty,[3] respectively. Alternative medications, such as nonsteroidal antiinflammatory drugs (NSAIDs) and acetaminophen, should be used as appropriate to minimize the use of narcotics. Less frequently used analgesics, such as

α_2-agonists, have also been used and may improve long-term outcomes, such as mortality.[49] The α_2-agonists have been shown to decrease postoperative opioid use and side effects and lessen pain.[50,51] Lastly, nonpharmacologic strategies, such as transcutaneous electrical nerve stimulation (TENS), which may have analgesic properties similar to opioids without respiratory effects, should be considered.

Monitoring

Data suggest that a majority of postoperative complications occur within the first 24 hours after surgery. There are no specific guidelines as to the duration, location, or type of monitoring that should occur peri/postoperatively. Perhaps this is because the degree of monitoring required may correlate with the severity of a patient's OSA, the risk of the procedure (higher risk for thoracic/abdominal surgery), and the amount of postoperative narcotic used. A recent Cochrane review showed no improvement in perioperative outcomes using routine pulse oximetry monitoring.[52] Most expert opinion, however, supports the use of continuous oximetry as a strategy to reduce complications for patients in whom there is a concern for or a diagnosis of OSA.[18]

Other protocols cited in the literature include telemetry for 24 hours postoperative, head of bed (HOB) elevation greater than or equal to 30° as able, and/or capnography. There have been some concerns raised about the accuracy of capnography, but Kasuya and colleagues[53] report that mainstream capnography with an oral guide nasal cannula performed well even in patients with obesity and/or OSA and better than sidestream capnography; and it has been shown to improve postoperative outcomes when patient-controlled analgesia is administered.[54] In a protocol by Karan and colleagues,[55] ODI was suggested in patients receiving narcotics with escalation to CPAP if needed. This approach is supported by the finding that PACU respiratory events, including an elevated ODI, are independent predictors of postoperative respiratory complications.[56]

Management

The literature supports the use of supplemental oxygen after extubation to maintain appropriate oxygen saturation, but the efficacy of noninvasive positive pressure ventilation (NIPPV) in the postoperative setting, especially in those not previously treated, is less clear.[18] Expert recommendations have ranged from using PAP in the PACU (may use patient's own mask/machine if available), especially if opioids have been given,[57,58] to using autotitrating PAP devices. One study found that autotitrating PAP can reduce postoperative AHI but compliance in this setting may be poor,[59] and additional studies are needed to assess the impact of autotitrating CPAP on postoperative cardiopulmonary complications. The supine position should be avoided and use of nasopharyngeal airways may also be of some benefit in patients with respiratory complications who cannot tolerate PAP. Postoperative management recommendations from several experts are summarized in **Box 2**.

Complications

Complications related to OSA later (within the first 72 hours) in the postoperative period are thought secondary to rapid eye movement sleep rebound (after suppression from anesthesia and opioids). Chung has reported a higher AHI and ODI for OSA patients on the third postoperative night compared with the preoperative or first postoperative night, which is likely related to this phenomenon.[60] There was no significant correlation between the opioid requirements and severity of SDB in OSA patients evaluated. In addition, opioids have been shown to induce central respiratory depression through μ- and κ-opioid receptors and also to "inhibit central tonic outflow to the primary upper airway dilator, the genioglossus muscle."[61,62]

Box 2
Postoperative management of suspected or confirmed obstructive sleep apnea

- Consider hospital admission for continuous cardiorespiratory monitoring for 24 hours or until oxygen saturation is at baseline.[45]
- Titrate supplemental oxygen to maintain oxygen saturation greater than 90% or patient's baseline during sleep.[18,45]
- Minimize use of systemic opioid analgesics and sedatives[18] and use alternative pharmacologic (ie, NSAIDS, ketamine, and tramadol) and nonpharmacologic (ie, ice and TENS) as appropriate[45]; regional analgesics are preferred over systemic administration.[18]
- Use NIPPV in the postoperative period in patients previously treated; consider using a patient's own mask/equipment.[18]
- Avoid the supine position[18]; elevate HOB greater than 30°–40° if no contraindications.[45]
- Consider continuous capnography monitoring to identify hypoventilation and early intervention (especially in patients who are/have received opioids).[45]

Disposition After Surgery

Few institutions have a formal policy for admission/discharge of postoperative patients with known or suspected OSA.[63] For patients who are admitted, standards of care for the type of unit and degree of monitoring are also lacking. In lieu of specific standards, practitioners report that postoperative disposition is based on many patient factors, including severity of OSA, type of surgery, age, comorbidities, type of anesthesia used, presence of PACU events, and need for postoperative medications (especially narcotics). One study's investigators looked at a change in their facility to limit postoperative laporascopic gastric bypass ICU admissions to only patients with BMI greater than 60 and severe OSA, and there were no differences or increase in complications or length of hospital stay.[64] After bariatric surgery, up to 25% of patients may need ICU care and the need is higher in those with a BMI greater than 60 and those with complications requiring reoperation. OSA and other pulmonary comorbidities may have played a role in extended mechanical ventilation but this was not significant in multivariate logistic regression.[65] Another study found that after bariatric surgery, 8% of patients were admitted to the ICU with a majority of those planned admissions.[66] In a study by Gali and colleagues,[56] the combination of preoperative screening with PACU evaluation predicted postoperative complications. Specifically, they looked at PACU events (3 episodes of bradypnea of <8 respirations per minute, 1 apnea of ≥10 seconds, 3 episodes of desaturation to <90%, or a pain sedation mismatch using the Richmond Agitation-Sedation Scale and pain scale scores) and if these events recurred over 90 minutes of evaluation. They found a high score (combining the preoperative screening and the PACU events) was associated with increased perioperative respiratory events, such as ICU admission for respiratory reasons, intensive respiratory therapy, and noninvasive ventilator support. This kind of prediction tool could be helpful in stratifying the need for higher level of monitoring postanesthesia. Implementing a protocol for post-PACU care should be considered at individual institutions.

SPECIAL GROUPS
Children

The prevalence of OSA in the pediatric population is 1% to 4%.[67] Unlike in the adult population, however, a diagnosis of SDB in children is often made by clinical assessment (including evaluation for adenotonsillar hypertrophy) as opposed to PSG studies. The management of SDB in the pediatric population often involves adenotonsillectomy (AT). AT is typically performed in the outpatient setting, but in pediatric patients with complicated medical histories/comorbidities, including obesity and/or OSA, consideration should be given to inpatient postoperative management. A study from Baugh and colleagues[67] support inpatient management, at least overnight, of children with medical comorbidities and those less than 3 years of age with PSG-proved OSA because they report an increased risk of postoperative respiratory complications in these groups.

Because an increased risk for respiratory complications (oxygen desaturations, apnea, and hypercarbia) may alter the postoperative management of these children, it is important to identify these patients prior to surgery. The literature for preoperative SDB screening tools in the pediatric populations is less well described than in adults. The sleep-related breathing disorder scale, a subscale of the pediatric sleep questionnaire, is a well-accepted pediatric OSA questionnaire, with 85% sensitivity and 81% specificity for the diagnosis of OSA.[21,68] It is a detailed questionnaire (22 items), however, and is not ideal for preoperative screening. Shorter, more user-friendly questionnaires are being developed, such as the I'M SLEEPY questionnaire (**Box 3**), which seems most accurate when completed by a child's parent or guardian (sensitivity 82% and specificity 50%).[68] As of the writing of this review, however, the questionnaire has not been validated as a preoperative screening tool.

A relationship between OSA and peri/postoperative complications has not been demonstrated in all studies and seems to depend on the type of surgery and age group evaluated. Additional predictors of postoperative complications in children, however, have been identified and include age less than 2 years, AHI greater than 24, intraoperative laryngospasm requiring treatment, oxygen saturations less than 90% on room air in the PACU, and PACU stay greater than 100 minutes.[69] As with adult cohorts, it is unclear if children should be observed on the pediatric floor or a monitored-step down unit or if they are better served in the pediatric ICU (PICU). A recent study by Theilhaber and colleagues[70] attempted to provide some additional insight. Their study found that children without a PACU event, after prolonged PACU monitoring (2 hours), were unlikely to later develop an adverse event and in those patients routine postoperative PICU care could likely be avoided.

Box 3
I'M SLEEPY (parental questionnaire)

I—Is your child often irritated or angry during the day?

M—BMI greater than 85%

S—Does your child usually snore?

L—Does your child sometimes have labored breathing at night?

E—Ever noticed a stop in your child's breathing at night?

E—Does your child have enlarged tonsils and/or adenoids?

P—Does your child have problems with concentration?

Y—Does your child often yawn or is often tired/sleepy during the day?

A child at high risk for OSA was defined as a child with a score of greater than 3.

Adapted from Kadmon G, Chung SA, Shapiro CM. I'M SLEEPY: a short pediatric sleep apnea questionnaire. Int J Pediatr Otorhinolaryngol 2014;78(12):2119; with permission.

In patients with OSA, it is important to be cognizant of the medication used in the preoperative setting because medications, such as benzodiazepines, barbiturates, propofol, and opioids, can persist into the recovery period and contribute to airway collapse and respiratory depression.[71] Anesthetic agents, such as ketamine and dexmedetomidine, may be less likely to contribute to airway obstruction and, thus, postoperative complications. The use of ketamine may help preserve pharyngeal muscle tone and airway reflexes.[72] In the peri/postoperative period, opioid-sparing anesthetic and analgesic approaches should be used, including regional anesthesia (local infiltration, peripheral nerve blocks, and central neuraxial blocks)[73] and acetaminophen and/or NSAIDs as appropriate. These strategies help avoid opioid-associated respiratory depression and sedation. Use of tramadol in children with OSA undergoing AT has been associated with fewer desaturation episodes in the perioperative period.[74] If opioid drugs are used, continuous monitoring with pulse oximetry is recommended. Other options to assess for respiratory complications in the pediatric population include the use of transthoracic impedance and nasal capnography.[73]

Pregnancy

Elevating HOB to 45° can improve AHI in pregnancy-associated SDB and may be a helpful management strategy in these women in the postoperative setting.[75]

Endoscopy

Performing endoscopic procedures on patients with OSA presents some unique challenges. First there is concern that patients with OSA are more sensitive to the effects of sedation and anesthesia compared with unaffected controls,[76] which can result in a more collapsible upper airway. Second, several endoscopic procedures require that the upper airway space be shared with the procedural scope. ASA guidelines from 2006[18] recommend general anesthesia with a secure airway over deep sedation. Despite the theoretic concerns of increased risk for complications in patients with sleep apnea, however, conscious sedation for endoscopy procedures has not clearly demonstrated an increased risk for cardiorespiratory complications.[77] This finding suggests that sleep apnea patients can undergo routine endoscopic procedures safely with standard monitoring procedures.

SUMMARY

SDB has an increased prevalence in surgical patients compared with the general population and in some surgical subgroups the frequency can be high. The true risk of postoperative complications in patients with OSA has not been clearly defined despite multiple studies and meta-analysis to assess this risk. Ongoing evaluation to identify which patient groups with OSA are at the greatest risk of peri/postoperative complications is important because this is a patient population that can have serious yet preventable complications. SDB in the perioperative setting remains an important area of investigation as medical providers strive to provide the best medical care possible to each and every patient.

REFERENCES

1. Punjabi NM. The epidemiology of adult obstructive sleep apnea. Proc Am Thorac Soc 2008;5(2):136–43.
2. Lyons PG, Mokhlesi B. Diagnosis and management of obstructive sleep apnea in the perioperative setting. Semin Respir Crit Care Med 2014;35(5):571–81.

3. Berend KR, Ajluni AF, Nunez-Garcia LA, et al. Prevalence and management of obstructive sleep apnea in patients undergoing total joint arthroplasty. J Arthroplasty 2010;25(6 Suppl):54–7.

4. Kulkarni GV, Horst A, Eberhardt JM, et al. Obstructive sleep apnea in general surgery patients: is it more common than we think? Am J Surg 2014;207(3):436–40 [discussion: 439–40].

5. Finkel KJ, Searleman AC, Tymkew H, et al. Prevalence of undiagnosed obstructive sleep apnea among adult surgical patients in an academic medical center. Sleep Med 2009;10(7):753–8.

6. Singh M, Liao P, Kobah S, et al. Proportion of surgical patients with undiagnosed obstructive sleep apnoea. Br J Anaesth 2013;110(4):629–36.

7. Payne RJ, Hier MP, Kost KM, et al. High prevalence of obstructive sleep apnea among patients with head and neck cancer. J Otolaryngol 2005;34(5):304–11.

8. Kolotkin RL, LaMonte MJ, Walker JM, et al. Predicting sleep apnea in bariatric surgery patients. Surg Obes Relat Dis 2011;7(5):605–10.

9. Malbois M, Giusti V, Suter M, et al. Oximetry alone versus portable polygraphy for sleep apnea screening before bariatric surgery. Obes Surg 2010;20(3):326–31.

10. Lopez PP, Stefan B, Schulman CI, et al. Prevalence of sleep apnea in morbidly obese patients who presented for weight loss surgery evaluation: more evidence for routine screening for obstructive sleep apnea before weight loss surgery. Am Surg 2008;74(9):834–8.

11. Gaddam S, Gunukula SK, Mador MJ. Post-operative outcomes in adult obstructive sleep apnea patients undergoing non-upper airway surgery: a systematic review and meta-analysis. Sleep Breath 2014;18(3):615–33.

12. Kaw R, Pasupuleti V, Walker E, et al. Postoperative complications in patients with obstructive sleep apnea. Chest 2012;141(2):436–41.

13. Auckley D, Cox R, Bolden N, et al. Attitudes regarding perioperative care of patients with OSA: a survey study of four specialties in the United States. Sleep Breath 2015;19(1):315–25.

14. Mokhlesi B, Hovda MD, Vekhter B, et al. Sleep-disordered breathing and postoperative outcomes after elective surgery: analysis of the nationwide inpatient sample. Chest 2013;144(3):903–14.

15. Mutter TC, Chateau D, Moffatt M, et al. A matched cohort study of postoperative outcomes in obstructive sleep apnea: could preoperative diagnosis and treatment prevent complications? Anesthesiology 2014;121(4):707–18.

16. Mador MJ, Goplani S, Gottumukkala VA, et al. Postoperative complications in obstructive sleep apnea. Sleep Breath 2013;17(2):727–34.

17. Liao P, Yegneswaran B, Vairavanathan S, et al. Postoperative complications in patients with obstructive sleep apnea: a retrospective matched cohort study. Can J Anaesth 2009;56(11):819–28.

18. Gross JB, Bachenberg KL, Benumof JL, et al. Practice guidelines for the perioperative management of patients with obstructive sleep apnea: a report by the American Society of Anesthesiologists Task Force on Perioperative Management of patients with obstructive sleep apnea. Anesthesiology 2006;104(5):1081–93 [quiz: 1117–8].

19. Johns MW. Reliability and factor analysis of the Epworth Sleepiness Scale. Sleep 1992;15(4):376–81.

20. Johns MW. A new method for measuring daytime sleepiness: the Epworth sleepiness scale. Sleep 1991;14(6):540–5.

21. Chung F, Yegneswaran B, Liao P, et al. STOP questionnaire: a tool to screen patients for obstructive sleep apnea. Anesthesiology 2008;108(5):812–21.

22. Takegami M, Hayashino Y, Chin K, et al. Simple four-variable screening tool for identification of patients with sleep-disordered breathing. Sleep 2009;32(7): 939–48.

23. Netzer NC, Stoohs RA, Netzer CM, et al. Using the Berlin Questionnaire to identify patients at risk for the sleep apnea syndrome. Ann Intern Med 1999;131(7): 485–91.

24. Silva GE, Vana KD, Goodwin JL, et al. Identification of patients with sleep disordered breathing: comparing the four-variable screening tool, STOP, STOP-Bang, and Epworth Sleepiness Scales. J Clin Sleep Med 2011;7(5):467–72.

25. Chung F, Yegneswaran B, Liao P, et al. Validation of the Berlin questionnaire and American Society of Anesthesiologists checklist as screening tools for obstructive sleep apnea in surgical patients. Anesthesiology 2008;108(5):822–30.

26. Chung F, Subramanyam R, Liao P, et al. High STOP-Bang score indicates a high probability of obstructive sleep apnoea. Br J Anaesth 2012;108(5):768–75.

27. Nunes FS, Danzi-Soares NJ, Genta PR, et al. Critical evaluation of screening questionnaires for obstructive sleep apnea in patients undergoing coronary artery bypass grafting and abdominal surgery. Sleep Breath 2015;19(1):115–22.

28. Kunisaki KM, Brown KE, Fabbrini AE, et al. STOP-BANG questionnaire performance in a Veterans Affairs unattended sleep study program. Ann Am Thorac Soc 2014;11(2):192–7.

29. Chung F, Chau E, Yang Y, et al. Serum bicarbonate level improves specificity of STOP-Bang screening for obstructive sleep apnea. Chest 2013;143(5):1284–93.

30. Ursavas A, Guven T, Coskun F, et al. Association between self reported snoring, STOP questionnaire and postoperative pulmonary complications in patients submitted to ortophaedic surgery. Multidiscip Respir Med 2013;8(1):3.

31. Vasu TS, Doghramji K, Cavallazzi R, et al. Obstructive sleep apnea syndrome and postoperative complications: clinical use of the STOP-BANG questionnaire. Arch Otolaryngol Head Neck Surg 2010;136(10):1020–4.

32. Proczko MA, Stepaniak PS, de Quelerij M, et al. STOP-Bang and the effect on patient outcome and length of hospital stay when patients are not using continuous positive airway pressure. J Anesth 2014;28(6):891–7.

33. Chia P, Seet E, Macachor JD, et al. The association of pre-operative STOP-BANG scores with postoperative critical care admission. Anaesthesia 2013;68(9):950–2.

34. Corso RM, Cattano D. Does STOP-BANG really predict postoperative critical care admission? Anaesthesia 2013;68(11):1200.

35. Toshniwal G, McKelvey GM, Wang H. STOP-Bang and prediction of difficult airway in obese patients. J Clin Anesth 2014;26(5):360–7.

36. Joshi GP, Ankichetty SP, Gan TJ, et al. Society for Ambulatory Anesthesia consensus statement on preoperative selection of adult patients with obstructive sleep apnea scheduled for ambulatory surgery. Anesth Analg 2012;115(5):1060–8.

37. Hwang D, Shakir N, Limann B, et al. Association of sleep-disordered breathing with postoperative complications. Chest 2008;133(5):1128–34.

38. Teferra RA, Grant BJ, Mindel JW, et al. Cost minimization using an artificial neural network sleep apnea prediction tool for sleep studies. Ann Am Thorac Soc 2014; 11(7):1064–74.

39. Chong CT, Tey J, Leow SL, et al. Management plan to reduce risks in perioperative care of patients with obstructive sleep apnoea averts the need for presurgical polysomnography. Ann Acad Med Singapore 2013;42(3):110–9.

40. Neligan PJ, Porter S, Max B, et al. Obstructive sleep apnea is not a risk factor for difficult intubation in morbidly obese patients. Anesth Analg 2009;109(4): 1182–6.

41. Sato Y, Ikeda A, Ishikawa T, et al. How can we improve mask ventilation in patients with obstructive sleep apnea during anesthesia induction? J Anesth 2013;27(1):152–6.
42. Eikermann M, Garzon-Serrano J, Kwo J, et al. Do patients with obstructive sleep apnea have an increased risk of desaturation during induction of anesthesia for weight loss surgery? Open Respir Med J 2010;4:58–62.
43. Kapala M, Meterissian S, Schricker T. Neuraxial anesthesia and intraoperative bilevel positive airway pressure in a patient with severe chronic obstructive pulmonary disease and obstructive sleep apnea undergoing elective sigmoid resection. Reg Anesth Pain Med 2009;34(1):69–71.
44. Dholakia C, Beverstein G, Garren M, et al. The impact of perioperative dexmedetomidine infusion on postoperative narcotic use and duration of stay after laparoscopic bariatric surgery. J Gastrointest Surg 2007;11(11):1556–9.
45. Gammon BT, Ricker KF. An evidence-based checklist for the postoperative management of obstructive sleep apnea. J Perianesth Nurs 2012;27(5):316–22.
46. Boushra NN. Anaesthetic management of patients with sleep apnoea syndrome. Can J Anaesth 1996;43(6):599–616.
47. Loadsman JA, Hillman DR. Anaesthesia and sleep apnoea. Br J Anaesth 2001; 86(2):254–66.
48. Zotou A, Siampalioti A, Tagari P, et al. Does epidural morphine loading in addition to thoracic epidural analgesia benefit the postoperative management of morbidly obese patients undergoing open bariatric surgery? A pilot study. Obes Surg 2014;24(12):2099–108.
49. Porhomayon J, El-Solh A, Chhangani S, et al. The management of surgical patients with obstructive sleep apnea. Lung 2011;189(5):359–67.
50. Tan M, Law LS, Gan TJ. Optimizing pain management to facilitate Enhanced Recovery After Surgery pathways. Can J Anaesth 2014;62(2):203–18.
51. Blaudszun G, Lysakowski C, Elia N, et al. Effect of perioperative systemic alpha2 agonists on postoperative morphine consumption and pain intensity: systematic review and meta-analysis of randomized controlled trials. Anesthesiology 2012; 116(6):1312–22.
52. Pedersen T, Nicholson A, Hovhannisyan K, et al. Pulse oximetry for perioperative monitoring. Cochrane Database Syst Rev 2014;(3):CD002013.
53. Kasuya Y, Akca O, Sessler DI, et al. Accuracy of postoperative end-tidal Pco2 measurements with mainstream and sidestream capnography in non-obese patients and in obese patients with and without obstructive sleep apnea. Anesthesiology 2009;111(3):609–15.
54. McCarter T, Shaik Z, Scarfo K, et al. Capnography monitoring enhances safety of postoperative patient-controlled analgesia. Am Health Drug Benefits 2008;1(5):28–35.
55. Karan S, Black S, Mouton F. Perioperative Implementation of continuous positive airway pressure: a review of the considerations. Open Anesthesiol J 2011; 5(Supplement 1-M4):14–8.
56. Gali B, Whalen FX, Schroeder DR, et al. Identification of patients at risk for postoperative respiratory complications using a preoperative obstructive sleep apnea screening tool and postanesthesia care assessment. Anesthesiology 2009; 110(4):869–77.
57. Schumann R, Jones SB, Cooper B, et al. Update on best practice recommendations for anesthetic perioperative care and pain management in weight loss surgery, 2004–2007. Obesity 2009;17(5):889–94.
58. Alvarez A, Singh PM, Sinha AC. Postoperative analgesia in morbid obesity. Obes Surg 2014;24(4):652–9.

59. Liao P, Luo Q, Elsaid H, et al. Perioperative auto-titrated continuous positive airway pressure treatment in surgical patients with obstructive sleep apnea: a randomized controlled trial. Anesthesiology 2013;119(4):837–47.
60. Chung F, Liao P, Yegneswaran B, et al. Postoperative changes in sleep-disordered breathing and sleep architecture in patients with obstructive sleep apnea. Anesthesiology 2014;120(2):287–98.
61. Macintyre PE, Loadsman JA, Scott DA. Opioids, ventilation and acute pain management. Anaesth Intensive Care 2011;39(4):545–58.
62. Hajiha M, DuBord MA, Liu H, et al. Opioid receptor mechanisms at the hypoglossal motor pool and effects on tongue muscle activity in vivo. J Physiol 2009;587(Pt 11):2677–92.
63. Dhanda Patil R, Patil YJ. Perioperative management of obstructive sleep apnea: a survey of Veterans Affairs health care providers. Otolaryngol Head Neck Surg 2012;146(1):156–61.
64. El Shobary H, Backman S, Christou N, et al. Use of critical care resources after laparoscopic gastric bypass: effect on respiratory complications. Surg Obes Relat Dis 2008;4(6):698–702.
65. Helling TS, Willoughby TL, Maxfield DM, et al. Determinants of the need for intensive care and prolonged mechanical ventilation in patients undergoing bariatric surgery. Obes Surg 2004;14(8):1036–41.
66. van den Broek RJ, Buise MP, van Dielen FM, et al. Characteristics and outcome of patients admitted to the ICU following bariatric surgery. Obes Surg 2009;19(5): 560–4.
67. Baugh RF, Archer SM, Mitchell RB, et al. Clinical practice guideline: tonsillectomy in children. Otolaryngol Head Neck Surg 2011;144(1 Suppl):S1–30.
68. Kadmon G, Chung SA, Shapiro CM. I'M SLEEPY: a short pediatric sleep apnea questionnaire. Int J Pediatr Otorhinolaryngol 2014;78(12):2116–20.
69. Hill CA, Litvak A, Canapari C, et al. A pilot study to identify pre- and peri-operative risk factors for airway complications following adenotonsillectomy for treatment of severe pediatric OSA. Int J Pediatr Otorhinolaryngol 2011;75(11):1385–90.
70. Theilhaber M, Arachchi S, Armstrong DS, et al. Routine post-operative intensive care is not necessary for children with obstructive sleep apnea at high risk after adenotonsillectomy. Int J Pediatr Otorhinolaryngol 2014;78(5):744–7.
71. Connolly LA. Anesthetic management of obstructive sleep apnea patients. J Clin Anesth 1991;3(6):461–9.
72. Drummond GB. Comparison of sedation with midazolam and ketamine: effects on airway muscle activity. Br J Anaesth 1996;76(5):663–7.
73. Patino M, Sadhasivam S, Mahmoud M. Obstructive sleep apnoea in children: perioperative considerations. Br J Anaesth 2013;111(Suppl 1):i83–95.
74. Hullett BJ, Chambers NA, Pascoe EM, et al. Tramadol vs morphine during adenotonsillectomy for obstructive sleep apnea in children. Paediatr Anaesth 2006; 16(6):648–53.
75. Jung S, Zaremba S, Heisig A, et al. Elevated body position early after delivery increased airway size during wakefulness, and decreased apnea hypopnea index in a woman with pregnancy related sleep apnea. J Clin Sleep Med 2014; 10(7):815–7.
76. Chung SA, Yuan H, Chung F. A systemic review of obstructive sleep apnea and its implications for anesthesiologists. Anesth Analg 2008;107(5):1543–63.
77. Mador MJ, Abo Khamis M, Nag N, et al. Does sleep apnea increase the risk of cardiorespiratory complications during endoscopy procedures? Sleep Breath 2011;15(3):393–401.

Seizures in Sleep
Clinical Spectrum, Diagnostic Features, and Management

Dawn Eliashiv, MD[a], Alon Y. Avidan, MD, MPH[b],*

KEYWORDS

- Seizures • Epilepsy • Epilepsy syndrome • Antiepileptic drugs

KEY POINTS

- Epilepsy and antiepileptic agents influence sleep.
- Sleep, arousal, and sleep deprivation influence epilepsy.
- Sleep state modulates epileptic seizures and interictal epileptiform discharges.
- Hypersomnolence may be frequent among patients suffering from epilepsy.
- Successful amelioration of coexisting sleep disorders may improve seizure control.

INTRODUCTION: THE RELATIONSHIP BETWEEN SLEEP AND EPILEPSY

Sleep and epilepsy have a reciprocal relationship. Sleep can affect the distribution and frequency of epileptiform discharges, and epileptic discharges can change sleep regulation and provoke sleep disruption.[1] Patients with epilepsy frequently complain of symptoms such as hypersomnia, insomnia, and breakthrough seizures, which are owed to disturbed sleep.[2] These symptoms commonly indicate an underlying sleep disorder rather than the effect of epilepsy or medication on sleep. Clinicians must be able to identify and differentiate between potential sleep disorders related to epilepsy, and direct therapy to improve the patient's symptoms.[3] Sleep deprivation, which is a very common problem in the intensive care unit (ICU), is known to facilitate interictal discharges in patients with epilepsy with a more prominent increase noted in generalized-onset epilepsy.[4] Indeed a recent review by Foldvary-Schaefer and colleagues[5] demonstrates that total sleep deprivation activates interictal epileptiform discharges in 23% to 93% of patients with definite or suspected seizures.

Disclosures: Dr Eliashiv: UCB, Sunovion, Cyberonics; Dr Avidan: Xenoport, Merck.
[a] UCLA, Department of Neurology, UCLA Seizure Disorders Center, David Geffen School of Medicine at UCLA, 710 Westwood Boulevard, Room 1-250, RNRC, Los Angeles, CA 90095-1769, USA; [b] UCLA, Department of Neurology, UCLA Neurology Clinic, UCLA Sleep Disorders Center, David Geffen School of Medicine at UCLA, 710 Westwood Boulevard, Room 1-145, RNRC, Los Angeles, CA 90095-1769, USA
* Corresponding author.
E-mail address: avidan@mednet.ucla.edu

Crit Care Clin 31 (2015) 511–531
http://dx.doi.org/10.1016/j.ccc.2015.03.009
criticalcare.theclinics.com

Some antiseizure medications are associated with weight gain and increased body mass index (BMI). Increased BMI is associated with an increased risk of obstructive sleep apnea (OSA). In fact, up to one-third of patients with medically refractory epilepsy show evidence of OSA, and treatment of the underlying OSA may reduce seizure frequency.[6,7]

INTRODUCTION TO EPILEPSY

A seizure is an event characterized by excessive or hypersynchronized discharges of neurons. Epilepsy is defined as a disorder characterized by either 2 unprovoked seizures occurring during a time interval more than 24 hours apart or a 60% increased risk of recurrence after 1 unprovoked seizure.[8] During an epileptic spell, there are recurrent episodes of altered cerebral function associated with abnormal, excessive, paroxysmal, hypersynchronous discharge of cerebral neurons. The International League against Epilepsy (ILAE) has recently revised the seizure classification. Seizures are now classified as either focal or generalized.[9] **Box 1** depicts a seizure classification scheme according to the updated ILAE, which was designed to ensure that concepts and terminology are in place to reflect the advances in understanding and knowledge of these disorders.

EPIDEMIOLOGY OF EPILEPSY AND IMPACT ON SLEEP DISORDERS

According to the Institute of Medicine report in 2012, 2.2 million people in the United States are afflicted with epilepsy. The lifetime prevalence is 1 in 26 and 150,000 cases

---

Box 1
The classification of seizures

- Generalized seizures
  - Tonic-clonic
    - Absence
    - Typical
    - Atypical
    - Absence with special features
      - Myoclonic absence
      - Eyelid myoclonia
  - Myoclonic
    - Myoclonic
    - Myoclonic atonic
    - Myoclonic tonic
  - Clonic
  - Tonic
  - Atonic
- Focal seizures
- Unknown
  - Epileptic spasms

From Berg AT, Berkovic SF, Brodie MJ, et al. Revised terminology and concepts for organization of seizures and epilepsies: report of the ILAE Commission on Classification and Terminology, 2005–2009. Epilepsia 2010;51(4):676–85; with permission.

of epilepsy are diagnosed annually.[10] Approximately 1 in 10 individuals will have a seizure at some point in their lives. Approximately 25% to 35% of patients with epilepsy have seizures despite the use of antiepileptic drugs. Most patients with epilepsy (75%) have seizures while asleep and awake; 20% of patients with epilepsy have seizures solely while asleep. Xu and colleagues[11] surveyed 201 patients with focal seizures on at least 2 antiseizure drugs and reported that 34% had sleep disturbances and 10% had been prescribed sleep medications. Depression is a known comorbidity of epilepsy, which may occur in up to 50% of patients, and also can affect sleep patterns.[12]

THE EFFECTS OF SEIZURE DRUGS ON SLEEP ORGANIZATION AND ARCHITECTURE

Antiepileptic drugs (AEDs) may have a significant impact on sleep architecture and sleep disturbances, as summarized in **Table 1**.[13] The ICU attending physician, ICU trainees, and other health care providers need to be aware of the major side effects, as many can lead to sedation, insomnia, and predisposition for sleep disorders, whereas others may improve sleep quality.

Examples of the effects of AED on sleep are multiple. Barbiturates and benzodiazepines generally shorten sleep latency and reduce arousals from sleep. Benzodiazepines also decrease sleep latency and reduce slow-wave sleep (SWS; as demarcated by stage N3 non–rapid eye movement [REM] sleep).[14] Phenobarbital decreases the overall REM sleep percentage. Phenytoin increases the amount of non-REM sleep, decreases sleep efficiency, and reduces sleep latency.[15] Carbamazepine increases the number of sleep-stage shifts and decreases the amount of REM sleep.[16] Gabapentin has been shown to improve sleep efficiency, increase SWS, and increase REM sleep.[17,18] Similarly Bazil and colleagues[19,20] demonstrated that pregabalin increases SWS and improves daytime attention in patients with focal epilepsy and insomnia. Conversely Lacosamide is associated with insomnia. In clinical practice, understanding the unique effects of these AEDs may offer the clinician an opportunity to improve sleep and wakefulness; medications that improve sleep disorders may require tailored dosing schedules to maximize their benefit.[3] Foldvary and colleagues[21] found that lamotrigine decreased stage shifts and arousals and increased REM sleep, without affecting sleep efficiency and sleep latency or suppressing REM sleep. Insomnia has been reported in association with felbamate, lamotrigine,[21] and lacosamide.[19] Complaints of insomnia also have been reported to occur during withdrawal of antiepileptic medication.[22–24]

ELECTROPHYSIOLOGICAL CONSIDERATIONS IN THE DIAGNOSIS OF SEIZURE DISORDERS

Polysomnographic electroencephalogram (EEG) channels are often limited with some routine polysomnography (PSG) including only 2 channels, C3-A1 and C4-A2, as opposed to standard full EEG montage used during routine EEG and continuous EEG recordings (full 21-channel array). The limited polysomnographic montage may limit the ability to capture focal epileptiform activity. In one study comparing the ability of polysomnographers to correctly identify seizures by using 4, 7, and 18 channels of EEG at both 30-mm/s and 10-mm/s epochs, the yield was 70%, 74%, 81%, respectively.[25] Another study determined a significant increase in the ability to differentiate seizures from psychogenic nonepileptic seizures when 18-channel EEGs were used when compared with 8-channel EEG recordings.[26] It is therefore recommended that in patients with suspected epilepsy, a full EEG montage be

Table 1
Contribution of AED on sleep disorders and sleep architecture

AED	Sleep Disorders		Sleep Architecture	
	Positive Effects	Negative Effects	Positive Effects	Negative Effects
Phenobarbital	Insomnia	Obstructive sleep apnea	↓SL	↓REM
Benzodiazepines	Insomnia, Willis Ekbom disease, REM sleep disorder	Obstructive sleep apnea	↓SL, ↓arousals, ↓CAP rate	↓REM ↓N3
Carbamazepine	Willis Ekbom disease	None	None	↓REM, ↑Sleep stage shifts
Valproate	Willis Ekbom disease	Obstructive sleep apnea	Sometimes no effect	↑1N Reduction in REM
Gabapentin	Willis Ekbom disease, insomnia	Obstructive sleep apnea	↑N3, ↓arousals ↑sleep efficiency	None
Lamotrigine	Consolidating sleep reducing arousals stage shifts	Insomnia; REM sleep behavior disorder	↓Sleep stage shifts, ↓arousals, ↑REM	↓N3(possible)
Levetiracetam	Willis Ekbom disease (case reports)	Insomnia	↑N3 Stage shifts and wake after sleep onset were significantly decreased	None
Pregabalin	Willis Ekbom disease, insomnia, daytime attention	Obstructive sleep apnea	↑N3, ↑REM, ↓arousals	None
Topiramate	Weight loss, Obstructive sleep apnea	Willis Ekbom disease	No changes	No changes
Zonisamide	Obstructive sleep apnea	Willis Ekbom disease	No changes	No changes

Abbreviations: AED, anti epileptic drugs; CAP, cyclic alternating pattern (A marker of sleep insta-bility); N1, Stage 1 non-REM sleep; N3, Stage III or slow wave sleep (SWS); REM, rapid eye move-ment sleep; SL, sleep latency (timing from lights out to sleep onset); X, no/unknown effect; ↑, increased; ↓, decreased.

Adapted from Zucconi M, Maestri M. Sleep and epilepsy. In: Kryger M, Avidan AY, Berry R, editors. Atlas of clinical sleep medicine, 2nd edition. Philadelphia: Elsevier/Saunders; 2013; with permission.

used. This is especially true in patients with suspected nonconvulsive status epilep-ticus (NCSE), which refers to a prolonged seizure that manifests primarily as altered mental status as opposed to the dramatic convulsions classically seen in generalized tonic-clonic (GTC) status epilepticus.[27] Patients who present with NCSE, often pre-sent with confusion or behavioral abnormalities, suggesting the diagnosis of absence status epilepticus or complex partial status epilepticus.[27] The second type of NCSE (subtle status epilepticus [SSE]), is critical to evaluate and consider in comatose ICU patients who present after a prolonged GTC seizure (GTCS) and who may exhibit subtle motor manifestations of a seizure, such as hand or facial twitching, as the mortality associated with SSE can exceed 30% if the seizure duration is longer than 60 minutes.[27] In this setting, continuous EEG monitoring is very helpful when consciousness or alteration of alertness persist after initial treatment.[28]

In the setting of the ICU (and in the epilepsy monitoring unit), where continuous EEG monitoring is often used, dedicated respiratory channels monitoring for hypopnea, desaturations, and pulse oximetry are generally absent.[29] This shortcoming is of paramount importance, as seizures may be associated with sleep-disordered breathing.[29] Lately there has been an increased interest in SUDEP (sudden unexplained death in epilepsy) with a risk of 1% per decade in patients with uncontrolled epilepsy. Potential etiologic factors are postulated by some to cardiac arrhythmia, due to myocardial ischemia, electrolyte disturbances, arrhythmogenic medications, or transmission of the epileptic activity via the autonomic nervous system to the heart, and central or obstructive apnea (**Fig. 1**).[30,31] Lately, this has led some centers to routinely advocate adding respiratory channels and pulse oximetry when monitoring patients with suspected seizures in this setting.[29,32] Some have advocated the use of simultaneous video-PSG in the differentiation between parasomnias and seizures.[1] The 2005 American Academy of Sleep Medicine practice parameter advocates the use of video-EEG–PSG in atypical parasomnias and in paroxysmal disorders suspected of representing an ictal process, in situations in which the routine EEG is inconclusive.

Another challenge facing the sleep physician when evaluating sleep studies in the setting of the ICU is differentiating between epileptiform transients, benign normal variants, and external artifacts that may come from the monitoring environment

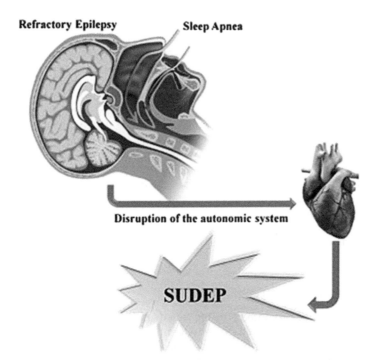

Fig. 1. SUDEP. The hypothesis that disruption of the autonomic system and SUDEP could be related to the occurrence of OSA in people with refractory epilepsy. (*From* Andersen ML, Tufik S, Cavalheiro EA, et al. Lights out! It is time for bed. Warning: obstructive sleep apnea increases risk of sudden death in people with epilepsy. Epilepsy Behav 2012;23(4):510–1.)

(respirators, 60 Hz, pumps, noise, from nursing activities, and other electrical devices). Epileptiform transients consist either of spikes with duration between 20 and 70 µs or sharp waves of 70 to 200 µs and distort the background activity. These patterns are often polyphasic, occurring at all stages of wakefulness and sleep and are followed by a slow wave. Benign variants are often biphasic, do not distort the background activity, are not followed by a slow wave after the spike-wave discharges, and occur predominantly during drowsiness.[33]

Common benign transients include positive occipital sharp transients of sleep (POSTS), Lambda waves, and rhythmic midtemporal theta bursts of drowsiness (RMTDs). POSTS are symmetric occipital surface *positive* transients with duration of 200 to 300 ms and an amplitude 20 to 50 µV (in comparison, epileptiform transients are typically surface *negative*). They are restricted to drowsiness and stage N2 sleep and do not persist typically beyond young adulthood. There is also no associated focal slowing of the background activity.[34]

Lambda waves are seen in association with saccadic eye movements during the wake state during visual exploration. These surface positive waves are biphasic, less than 50 µV in amplitude over the occipital regions, and may be sharply contoured. Eliminating the visual trigger by placing a white sheet of paper in front of the patient ameliorates this activity.[34] RMTDs are characterized by brief runs of sharply contoured theta that may be unilateral or asymmetric. This pattern is also restricted to drowsiness with a typical morphology, but may be mistaken for epileptiform activity.[35]

Recognition of artifacts also may present a challenge for the sleep physician who monitors patents with epilepsy. In the ICU setting, one of the most frequent artifacts includes 60 Hz due to electrical wires, and devices in the recording environment, electrode pop artifact (recognized by the morphology and it being limited to one electrode), and a pulse artifact.[36]

The hallmark of subclinical or clinical ictal activity is the appearance of rhythmic evolving activity,[37] which may be challenging to appreciate on a routine PSG montage. Arousal patterns, such as occipital rhythmic activity in infancy and frontal arousal rhythm in childhood, may mimic ictal rhythmic activity.[38] In older adults, a subclinical rhythmic electrographic discharges of adults pattern may also be confused as an ictal pattern, although it does not posses the characteristic evolution of activity spatially and temporally and is considered a benign variant.[39] Vertex waves also may be confused as abnormal sharp waves. These are more easy to differentiate in an extended array of EEG electrodes, as they often have a clear negativity over central electrodes. Vertex sharp waves typically have a duration of 200 ms but in children they are particularly likely to assume high-voltage, sharply contoured morphology with asymmetric features that could be mistaken for right or left central epileptiform sharp waves.[38] The sleep technologist may be able to demonstrate that these are vertex sharp waves by arousing the patient briefly and demonstrating their dissipation.

SLEEP STATE AS A FACILITATOR OF EPILEPSY

Some seizures are promoted or facilitated preferentially by sleep.[2,3,5,40,41] **Fig. 2** provides a diagrammatic presentation of seizure distribution and epileptiform discharges across a 24-hour sleep cycle, demonstrating the high likelihood of patients with frontal lobe and extratemporal lobe epilepsy to have mostly nighttime epileptic events.

Several explanations for this relationship have been proposed. One theory is that non-REM sleep is a physiologic state of relative neuronal synchronization. During

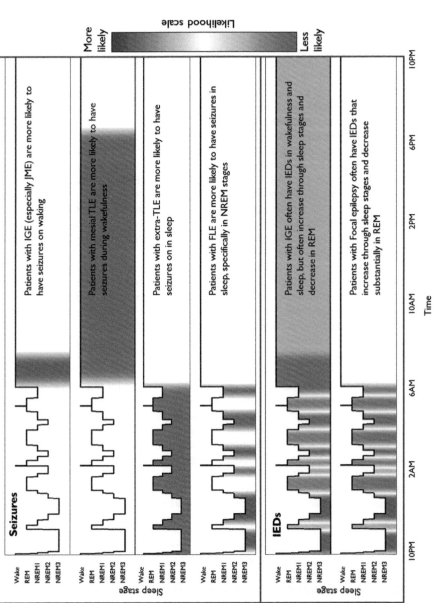

Fig. 2. Diagrammatic presentation of seizure distribution and corresponding ictal and interictal epileptiform discharges across a 24-hour sleep cycle for generalized and focal epilepsies. The sleep stages are scored based on normal sleep cycling between non-REM sleep stages N1 to N3 and REM sleep cycle during the night. FLE, frontal lobe epilepsy; IEDs, interictal discharges; IGE, idiopathic generalized epilepsy; TLE, temporal lobe epilepsy. (*From* Badawy RA, Freestone DR, Lai A, et al. Epilepsy: ever-changing states of cortical excitability. Neuroscience 2012;222:89–99.)

this sleep state, there is a greater likelihood of recruiting the neurons needed to initiate and sustain a seizure.[2,5] Non-REM sleep can be viewed as a state of relative synchronization within the thalamocortical neurons. This mode of hyperpolarization results from a progressive reduction in the firing rates of brainstem afferent neurons. This synchronization is reflected in the EEG of non-REM sleep, as seen by the presence of sleep spindles and high-amplitude delta waves. In contrast, REM sleep is characterized by increased brainstem cholinergic input to thalamocortical neurons, producing a relative state of cortical activation. Although there is an increase in both the frequency and the area generating interictal spikes during non-REM sleep, the residual spikes during REM sleep are more predictive of the regions involved in the epileptogenic zone.[42] A recent review of the literature postulated that non-REM sleep may be less epileptogenic than periods of REM sleep accompanied by theta oscillations, but more epileptogenic than REM sleep when theta is absent.[43]

A second theory proposes that sudden synchronous excitatory input from the posterior hypothalamus projects to the neocortical mantle, and may facilitate seizures via exacerbation of cortical hyperexcitability.[44] The strongest clinical examples supporting this theory come from juvenile myoclonic epilepsy (JME) and GTCSs on awakening, in which seizures occur shortly after awakening.[45]

Several of the sleep-related epilepsy syndromes involve seizures of frontal lobe origin. Crespel and coworkers[46] compared patients with frontal lobe and mesial temporal lobe epilepsy and found significant differences between the 2 groups in the occurrence of seizures. In patients with frontal lobe epilepsy, most seizures occurred during sleep, whereas in temporal lobe epilepsy, most seizures occurred while the patients were awake. These findings suggest that changes in neuronal excitability associated with sleep are different in frontal and temporal structures. The frontal lobe receives ascending input from the thalamus and has rich interconnections, which may explain its propensity to facilitate seizures during sleep.

EPILEPSY SYNDROMES ASSOCIATED WITH SLEEP

In the differentiation of nocturnal spells, video-PSG is required for the diagnosis, but for practical reasons this may not always be feasible in the ICU in centers in which formal epilepsy monitoring units are absent. However, even when formal recordings take place, a small population of patients remains without a definitive diagnosis despite an extensive workup. Briefly, natural history of the episodes (that appear or increase in frequency after childhood), occurrence of more than 1 episode per night and semiology of the attacks (stereotypy, dyskinetic and dystonic components, clear onset and offset) are generally more indicative of epileptic seizures than disorders of arousal. Nocturnal seizures often have bizarre clinical manifestations. As a general rule, during a spell, patients have preservation of consciousness with rapid recovery.[47,48] Scalp EEG monitoring reveals the absence of epileptic activity, which makes diagnosis of nocturnal seizures and distinguishing them from other parasomnias challenging.[49] **Table 2** highlights some of the salient features differentiating parasomnias from nocturnal frontal lobe seizures.[50–52] Observers may not be present to corroborate the episode; therefore, the description of these spells is often lacking or ambiguous. Unlike seizures that occur while awake, nocturnal seizures have auras and postictal periods that tend to be masked by sleep. However, all in all, *stereotypy* is the key in the clinical presentation and is often the one element in the history that leads the clinician toward the diagnosis of nocturnal seizures. Behavioral manifestations during nocturnal seizures are often complex, and patients may exhibit any of the following: fighting; sensation of fear and tachycardia; running spells; bicycling,

Table 2
Comparative features of non-REM parasomnia versus NFLE

	NFLE	Non-REM Parasomnias
Length of event	Typically brief (<1 min)	Longer in duration (5–15 min)
Motor activity	Generally stereotyped	More likely to be complex, variable
Onset	Within 30 min of sleep onset	Within 2 h of sleep onset
Frequency	Generally more likely to occur nightly and multiple times per night	Usually <3 times per a month, rarely more than several times per week
Recall	Can have lucid recall	Amnestic of event. Partial recall with complex partial seizures
Age of onset, y	14 ± 10	<10
Family history	39% more likely, especially in NFLE	Frequently positive 62%–96%
Triggering factors	Not typical, but may be precipitated by sleep deprivation	Yes: sleep deprivation, febrile illness, anxiety, stress, sleep apnea, motor disorders of sleep
Other	Presence of aura, dystonic or tonic posturing, abrupt offset	Interaction with environment, wander outside bedroom, slow offset or ending of event
Common features of both	Commonly start in childhood, may have vocalizations, motor artifact seen on EEG	

Abbreviations: EEG, electroencephalogram; NFLE, nocturnal frontal lobe epilepsy; REM, rapid eye movement sleep.

kicking, and thrashing movements; and episodes of shouting, screaming, or laughing.[47,48,53]

SLEEP-RELATED EPILEPSY SYNDROMES

Sleep physicians, whether trained in primary neurology residency or not, should become familiar with some of the most common sleep-related epilepsy syndromes, especially in the setting of the ICU. These syndromes are heterogeneous and include both generalized and focal-onset seizures, with specific predilection to occur during sleep. Specific syndromes include nocturnal temporal lobe epilepsy, benign epilepsy of childhood with centrotemporal spikes, nocturnal paroxysmal dystonia (NPD), supplementary sensorimotor seizures, autosomal-dominant nocturnal frontal lobe epilepsy, epilepsy with continuous-spike slow-wave activity during sleep, JME, and GTCSs on awakening.[54] In a well-designed prospective study by Herman and colleagues[55] analyzing 613 seizures in 133 patients with focal seizures over a 2-year period, 43% occurred out of sleep (I 23%, II 68%). Seizures were rare in SWS and no seizures were seen during REM sleep. Temporal lobe complex partial seizures were more likely to secondarily generalize during sleep (31%) than during wakefulness (15%), but frontal lobe seizures were less likely to secondarily generalize during sleep (10% vs 26%; P<.005).

Nocturnal Temporal Lobe Epilepsy

Although frontal lobe seizures commonly occur during sleep, temporal lobe epilepsy is the most common type of sleep-related focal epilepsy in adults.[46] This is not surprising, as seizures during sleep are commonly of temporal lobe origin.[56] Many patients with seizures during the day may also have unrecognized seizures during sleep for several reasons. Patients may lack an aura or not recall the event.[57] Also, patients who sleep alone will not have observers to witness their seizures. Finally, patients with subtle arousals from sleep may not sufficiently awaken their bed partners, and thus the description may be vague.

Nocturnal seizures also may be mistaken for a non-REM arousal disorder, REM sleep behavior disorder, panic disorder, sleep terrors, and psychogenic seizures, especially if motor manifestations are prominent and the EEG is normal. Bernasconi and colleagues[56] identified a group of 26 patients with nonlesional refractory temporal lobe epilepsy in whom seizures occurred exclusively or predominantly (>90%) after they fell asleep or before they awakened. Simple partial seizures (focal nondyscognitive seizures) occurred in 69% of patients and woke the patients; these seizures had experiential, autonomic, or special sensory components. Brief periods of impaired consciousness with motionless staring or automatisms dominated, although sleepwalking was reported in 5 patients. Eighty-one percent had secondary generalization of the partial attacks.[56] This group of patients was compared with an age-matched group of patients with nonlesional temporal lobe epilepsy and predominantly diurnal seizures; the patients with nocturnal seizures differed in that they had infrequent and nonclustered seizures, rarely had a family history of epilepsy, and had a low prevalence of childhood febrile convulsions. All 8 patients who underwent epilepsy surgery became seizure free for at least 1 year. This subset of patients with nocturnal temporal lobe epilepsy is especially important to recognize because of their favorable surgical outcome.[56]

Benign Epilepsy of Childhood with Centrotemporal Spikes

Benign epilepsy of childhood with centrotemporal spikes (BECT), also called *rolandic epilepsy* or *sylvian seizure syndrome*, is the most common form of partial epilepsy in children.[58] BECT displays a strong genetic, and at times autosomal-dominant, predisposition[59] and appears in healthy persons with no evidence of brain lesions. Seizures begin in the early school years, at approximately 7 years of age (ranging between 3 and 13 years). Sleep is an important activating state of seizures; in 70% to 80% of cases, seizures are confined to sleep. Seizures are often rare, and tend to occur in clusters with prolonged seizure-free intervals. Owing to their rarity and to their occurrence exclusively or predominantly during sleep, seizures may remain unnoticed by parents for years.[60–62]

A typical BECT case is characterized by paresthesias in one-half of the face, sometimes involving the tongue and lips, followed by clonic jerks involving the face, tongue, lips, larynx, and pharynx. These clonic jerks may provoke speech impairment. Clonic movements cause a feeling of suffocation and dysphagia with hypersalivation.[53,55] Consciousness is usually preserved. Patients may be awakened by the seizures. The typical hemifacial seizure may spread to the ipsilateral arm (brachiofacial convulsion) and, rarely, to the leg, producing a hemiconvulsive seizure, which may involve loss of consciousness. A postictal Todd paresis is observed in 7% to 16% of cases.[60]

GTCSs are rare. The EEG reveals characteristic high-amplitude interictal spikes followed by slow waves in the midtemporal region and central broad spikes or sharp waves, particularly during sleep.[63] The EEG pattern is inherited as an autosomal-dominant trait; only 25% of persons with this EEG pattern actually have the seizures.[64] The EEG spike activity is enhanced during sleep; in approximately 30% of cases, this activity appears only during sleep. Spikes can remain unilateral or can spread to the contralateral hemisphere (50% of the cases). Epileptiform discharges sometimes occur outside the centrotemporal region in children who exhibit symptoms consistent with BECT.[65]

The prognosis for a patient with these spells is excellent, with response to antiepileptic medications the rule. If there are atypical features or abnormal examination findings, a brain MRI is mandatory to exclude an underlying lesion. The seizures of BECT are usually easily distinguishable from movement disorders and psychogenic disorders on the basis of the history, EEG, and the response to medications. Treatment may or may not be given and includes the use of AEDs, such as phenytoin, phenobarbital, valproic acid, or carbamazepine, and more recently levetiracetam.[59,66] The medication may be withdrawn after a seizure-free interval of 3 years. Interestingly, the EEG pattern may persist even after treatment. Cognitive abnormalities have been described with BECT.[67]

Nocturnal Paroxysmal Dystonia

NPD is still listed as a motor disorder of sleep in the *International Classification of Sleep Disorders*, although most regard this disorder as a form of frontal lobe epilepsy (nocturnal frontal lobe epilepsy [NFLE]). It may also be considered as an non rapid eye movement sleep arousal parasomnia.[59,68] NPD consists of a sudden arousal associated with a complex sequence of movements, repeated dystonia, or dyskinesia (ballistic or choreoathetotic).[69] Patients may also move their legs and arms with cycling or kicking movements, rock their trunks, and show tonic asymmetric or dystonic posture of the limbs. A few cases are characterized by a violent ballistic pattern with flailing of the limbs.[69] Consciousness is often preserved. These spells are stereotyped and occur during non-REM sleep. They are short episodes, lasting 15 to 60 seconds, and recur up to 15 times per night, usually preceded by clinical and EEG arousal; these episodes occur nearly every night. The patient's eyes are often open, and almost immediately there is dystonic posturing associated with ballistic or choreoathetotic movements often associated with localization. At the end of the episode, the patient is coherent and if left undisturbed, usually resumes sleep. Prolonged episodes may last up to 60 minutes.[69–72]

Evidence supporting the epileptic etiology of NPD includes the following: (1) the stereotyped nature of the spells; (2) the observation that seizures originating in deep mesial frontal generators often lack interictal and ictal correlates and require invasive monitoring for definitive diagnosis; (3) the occurrence of cases in which convulsive seizures, with epileptiform EEG patterns, have followed typical NPD episodes; and (4) the similarity in clinical features in patients with NPD, daytime frontal lobe seizures, and nocturnal epilepsy.[71]

The differential diagnosis includes REM sleep behavior disorder, sleep terrors, and epilepsy, especially frontal lobe epilepsy.[73] Criteria for diagnosis include dystonic and dyskinetic attacks during sleep, onset during non-REM sleep, absence of ictal epileptic EEG activity, and normal neurologic imaging (including brain computed tomography and MRIs). When the episodes are short (<1 to 2 minutes), carbamazepine is often the agent of choice and provides an excellent response. Carbamazepine therapy begins at a low dose (ie, 200 mg before bedtime) and increases progressively by 200 mg/d every week until the attacks are controlled. If there is an adverse reaction or no response, the second agent of choice is phenytoin.[42] For prolonged episodes, treatment is not very effective.[69,72,74]

Nocturnal Frontal Lobe Epilepsy and Supplementary Sensorimotor Seizures

In NFLE including supplementary motor-area seizures, episodes have predominantly motor manifestations and a nocturnal preponderance.[75] Frequent seizures often occur in clusters with many per day. These are brief seizures (<1 minute) that occur suddenly with little or no ictal confusion. There is often vocalization of variable complexity; there is frequently a warning, usually nonspecific; the attacks appear to be bizarre and hysterical.[76] The unique feature is a stereotypical pattern. The inter-ictal and ictal surface EEGs are often normal. These episodes can be misdiagnosed during wakefulness as psychogenic nonepileptic seizures, and during sleep as move-ment disorders or sleep disturbance, such as NPD or epileptic nocturnal wandering.[77]

Supplementary sensorimotor seizures are associated with bilateral, contralateral, and ipsilateral somatosensory sensations of numbness or tingling.[78] Seizures origi-nate in or spread to involve area 6 on the medial surface of the cerebral hemisphere. There is an abrupt onset of fixed posture, classically with the arm contralateral to the side of seizure origin abducted at the shoulder, externally rotated, and flexed at the elbow. The head and eyes are deviated, as if the patient is looking at an upraised hand. Speech arrest or vocalizations may occur. Seizures are generally brief, lasting several seconds.[79] Flailing, thrashing movements of arms and legs, kicking, and tonic/dystonic posturing of the arms and legs may occur.[80] The surface EEG is often normal, although interictal epileptiform activity or ictal patterns may occur in elec-trodes at or adjacent to the midline. Withdrawal of antiepileptic medications to pro-mote GTCSs during inpatient evaluation with continuous video-EEG monitoring is a useful diagnostic maneuver.[81]

Autosomal-Dominant Nocturnal Frontal Lobe Epilepsy

The clinical manifestations of autosomal-dominant NFLE (ADNFLE) overlap with NPD and supplementary sensorimotor seizures.[82,83] The syndrome of ADNFLE was initially described in 47 individuals from 5 families. These individuals exhibited clusters of brief nocturnal motor seizures with hyperkinetic or tonic manifestations indistinguish-able from NPD. Many were misdiagnosed as having night terrors, nightmares, and hysteria. One large Australian kindred with frontal lobe epilepsy showed a missense mutation in the A4 subunit of the neuronal nicotinic acetylcholine receptor gene, located on chromosome 20q. Oldani and colleagues[84] reported on ADNFLE in 40 subjects from 30 unrelated Italian families. In addition to NPD, sleepwalking and sud-den awakenings with fear and tachycardia were exhibited. This group of investigators also determined that ADNFLE is a genetically heterogeneous disorder, in that their 5 families undergoing genetic sequencing did not show linkage to the long arm of chro-mosome 20. Other genetic abnormalities, including DEPDC5 mutations have been demonstrated.[85–87]

EPILEPTIC ENCEPHALOPATHY WITH CONTINUOUS SPIKE-AND-WAVE DURING SLEEP

Epileptic encephalopathy with continuous spike-waves during SWS (CSWS) has a heterogeneous clinical presentation. Some patients have rare partial motor or GTCSs in sleep, and others may lack seizures during sleep.[88] Still others may not have clini-cally apparent seizures at all. The defining feature of CSWS is an EEG pattern consist-ing of generalized slow spike-wave discharges, which are present for 85% to 90% of SWS and relatively suppressed during REM sleep and wakefulness. The syndrome used to be called *electrical status epilepticus of sleep*, but the name was changed because that term implied frequent seizures, which may not capture the variability of this syndrome. There is no consensus as to the preferred treatment, but most com-mon treatments include high-dose benzodiazepines, valproate, levetiracetam, and corticosteroids.[89,90] Clinical seizures are usually responsive to AEDs and remit by the middle teenage years. Cognitive disturbances, including Landau Kleffner, do not remit and are not improved by AEDs.[91]

Juvenile Myoclonic Epilepsy

JME is one of the most common forms of idiopathic generalized epilepsy. It consists of a triad of 3 seizure types: myoclonic jerks, GTCS, and absence seizures with myoclonic jerks that occur predominantly after awakening.[92–94] Absence seizures are present in 10% to 33% of patients with JME. The typical presentation is of GTCS; the patient may not acknowledge that myoclonic jerks are present unless specifically asked. However, jerks or absence seizures may precede GTCS or predominate throughout a patient's life span with only rare GTCS.[92] The seizures of JME are usually responsive to valproate or lamotrigine, although therapy is usually but not always lifelong.[95] The mean age of onset of JME is 14 years, with most presenting between 12 and 18 years of age. The percentage of patients with JME with a family history of epilepsy has been estimated at between 17% and 49%. There are numerous genetic abnormalities associated with JME.[96]

The jerks of JME are most prominent in the early morning, and are often accompanied by a history of GTCS and possibly absence seizures.[97] In addition, an EEG demonstrates polyspike-wave discharges, with photoparoxysmal responses common. These EEG discharges may be seen either during myoclonic jerks or in the interictal (between seizure) state.[98]

GENERALIZED TONIC-CLONIC SEIZURES ON AWAKENING

Another idiopathic generalized epilepsy syndrome associated with the sleep-wake cycle is GTCSs on awakening (generalized-onset "grand mal" seizures on awakening)[99] and is illustrated with the signature ictal EEG pattern in **Fig. 3**. Similar to JME, this syndrome typically begins in the second decade of life, may consist of absence and myoclonic seizures in addition to GTCSs,[100] has a genetic component, and has an EEG pattern seen in idiopathic generalized epilepsy, including a photoparoxysmal response. As with JME, the seizures respond well to treatment, but lifelong therapy is often necessary. A wide prevalence range is reported (10% to 53%), which varies depending on the number of GTCSs required for diagnosis, the presence of other seizure types, and the time of occurrence of GTCSs. When myoclonus is a prominent feature of this disorder, GTCSs on awakening may be confused with a movement disorder. However, as with JME, the characteristic EEG patterns and presence of GTCSs should allow differentiation from a movement disorder without difficulty. Sleep deprivation is a common trigger (see **Fig. 3**).[99]

The syndromes of GTCSs on awakening and JME show overlap, especially in seizure type and age of onset. In fact, JME may appear with GTCSs on awakening but, in this case, rhythmic myoclonic jerks often precede the tonic-clonic seizures. In general, a useful distinguishing feature is that relatively frequent myoclonic jerks and infrequent GTCSs characterize JME. Patients with "pure" GTCSs on awakening have had at least 6 GTCSs.

PROGNOSIS

The prognosis of nocturnal seizures depends on the seizure type. Certain epilepsy syndromes, such as BECT and JME, typically respond well to AEDs. Remission of BECT by the early adult years is the general rule. Other partial epilepsy syndromes predominating during sleep do not carry as favorable a prognosis. In fact, partial seizures that are limited to sleep frequently develop into waking seizures. Park and coworkers[101] retrospectively identified 63 patients with pure sleep epilepsy, 21 of whom had GTCSs during sleep and 42 of whom had partial seizures during sleep.

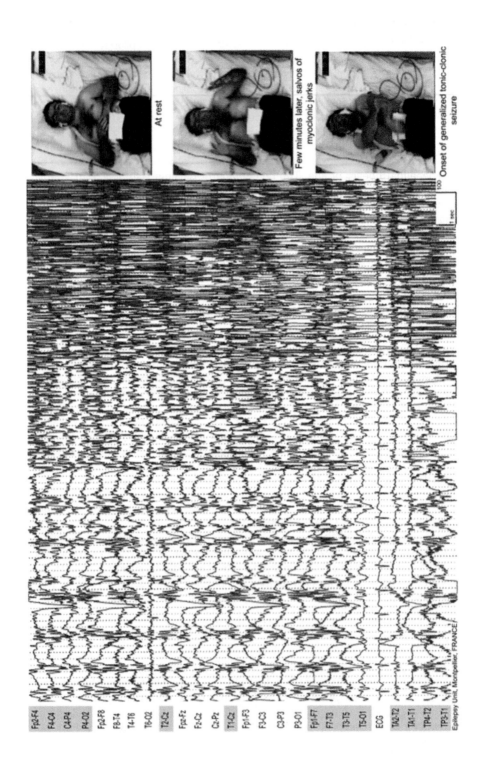

Two years later, 17 of the patients with GTCSs (81%) were seizure free, compared with 15 of the patients with partial seizures (36%). Seizures developed during wakefulness in 11 patients with partial seizures (26%), versus 1 patient with GTCS (5%). In NFLE, carbamazepine abolished seizures in 20% of cases and reduced seizures by 50% or more in another 48% of cases.[101] In approximately one-third of patients, however, seizures were refractory to AEDs. Cases responding to treatment relapsed when AEDs were withdrawn.

OBSTRUCTIVE SLEEP APNEA AND EPILEPSY

Sleep apnea may coexist with epilepsy.[102] Several mechanisms have been proposed to explain seizure facilitation in OSA. Some have proposed that sleep deprivation resulting from frequent arousals from sleep increases neuronal excitability.[6] Frequent arousals or stage shifts into and out of sleep thereby facilitate sleep-related seizures.[103] The treatment of OSA may improve seizure control,[104] daytime sleepiness, or both. Wyler and Weymuller[105] demonstrated that in patients with OSA and epilepsy who underwent tracheostomy, generalized seizures diminished. Later on, Devinsky and colleagues[6] showed that continuous positive airway pressure (PAP) or other therapy improved seizure control and daytime alertness in 6 of 7 patients with partial seizures. Vaughn and colleagues[103] found that continuous PAP or positional therapy improved seizure control in 7 of 10 patients with seizures and OSA, and antiepileptic medications were optimized in 3 of the 10 patients. A more recent study by Pornsriniyom and colleagues[106] looked into 76 patients with epilepsy and OSA. The group with PAP-treated OSA had 32.3 times the odds of having a seizure reduction of 50% or more compared with the group with untreated OSA, and 6.13 times compared with the group with no OSA. The same investigators separately reported a decrease in interictal epileptiform transients with CPAP.[107] As mentioned previously, the increase in BMI associated with some antiseizure medications, such as valproic acid and pregabalin, may also secondarily increase the risk for OSA.

EFFECT OF VAGAL NERVE STIMULATOR ON SLEEP

Neuromodulation is an increasing modality of treatment in patients with medically refractory focal epilepsy. Vagal nerve stimulation (VNS) has been in use since 1997 and has been associated with decreased REM sleep and increased awakenings, wake after sleep onset, and stage N1 non-REM sleep. Stimulation is also associated with decreases in airflow and effort coinciding with VNS activation.[108–110] There are insufficient data as to the effect of other recently approved devices, such as intracranial responsive nerve stimulation on sleep.

◀ ───────────────────────────────────

Fig. 3. EEG in GTCSs. A 38-year-old man undergoing a sleep-deprived EEG. Patient went to sleep at 2 AM, and was awakened at 6 AM. A few minutes after awakening, the patient began having myoclonic jerks. In the figure, there are bursts of generalized poly-spikes with vigorous myoclonic jerks. At second 8, the panel depicts the sudden onset of the GTCS with generalized recruiting spikes predominating anteriorly with marked superposition of electromyographic muscular artifacts. Key: Paper speed 15 mm/s; Amplitude (Voltage) of EEG waves 10 mV/mm; Electrode placement followed the International 10–20 electrode system with supplementary anterior/inferior temporal electrodes (TA1, T1, TP1, TA2, T2, and TP2). (*From* Serafini A, Rubboli G, Gigli GL, et al. Neurophysiology of juvenile myoclonic epilepsy. Epilepsy Behav 2013;28(Suppl 1):S30–9.)

SEIZURES IN THE INTENSIVE CARE UNIT ENVIRONMENT: PROGNOSIS

The ICU environment poses unique challenges. Patients often have a disruption in the wake-sleep cycling pattern. This is compounded by the noisy ICU environment, which increases noise and sleep deprivation.[111] Patients in the ICU are more susceptible to hypopnea and cardiac abnormalities, and receive medications, especially sedative agents such as propofol, versed, and barbiturates, which have a profound effect on sleep architecture.[111]

There have been many studies showing that in the neurointensive care unit there is a high prevalence of nonconvulsive seizures of 19% to 31%.[112,113] Oddo and colleagues[114] looked at 201 patients in the medical ICU (60% had sepsis) and found seizures in 10% (two-thirds were subclinical). The presence of seizures was predictive of a worse outcome. More recently, Kurtz and colleagues[115] reported an incidence of 16% of seizures in the surgical ICU. The recent neurocritical care guidelines published in 2012 advocate the use of continuous EEG (CEEG) in patients with a recent clinical seizure without return to baseline of longer than 10 minutes, coma including post–cardiac arrest, epileptiform activity in an initial EEG, intracranial hemorrhage, and suspected nonconvulsive seizures in patients with altered mental status.[116] The extended use of CEEG with or without additional polysomnographic channels presents unique opportunities and challenges, as both epileptologist and sleep physicians will be consulted as to the differentiation of paroxysmal episodes in the ICU as well as the recognition of clinical and subclinical seizures.

SUMMARY

The ICU is potentially an inhospitable location for patients with epilepsy and seizures, including subclinical seizures, which are common in the neurosurgical, surgical, and medical ICUs. Often overlooked exacerbating factors that are likely culprits may include noise levels, nursing activities, medications, and lack of or inappropriate light exposure. When sleep is disrupted, so is the potential to have breakthrough seizures. The sleep physician and pulmonary/neurocritical care provider should be aware of the differential diagnosis of sleep-related events in the ICU and have a low threshold to manage comorbid sleep disorders in patients with epilepsy on the unit, particularly in SSE. Although CEEG is becoming more frequently used, recent advances have helped clarify the value of recording PSG/EEG in diagnosing and localizing focal epilepsy and parasomnias. Sleep-related epilepsy, particularly NFLE, is better understood and is most likely to manifest at night.

REFERENCES

1. Foldvary-Schaefer N, Grigg-Damberger M. Sleep and epilepsy: what we know, don't know, and need to know. J Clin Neurophysiol 2006;23(1):4–20.
2. Malow BA. Sleep and epilepsy. Neurol Clin 2005;23(4):1127–47.
3. Vaughn BV, D'Cruz OF. Sleep and epilepsy. Semin Neurol 2004;24(3): 301–13.
4. Degen R, Degen HE. Sleep and sleep deprivation in epileptology. Epilepsy Res Suppl 1991;2:235–60.
5. Foldvary-Schaefer N, Grigg-Damberger M. Sleep and epilepsy. Semin Neurol 2009;29(4):419–28.
6. Devinsky O, Ehrenberg B, Barthlen GM, et al. Epilepsy and sleep apnea syndrome. Neurology 1994;44(11):2060–4.

7. Adusumalli VE, Wichmann JK, Kucharczyk N, et al. Drug concentrations in human brain tissue samples from epileptic patients treated with felbamate. Drug Metab Dispos 1994;22(1):168–70.
8. Fisher RS, Acevedo C, Arzimanoglou A, et al. ILAE official report: a practical clinical definition of epilepsy. Epilepsia 2014;55(4):475–82.
9. Berg AT, Berkovic SF, Brodie MJ, et al. Revised terminology and concepts for organization of seizures and epilepsies: report of the ILAE Commission on Classification and Terminology, 2005–2009. Epilepsia 2010;51(4):676–85.
10. England MJ, Liverman CT, Schultz AM, et al. Epilepsy across the spectrum: promoting health and understanding. A summary of the Institute of Medicine report. Epilepsy Behav 2012;25(2):266–76.
11. Xu X, Brandenburg NA, McDermott AM, et al. Sleep disturbances reported by refractory partial-onset epilepsy patients receiving polytherapy. Epilepsia 2006;47(7):1176–83.
12. Kanner AM. Depression in epilepsy: prevalence, clinical semiology, pathogenic mechanisms, and treatment. Biol Psychiatry 2003;54(3):388–98.
13. Zucconi M, Maestri M. Atlas of clinical sleep medicine. In: Kryger M, Avidan AY, Berry R, editors. Sleep and epilepsy. 2nd edition. Philadelphia: Elsevier/Saunders; 2013. p. 196–212.
14. Sammaritano M, Sherwin A. Effect of anticonvulsants on sleep. Neurology 2000; 54(5 Suppl 1):S16–24.
15. Wolf P, Roder-Wanner UU, Brede M. Influence of therapeutic phenobarbital and phenytoin medication on the polygraphic sleep of patients with epilepsy. Epilepsia 1984;25(4):467–75.
16. Gigli GL, Placidi F, Diomedi M, et al. Nocturnal sleep and daytime somnolence in untreated patients with temporal lobe epilepsy: changes after treatment with controlled-release carbamazepine. Epilepsia 1997;38(6):696–701.
17. Placidi F, Diomedi M, Scalise A, et al. Effect of anticonvulsants on nocturnal sleep in epilepsy. Neurology 2000;54(5 Suppl 1):S25–32.
18. Foldvary-Schaefer N, De Leon Sanchez I, Karafa M, et al. Gabapentin increases slow-wave sleep in normal adults. Epilepsia 2002;43(12):1493–7.
19. Wechsler RT, Li G, French J, et al. Conversion to lacosamide monotherapy in the treatment of focal epilepsy: results from a historical-controlled, multicenter, double-blind study. Epilepsia 2014;55(7):1088–98.
20. Bazil CW, Dave J, Cole J, et al. Pregabalin increases slow-wave sleep and may improve attention in patients with partial epilepsy and insomnia. Epilepsy Behav 2012;23(4):422–5.
21. Foldvary N, Perry M, Lee J, et al. The effects of lamotrigine on sleep in patients with epilepsy. Epilepsia 2001;42(12):1569–73.
22. Bidlack JM, Morris HH 3rd. Phenobarbital withdrawal seizures may occur over several weeks before remitting: human data and hypothetical mechanism. Seizure 2009;18(1):79–81.
23. Shvarts V, Chung S. Epilepsy, antiseizure therapy, and sleep cycle parameters. Epilepsy Res Treat 2013;2013:670682.
24. De Paolis F, Colizzi E, Milioli G, et al. Effects of antiepileptic treatment on sleep and seizures in nocturnal frontal lobe epilepsy. Sleep Med 2013;14(7):597–604.
25. Foldvary N, Caruso AC, Mascha E, et al. Identifying montages that best detect electrographic seizure activity during polysomnography. Sleep 2000;23(2):221–9.
26. Foldvary-Schaefer N, De Ocampo J, Mascha E, et al. Accuracy of seizure detection using abbreviated EEG during polysomnography. J Clin Neurophysiol 2006;23(1):68–71.

27. Chang AK, Shinnar S. Nonconvulsive status epilepticus. Emerg Med Clin North Am 2011;29(1):65–72.
28. Andre-Obadia N, Parain D, Szurhaj W. Continuous EEG monitoring in adults in the intensive care unit (ICU). Neurophysiol Clin 2015;45(1):39–46.
29. Phillips MC, Costello CA, White EJ, et al. Routine polysomnography in an epilepsy monitoring unit. Epilepsy Res 2013;105(3):401–4.
30. Stollberger C, Finsterer J. Cardiorespiratory findings in sudden unexplained/unexpected death in epilepsy (SUDEP). Epilepsy Res 2004;59(1):51–60.
31. Sperling MR. Sudden unexplained death in epilepsy. Epilepsy Curr 2001;1(1):21–3.
32. Foldvary-Schaefer N, Alsheikhtaha Z. Complex nocturnal behaviors: nocturnal seizures and parasomnias. Continuum (Minneap Minn) 2013;19(1 Sleep Disorders):104–31.
33. Ebersole JS, Nordli DR, Husain AM. Current practice of clinical electroencephalography. 4th edition. Philadelphia: Lippincott Williams & Wilkins; 2014.
34. Egawa I, Yoshino K, Hishikawa Y. Positive occipital sharp transients in the human sleep EEG. Folia Psychiatr Neurol Jpn 1983;37(1):57–65.
35. Tatum WO 4th, Husain AM, Benbadis SR, et al. Normal adult EEG and patterns of uncertain significance. J Clin Neurophysiol 2006;23(3):194–207.
36. Tatum WO, Dworetzky BA, Schomer DL. Artifact and recording concepts in EEG. J Clin Neurophysiol 2011;28(3):252–63.
37. Blume WT, Young GB, Lemieux JF. EEG morphology of partial epileptic seizures. Electroencephalogr Clin Neurophysiol 1984;57(4):295–302.
38. Mizrahi EM. Avoiding the pitfalls of EEG interpretation in childhood epilepsy. Epilepsia 1996;37(Suppl 1):S41–51.
39. O'Brien TJ, Sharbrough FW, Westmoreland BF, et al. Subclinical rhythmic electrographic discharges of adults (SREDA) revisited: a study using digital EEG analysis. J Clin Neurophysiol 1998;15(6):493–501.
40. Romigi A, Bonanni E, Maestri M. Sleep and epilepsy. Epilepsy Res Treat 2013; 2013:483248.
41. Derry CP, Duncan S. Sleep and epilepsy. Epilepsy Behav 2013;26(3):394–404.
42. Malow BA, Aldrich MS. Localizing value of rapid eye movement sleep in temporal lobe epilepsy. Sleep Med 2000;1(1):57–60.
43. Ahmed OJ, Vijayan S. The roles of sleep-wake states and brain rhythms in epileptic seizure onset. J Neurosci 2014;34(22):7395–7.
44. Shouse MN, da Silva AM, Sammaritano M. Circadian rhythm, sleep, and epilepsy. J Clin Neurophysiol 1996;13(1):32–50.
45. Janz D. The grand Mal epilepsies and the sleeping-waking cycle. Epilepsia 1962;3(1):69–109.
46. Crespel A, Baldy-Moulinier M, Coubes P. The relationship between sleep and epilepsy in frontal and temporal lobe epilepsies: practical and physiopathologic considerations. Epilepsia 1998;39(2):150–7.
47. Provini F, Montagna P, Plazzi G, et al. Nocturnal frontal lobe epilepsy: a wide spectrum of seizures. Mov Disord 2000;15(6):1264.
48. Bazil CW. Nocturnal seizures. Semin Neurol 2004;24(3):293–300.
49. Derry CP, Duncan JS, Berkovic SF. Paroxysmal motor disorders of sleep: the clinical spectrum and differentiation from epilepsy. Epilepsia 2006;47(11):1775–91.
50. Nobili L. Nocturnal frontal lobe epilepsy and non-rapid eye movement sleep parasomnias: differences and similarities. Sleep Med Rev 2007;11(4):251–4.
51. Bisulli F, Vignatelli L, Provini F, et al. Parasomnias and nocturnal frontal lobe epilepsy (NFLE): lights and shadows–controversial points in the differential diagnosis. Sleep Med 2011;12(Suppl 2):S27–32.

52. Derry C. Nocturnal frontal lobe epilepsy vs parasomnias. Curr Treat Options Neurol 2012;14(5):451–63.
53. Boursoulian LJ, Schenck CH, Mahowald MW, et al. Differentiating parasomnias from nocturnal seizures. J Clin Sleep Med 2012;8(1):108–12.
54. Bazil CW. Sleep-related epilepsy. Curr Neurol Neurosci Rep 2003;3(2):167–8.
55. Herman ST, Walczak TS, Bazil CW. Distribution of partial seizures during the sleep–wake cycle: differences by seizure onset site. Neurology 2001;56(11): 1453–9.
56. Bernasconi A, Andermann F, Cendes F, et al. Nocturnal temporal lobe epilepsy. Neurology 1998;50(6):1772–7.
57. Hoppe C, Poepel A, Elger CE. Epilepsy: accuracy of patient seizure counts. Arch Neurol 2007;64(11):1595–9.
58. Kramer U, Zelnik N, Lerman-Sagie T, et al. Benign childhood epilepsy with centrotemporal spikes: clinical characteristics and identification of patients at risk for multiple seizures. J Child Neurol 2002;17(1):17–9.
59. Verrotti A, Coppola G, Manco R, et al. Levetiracetam monotherapy for children and adolescents with benign rolandic seizures. Seizure 2007;16(3):271–5.
60. Wirrell EC. Benign epilepsy of childhood with centrotemporal spikes. Epilepsia 1998;39(Suppl 4):S32–41.
61. Tovia E, Goldberg-Stern H, Ben Zeev B, et al. The prevalence of atypical presentations and comorbidities of benign childhood epilepsy with centrotemporal spikes. Epilepsia 2011;52(8):1483–8.
62. Stephani U. Typical semiology of benign childhood epilepsy with centrotemporal spikes (BCECTS). Epileptic Disord 2000;2(Suppl 1):S3–4.
63. Beaussart M. Benign epilepsy of children with rolandic (centro-temporal) paroxysmal foci. A clinical entity. Study of 221 cases. Epilepsia 1972;13(6):795–811.
64. Bali B, Kull LL, Strug LJ, et al. Autosomal dominant inheritance of centrotemporal sharp waves in rolandic epilepsy families. Epilepsia 2007;48(12):2266–72.
65. Beydoun A, Garofalo EA, Drury I. Generalized spike-waves, multiple loci, and clinical course in children with EEG features of benign epilepsy of childhood with centrotemporal spikes. Epilepsia 1992;33(6):1091–6.
66. Hughes JR. Benign epilepsy of childhood with centrotemporal spikes (BECTS): to treat or not to treat, that is the question. Epilepsy Behav 2010; 19(3):197–203.
67. Fonseca LC, Tedrus GM, Pacheco EM, et al. Benign childhood epilepsy with centro-temporal spikes: correlation between clinical, cognitive and EEG aspects. Arq Neuropsiquiatr 2007;65(3A):569–75.
68. Kaleyias J, Arora R, Kothare SV. Nocturnal paroxysmal dystonia. Parasomnias. New York: Springer; 2013. p. 249–70.
69. Sellal F, Hirsch E. Nocturnal paroxysmal dystonia. Mov Disord 1993;8(2):252–3.
70. Borrow S, Tattersall ML, Hartman D, et al. Sleep disorders. Consider nocturnal paroxysmal dystonia. BMJ 1993;306(6890):1476–7.
71. Meierkord H, Fish DR, Smith SJ, et al. Is nocturnal paroxysmal dystonia a form of frontal lobe epilepsy? Mov Disord 1992;7(1):38–42.
72. Lugaresi E, Cirignotta F, Montagna P. Nocturnal paroxysmal dystonia. Epilepsy Res Suppl 1991;2:137–40.
73. Zucconi M, Ferini-Strambi L. NREM parasomnias: arousal disorders and differentiation from nocturnal frontal lobe epilepsy. Clin Neurophysiol 2000;111(Suppl 2):S129–35.
74. Provini F, Plazzi G, Lugaresi E. From nocturnal paroxysmal dystonia to nocturnal frontal lobe epilepsy. Clin Neurophysiol 2000;111(Suppl 2):S2–8.

75. Jobst BC, Siegel AM, Thadani VM, et al. Intractable seizures of frontal lobe origin: clinical characteristics, localizing signs, and results of surgery. Epilepsia 2000;41(9):1139–52.

76. Bonini F, McGonigal A, Trébuchon A, et al. Frontal lobe seizures: from clinical semiology to localization. Epilepsia 2014;55(2):264–77.

77. Crompton DE, Berkovic SF. The borderland of epilepsy: clinical and molecular features of phenomena that mimic epileptic seizures. Lancet Neurol 2009; 8(4):370–81.

78. Connolly MB, Langill L, Wong PK, et al. Seizures involving the supplementary sensorimotor area in children: a video-EEG analysis. Epilepsia 1995;36(10): 1025–32.

79. Ohara S, Ikeda A, Kunieda T, et al. Propagation of tonic posturing in supplementary motor area (SMA) seizures. Epilepsy Res 2004;62(2–3):179–87.

80. King DW, Smith JR. Supplementary sensorimotor area epilepsy in adults. Adv Neurol 1996;70:285–91.

81. Laich E, Kuzniecky R, Mountz J, et al. Supplementary sensorimotor area epilepsy. Seizure localization, cortical propagation and subcortical activation pathways using ictal SPECT. Brain 1997;120(Pt 5):855–64.

82. di Corcia G, Blasetti A, De Simone M, et al. Recent advances on autosomal dominant nocturnal frontal lobe epilepsy: "understanding the nicotinic acetylcholine receptor (nAChR)". Eur J Paediatr Neurol 2005;9(2):59–66.

83. Motamedi GK, Lesser RP. Autosomal dominant nocturnal frontal lobe epilepsy. Adv Neurol 2002;89:463–73.

84. Oldani A, Zucconi M, Asselta R, et al. Autosomal dominant nocturnal frontal lobe epilepsy. A video-polysomnographic and genetic appraisal of 40 patients and delineation of the epileptic syndrome. Brain 1998;121(Pt 2):205–23.

85. Steinlein OK. Genetic heterogeneity in familial nocturnal frontal lobe epilepsy. Prog Brain Res 2014;213:1–15.

86. Bazil CW, Legros B, Kenny E. Sleep structure in patients with psychogenic nonepileptic seizures. Epilepsy Behav 2003;4(4):395–8.

87. Picard F, Makrythanasis P, Navarro V, et al. DEPDC5 mutations in families presenting as autosomal dominant nocturnal frontal lobe epilepsy. Neurology 2014;82(23):2101–6.

88. Nishibayashi N, Oka E, Ohtsuka Y, et al. Clinical course of epilepsy with continuous spike-waves during slow wave sleep. Jpn J Psychiatry Neurol 1991;45(2):425–7.

89. Sanchez Fernandez I, Chapman K, Peters JM, et al. Treatment for continuous spikes and waves during sleep (CSWS): survey on treatment choices in North America. Epilepsia 2014;55(7):1099–108.

90. Veggiotti P, Pera MC, Teutonico F, et al. Therapy of encephalopathy with status epilepticus during sleep (ESES/CSWS syndrome): an update. Epileptic Disord 2012;14(1):1–11.

91. Raha S, Shah U, Udani V. Neurocognitive and neurobehavioral disabilities in epilepsy with electrical status epilepticus in slow sleep (ESES) and related syndromes. Epilepsy Behav 2012;25(3):381–5.

92. Genton P, Thomas P, Kasteleijn-Nolst Trenite DG, et al. Clinical aspects of juvenile myoclonic epilepsy. Epilepsy Behav 2013;28(Suppl 1):S8–14.

93. Montalenti E, Imperiale D, Rovera A, et al. Clinical features, EEG findings and diagnostic pitfalls in juvenile myoclonic epilepsy: a series of 63 patients. J Neurol Sci 2001;184(1):65–70.

94. Pedersen SB, Petersen KA. Juvenile myoclonic epilepsy: clinical and EEG features. Acta Neurol Scand 1998;97(3):160–3.

95. Koepp MJ, Thomas RH, Wandschneider B, et al. Concepts and controversies of juvenile myoclonic epilepsy: still an enigmatic epilepsy. Expert Rev Neurother 2014;14(7):819–31.

96. Delgado-Escueta AV, Koeleman BP, Bailey JN, et al. The quest for juvenile myoclonic epilepsy genes. Epilepsy Behav 2013;28(Suppl 1):S52–7.

97. Kasteleijn-Nolst Trenite DG, Schmitz B, Janz D, et al. Consensus on diagnosis and management of JME: from founder's observations to current trends. Epilepsy Behav 2013;28(Suppl 1):S87–90.

98. Grunewald RA, Panayiotopoulos CP. Juvenile myoclonic epilepsy. A review. Arch Neurol 1993;50(6):594–8.

99. Janz D. Epilepsy with grand mal on awakening and sleep-waking cycle. Clin Neurophysiol 2000;111(Suppl 2):S103–10.

100. Karlov VA, Ozherel'eva Iu V. Epilepsy with generalized convulsive seizures on awakening (epilepsy with generalized tonic-clonic seizures "around sleep"). Zh Nevrol Psikhiatr Im S S Korsakova 2008;108(4):12–8 [in Russian].

101. Park SA, Lee BI, Park SC, et al. Clinical courses of pure sleep epilepsies. Seizure 1998;7(5):369–77.

102. Malow BA, Levy K, Maturen K, et al. Obstructive sleep apnea is common in medically refractory epilepsy patients. Neurology 2000;55(7):1002–7.

103. Vaughn BV, D'Cruz OF, Beach R, et al. Improvement of epileptic seizure control with treatment of obstructive sleep apnoea. Seizure 1996;5(1):73–8.

104. Koh S, Ward SL, Lin M, et al. Sleep apnea treatment improves seizure control in children with neurodevelopmental disorders. Pediatr Neurol 2000;22(1):36–9.

105. Wyler AR, Weymuller EA Jr. Epilepsy complicated by sleep apnea. Ann Neurol 1981;9(4):403–4.

106. Pornsriniyom D, Kim H, Bena J, et al. Effect of positive airway pressure therapy on seizure control in patients with epilepsy and obstructive sleep apnea. Epilepsy Behav 2014;37:270–5.

107. Pornsriniyom D, Shinlapawittayatorn K, Fong J, et al. Continuous positive airway pressure therapy for obstructive sleep apnea reduces interictal epileptiform discharges in adults with epilepsy. Epilepsy Behav 2014;37:171–4.

108. Malow BA, Edwards J, Marzec M, et al. Effects of vagus nerve stimulation on respiration during sleep: a pilot study. Neurology 2000;55(10):1450–4.

109. Marzec M, Edwards J, Sagher O, et al. Effects of vagus nerve stimulation on sleep-related breathing in epilepsy patients. Epilepsia 2003;44(7):930–5.

110. Nagarajan L, Walsh P, Gregory P, et al. Respiratory pattern changes in sleep in children on vagal nerve stimulation for refractory epilepsy. Can J Neurol Sci 2003;30(3):224–7.

111. Weinhouse GL, Schwab RJ. Sleep in the critically ill patient. Sleep 2006;29(5):707–16.

112. Claassen J, Mayer S, Kowalski R, et al. Detection of electrographic seizures with continuous EEG monitoring in critically ill patients. Neurology 2004;62(10):1743–8.

113. Hirsch LJ. Continuous EEG monitoring in the intensive care unit: an overview. J Clin Neurophysiol 2004;21(5):332–40.

114. Oddo M, Carrera E, Claassen J, et al. Continuous electroencephalography in the medical intensive care unit. Crit Care Med 2009;37(6):2051–6.

115. Kurtz P, Gaspard N, Wahl AS, et al. Continuous electroencephalography in a surgical intensive care unit. Intensive Care Med 2014;40(2):228–34.

116. Brophy GM, Bell R, Claassen J, et al. Guidelines for the evaluation and management of status epilepticus. Neurocrit Care 2012;17(1):3–23.

Neuromuscular Disorders and Sleep in Critically Ill Patients

 CrossMark

Muna Irfan, MD[a,b], Bernardo Selim, MD[a],
Alejandro A. Rabinstein, MD[b], Erik K. St. Louis, MD, MS[a,b],*

KEYWORDS

- Neuromuscular disorders • Sleep • Sleep disorders • Critical care
- Intensive care unit • Management

KEY POINTS

- Sleep problems, especially sleep-disordered breathing (SDB), are frequent in neuromuscular patients and contribute significantly to morbidity and mortality.
- SDB usually manifests before any daytime respiratory symptoms evolve in patients with neuromuscular disorders.
- Nocturnal hypoventilation is particularly common, and obstructive sleep apnea and central sleep apnea are also common comorbidities in neuromuscular patients.
- During rapid eye movement (REM) sleep, respiration depends on diaphragmatic effort, and REM-related hypoventilation and SDB are early manifestations in neuromuscular patients with evolving diaphragmatic weakness.

Neuromuscular disorders are frequently associated with sleep-disordered breathing (SDB) abnormalities, although the cumulative prevalence is not well known and probably underestimated. Between 27% and 62% of children[1–3] and 36% and 53% of adults[4] with neuromuscular disorders have SDB, depending on the type of neuromuscular disorder involved, definition of respiratory impairment, and tools used to

Disclosures: None.

The project described was supported by the National Center for Research Resources and the National Center for Advancing Translational Sciences, National Institutes of Health, through Grant Number 1 UL1 RR024150-01. The content is solely the responsibility of the authors and does not necessarily represent the official views of the NIH.

a Department of Medicine, Mayo Center for Sleep Medicine, Mayo Clinic and Foundation, 200 First Street Southwest, Rochester, MN 55905, USA; b Department of Neurology, Mayo Center for Sleep Medicine, Mayo Clinic and Foundation, 200 First Street Southwest, Rochester, MN 55905, USA

* Corresponding author. Departments of Neurology and Medicine, Mayo Center for Sleep Medicine, Mayo Clinic and Foundation, 200 First Street Southwest, Rochester, MN 55905.

E-mail address: StLouis.Erik@mayo.edu

measure SDB. Forty percent of patients followed at a Mexican neuromuscular clinic had sleep or SDB abnormalities.[4] SDB with or without nocturnal hypercapnic hypoventilation is a common complication of respiratory muscle weakness in childhood neuromuscular disorders. SDB was found in 35 of 49 patients (71%), and 24 (49%) had SDB with nocturnal hypercapnic hypoventilation.[3] Patients suffering from neuromuscular disorders may present with impairment at the levels of the upper motor neuron, lower motor neuron, nerve roots, brachial plexus, peripheral nerve, neuromuscular junction, or muscle, causing weakness of respiratory muscles that may result in SDB.

SDB often precedes daytime respiratory symptoms and may be the presenting manifestation in patients with neuromuscular disorders. Hence, untreated SDB may result in acute or chronic respiratory failure, the most common cause of morbidity and mortality in up to 80% of patients with neuromuscular diseases.[5] The risk of respiratory infections is increased by impairment of cough because of respiratory muscle or bulbar weakness, and death is frequently due to respiratory failure. In addition to diaphragmatic and respiratory muscle weakness, several other factors mediate disturbed sleep in patients with neuromuscular disorders, including those summarized in **Box 1**.

During sleep, particularly in rapid eye movement (REM) sleep, upper airway resistance increases, while chemosensitivity and skeletal muscle tone decrease (with the exception of the diaphragm), resulting in hypoventilation and leading to hypoxemic and hypercapnic failure. The most common form of SDB in patients with respiratory muscle weakness is hypoventilation due to reduced tidal volume, particularly during REM sleep, but nocturnal desaturation may occur due to nocturnal hypoventilation, periodic apneas and hypopneas, or ventilation/perfusion mismatching resulting from atelectasis in the supine posture. Secondary lung diseases, such as aspiration from pharyngeal muscles, impair deglutition and decrease cough reflex, predisposing to atelectasis and bronchiectasis, leading to long-term pulmonary fibrosis.

SDB leads to significant deterioration in both subjective and objective sleep quality, with specific common objective alterations in sleep architecture and polysomnographic parameters as outlined in **Box 2**.

SDB is more likely to occur in patients with rib cage and spinal deformities, obesity, and craniofacial abnormalities. Because neuromuscular disorders are most vulnerable to oxygen desaturation during REM sleep, suppression of REM sleep may represent a compensatory mechanism. The risk of respiratory infections including pneumonia is also increased, because of impairment of cough and clearing of secretions, given respiratory and/or bulbar weakness.

Box 1
Factors causing sleep-related difficulties in neuromuscular patients

Factors causing sleep disruption

a. Diaphragmatic and respiratory muscle weakness

b. Upper airway and craniofacial weakness

c. Difficulty with secretion clearance

d. Impairment of cough mechanism

e. Limitation of posture/discomfort due to weakness

f. Diminished ventilatory drive

Box 2
Common alterations in objective sleep parameters in neuromuscular patients

Alterations in sleep structure in neuromuscular patients

1. ↓ Total sleep time

2. ↓ Sleep efficiency

3. ↑ Sleep fragmentation

4. ↑ Arousals

5. ↑ Stage 1 sleep

6. ↓ REM sleep

When there are clinical signs or symptoms of sleep-related hypoventilation, polysomnographic evaluation and noninvasive positive pressure ventilation (NIPV) should be promptly considered. Typical signs of sleep-related hypoventilation include orthopnea, abdominal paradox in the supine position, daytime hypercapnia with $Paco_2$ greater than 45 mg Hg, impairment of pulmonary function tests (PFTs; forced vital capacity [FVC] <50%, maximal inspiratory pressure [MIP] <40 cm H_2O), waking oxyhemoglobin saturation less than 91%, or SpO_2 saturation less than 88% for 5 or more minutes.[6] Paradoxic breathing while supine is not obvious until the diaphragmatic strength is less than 25% of normal. Other typical alterations in PFTs in neuromuscular patients that suggest the need for objective assessment for SDB are summarized in **Table 1**.

Symptoms of alveolar hypoventilation include shortness of breath when sleeping supine or bending; nocturnal awakenings and difficulties to awaken in the morning hours; early morning or nocturnal headaches; decreased daytime stamina without change in weakness; shallow breathing or labored breathing, tachypnea or cyanosis while asleep; and red eyes due to conjunctival congestion. However, patients with neuromuscular disorders often fail to endorse symptoms of sleep-wake disturbance. In fact, sleep-wake symptoms poorly predict patients with neuromuscular disorders

---

Table 1
Pulmonary function and lung volume alterations accompanying neuromuscular weakness

Pulmonary Function/Lung Volume	Effect
Residual volume (RV)	↓ (With expiratory muscle weakness)
VC	Initially normal, ↓ after maximum pressures ↓ 50%
Total lung capacity (TLC)	↓ (Inspiratory weakness)
Functional residual capacity	↓ (Inspiratory weakness)
Forced expiratory volume in 1 second (FEV_1)/FVC	Normal (proportional ↓ FEV1 & FVC in inspiratory weakness)
RV	↑ (With expiratory muscle weakness)
Peak expiratory flow (PEF) maximum voluntary ventilation (MVV)	↓ (Neuromuscular weakness or effort)
Diffusing capacity	Normal (unless infiltrative/parenchymal process)
MIP	↓ (More than MEP in diaphragmatic weakness, effort)
MEP	↓ (Neuromuscular weakness, effort)

Abbreviations: MEP, maximal expiratory pressure; MIP, maximal inspiratory pressure; VC, vital capacity.

who have SDB. Signs of alveolar hypoventilation include paradoxic breathing and tachypnea in the supine position; rapid, shallow breathing and tachypnea while awake; use of accessory inspiratory respiratory muscles; and expiratory abdominal muscles to breathe. Pulmonary predictors of sleep hypoventilation include FVC less than 50% (<60% if obese, pulmonary disease comorbidity, or kyphoscoliosis); supine paradoxic breathing and tachypnea; greater than 25% decrease in FVC from sitting to supine; awake oxyhemoglobin saturation less than 91% on room air; daytime hypercapnia with $Paco_2$ greater than 45; and MIP less than 40 cm H_2O.

Because nocturnal hypoxemia is caused by hypoventilation in neuromuscular weakness, oxygen should not be used without ventilatory support. Patients with chronic hypercapnia are dependent on hypoxemic respiratory drive, and oxygen alone could further blunt the hypoxic drive to breathe, raising the risk for severe hypercapnia and respiratory failure.

Studies on sleep disorders in general and SDB in particular in neuromuscular patients hospitalized in the intensive care unit (ICU) are lacking. However, it is to be expected that the problems observed in less seriously ill neuromuscular patients will be magnified in those already exhibiting neuromuscular respiratory failure or critically ill because of intercurrent systemic disease. The pathophysiologic concepts presented above should therefore be carefully kept in mind when caring for neuromuscular patients in the ICU, especially the risk of worsening respiratory failure during the night, because patients lose respiratory muscle tone and develop more profound hypoventilation.

SLEEP-DISORDERED BREATHING MANIFESTATIONS IN SPECIFIC NEUROMUSCULAR DISORDERS
Motor Neuron Disorders

Amyotrophic lateral sclerosis
Amyotrophic lateral sclerosis (ALS), also called motor neuron disease or Lou Gehrig disease, is a fatal neurodegenerative disorder caused by fulminant degeneration of upper and lower motor neurons in motor cortex, brainstem, and spinal cord. ALS is characterized by progressive muscle weakness, atrophy, fasciculations, hyperreflexia, spasticity, and bulbar symptoms. The major cause of morbidity and mortality in ALS is denervation weakness of respiratory muscles, leading to respiratory failure. ALS exists in a sporadic form, which is most common, having onset in the sixth and seventh decades, and a familial form, comprising 5% to 10% of cases and typically evolving at a younger age.[7] ALS most frequently begins asymmetrically in the limbs (60% of cases), although bulbar variants (30%) are particularly devastating given their more rapidly progressive courses toward respiratory failure, and isolated involvement of the diaphragm and respiratory muscles also affects approximately 2% of cases at onset.[8] Nocturnal hypoventilation and oxyhemoglobin desaturation are the principal sleep-related abnormalities, and sleep apnea is most frequently described in bulbar involvement.[9]

Patients often experience frequent nocturnal awakenings, poor sleep quality often with daytime sleepiness, and morning headaches due to hypoventilation. The main cause of hypoxemia is REM sleep hypoventilation due to diaphragmatic weakness.[10] PFTs are prognostically valuable in monitoring disease progression.[11] Respiratory insufficiency during sleep can be treated with NIPV, bilevel positive airway pressure (BPAP), or tracheostomy ventilation. Objective respiratory parameters signaling the need for consideration of NIPV are shown in **Box 3**.[11,12]

NIPV improves nocturnal breathing, sleep quality, cognitive function,[13,14] quality of life, and median survival, especially in patients with normal or moderate bulbar impairment.[13] There is no demonstrated effect on certain objective polysomnographic

---

Box 3
Objective respiratory parameter thresholds suggestive of need for noninvasive positive pressure ventilation in amyotrophic lateral sclerosis

Indicators for NIPV initiation

FVC less than 50% (possibly even earlier)

Absolute MIP less than 60 CWP

SNIP less than 40 CWP

O_2 sat of $\leq$88%, 5 min

$Paco_2$ greater than 45 mm Hg

Abbreviations: CWP, centimeters of water pressure; SNIP, sniff nasal inspiratory pressure.

---

parameters, such as sleep efficiency or arousal index.[15] Mask intolerance may result from excessive sialorrhea or facial weakness and remains a challenge and potential barrier to adequate adherence to NIPV. Excessive salivation can be reduced by tricyclic antidepressants, scopolamine patches, or botulinum injection.[6] Diaphragmatic pacing stimulation to induce phrenic nerve function may delay chronic mechanical ventilation up to 24 months.[16] Goals of care need to be clarified regarding invasive mechanical ventilation by tracheostomy, which is a resource-intensive undertaking with a potentially high emotional toll. Air hunger in terminal stages is managed by palliative (hospice) care teams using morphine administration. In an epidemiologic setting, ALS survival after tracheostomy was less than 1 year.[17]

Spinal muscular atrophy/Kennedy disease

Spinal muscular atrophy (SMA) is characterized by deterioration of spinal cord anterior horn motor neurons and variable deterioration of bulbar cranial nerve nuclei. There are 4 subtypes according to age of onset. Kennedy disease (spinal muscular bulbar atrophy) is an autosomal-recessive neurodegenerative disorder associated with mutation of the androgen receptor gene. Patients may have intercostal and diaphragmatic muscle weakness with different degrees of bulbar symptoms, leading to respiratory dysfunction, hypoventilation, and SDB. Chest wall deformities and scoliosis may worsen ventilation, eventually leading to respiratory failure, especially in childhood onset forms. SDB in Kennedy disease is characterized by obstructive sleep apnea (OSA)/hypopnea, hypercapnia, and oxyhemoglobin desaturation during REM sleep. Sleep is disrupted by frequent arousals and sweating, morning headache, daytime sleepiness, and school performance difficulties in children and adolescents.[18] NIPV can improve subjective and objective symptoms of SDB. OSA is the most common sleep disorder in Kennedy disease. The sleep impairment could be induced both by OSA and by the neurodegenerative processes involving crucial areas regulating the sleep-wake cycle.[19]

Postpolio syndrome

Postpolio syndrome (PPS) may develop in patients with a history of remote acute poliomyelitis, most often occurring between 2 to 5 decades after the initial attack.[20] In primary acute poliomyelitis infection, poliovirus destroys spinal cord anterior horn motor neurons, causing denervation weakness. PPS is manifested by new weakness in previously involved and spared muscles. The process of ongoing chronic denervation due to aging-related motor neuron loss exceeds the capacity for reinnervation of the muscle by healthy neurons. Patients with bulbar forms may develop impaired respiration and swallowing.

In the PPS, central respiratory control and peripheral respiratory function might be simultaneously affected, especially in sleep. PSG most often demonstrates obstructive sleep apnea (OSA), nocturnal hypoventilation, or a combination of both, with delayed REM sleep latency and reduced REM time (probably due to pontomedullary dysfunction in bulbar form), recurrent arousals, and sleep fragmentation.[21] SDB in the form of central sleep apnea (CSA) or OSA may lead to excessive daytime sleepiness, and ultimately, respiratory insufficiency may occur. Patients with bulbar involvement have more frequent CSA, especially in non-REM sleep, suggesting reduction in forebrain control of compromised bulbar respiratory centers during non-REM sleep in PPS.[22] Patients with kyphoscoliosis secondary to polio may develop restrictive respiratory dysfunction with thoracoabdominal and accessory muscle weakness.[10,23] Therapeutic options include introduction of NIPV with pain control and physical therapy, and only rarely is tracheostomy with mechanical ventilation necessary.[20]

Spinal Cord Disorders

Spinal cord injury

Sleep disruption in patients with spinal cord injury is multifactorial, caused by location of trauma, pain, spasms, bladder distention, incontinence, medication, and restless legs syndrome, requiring a highly collaborative and integrative multidisciplinary approach. Altered sleep-wake regulation may occur if spinal cord injury extends to the brainstem and affects reticular formation functioning. Concomitant traumatic brain injury accompanying spinal cord injury may cause central posttraumatic hypersomnia by affecting hypocretinergic projections.[24] Reduced plasma melatonin concentration may also occur in these patients, with consequences including shortened total sleep duration, repeated arousals, longer wakefulness periods, and reduced REM percentage. OSA is more common in patients with spinal cord injury than in the general population.[24] One series showed that 77% of spinal cord–injured patients had SDB (apnea-hypopnea index >5 events/h), and that cervical spinal cord–injured patients had decreased variability in minute ventilation and increased end-tidal CO_2 during sleep relative to thoracic spinal cord–injured patients.[25] Sleep-related hypoventilation may occur given reduced activity of intercostal and respiratory accessory muscles, especially during REM sleep. CSA may appear after cervical spinal cord injury with involvement of brainstem respiratory centers and syringobulbia.

Defective melatonin secretion can be treated with replacement by 2 to 6 mg dosed before bedtime, and hypnotics can be used for insomnia.[24] Excessive daytime sleepiness resulting from head injuries can be treated with modafinil.[24] Treatment of SDB and central hypoventilation syndrome includes conservative approaches like positional control and minimizing respiratory suppressants, and more sophisticated strategies like NIPV, tracheostomy, and diaphragm pacing.[16]

Autoimmune/Inflammatory Neuropathies

Acute inflammatory demyelinating polyradiculoneuropathy (Guillain-Barré syndrome)

Acute inflammatory demyelinating polyradiculoneuropathy (Guillain-Barré syndrome) (AIDP/GBS) is an autoimmune process mediating rapid-onset weakness of the limbs, with varying involvement of bulbar and respiratory weakness and autonomic dysfunction. AIDP/GBS results from acute immune-mediated nerve dysfunction that is often triggered by an infectious process, especially *Campylobacter jejuni*, mycoplasma, and viral processes, such as cytomegalovirus, Epstein-Barr virus, and HIV.[26]

Progressive weakness of respiratory muscles leads to respiratory failure, whereas bulbar weakness and ineffective cough predispose to aspiration pneumonia and atelectasis (**Table 2**).

Treatment includes intravenous immunoglobulin (IVIg) or plasmapheresis with supportive measures. Serial negative inspiratory force (NIF) and FVC should be monitored with observation in ICU if vital capacity (VC) is less than 1 L/min. Intubation is indicated in 30%[27] of cases of GBS usually secondary to respiratory muscles weakness. Dysautonomia can induce severe hypotension or cardiac arrhythmias associated with the use of sedatives.

Sleep disturbances in GBS include abnormal sleep onset latency, sleep fragmentation, and reduced sleep duration. The severity of disruption correlates with anxiety, pain, paresthesia, severity of immobility, and degree of respiratory involvement. Sleep disturbances are frequent in GBS and impact more than 50% patients; in one series, symptoms of insomnia were present in 13.3%, and 51.6% had symptoms of poor sleep quality on the Richard-Campbell Sleep Questionnaire.[28] Abnormal sleep onset latency, sleep fragmentation, and reduced sleep duration were reported in 35% to 46.6% of GBS patients. Symptoms of sleep disturbance were severe during the first week of hospitalization and significantly correlated with anxiety, pain, paresthesias, and severity of immobility, and symptoms improved after discharge.[28]

NIPV is not a good option in patients with GBS because once these patients develop respiratory failure their respiratory muscle weakness will be prolonged. In addition, these patients can develop dangerous complications from dysautonomia while being treated with NIPV and particularly during emergency intubation following failure of NIPV.[29] However, NIPV is a good option in recovering patients who can be extubated, but are still weak and need overnight support.

Bilateral isolated phrenic neuropathies

Diaphragmatic palsy can develop in association with a variety of disorders causing isolated injury to bilateral phrenic nerves, resulting in respiratory insufficiency. Unilateral diaphragmatic palsy is usually asymptomatic, unless there are other comorbid restrictive or obstructive pulmonary factors impacting ventilation (ie, obesity, chronic obstructive pulmonary disease), whereas insufficiency is frequent in the setting of bilateral phrenic neuropathies.[30] Causes of diaphragmatic weakness, especially when bilateral, include inflammatory brachial neuritis (Parsonage-Turner syndrome, also known as neuralgic amyotrophy or immune brachial plexus neuropathy), or as part of a more diffuse systemic neuromuscular disorder with causes as diverse as diabetic polyradiculoneuropathy, GBS, large artery vasculitis, von Recklinghausen disease,[31] shrinking lung syndrome, or iatrogenic causes (most cases in the ICU are encountered after thoracic surgery). The poorly understood entity of bilateral

Table 2
Predictors for intubation and mechanical ventilation in acute inflammatory demyelinating polyradiculoneuropathy (Guillain-Barré syndrome)

Predictors of Mechanical Ventilation in AIDP/GBS	Indications for Intubation in AIDP/GBS
Rapidly progressive motor weakness	VC <15–20 mL/kg or with rapid decline
Involvement of limb and the axial muscles	NIF <25 cm H_2O
Ineffective cough	Hypoxemia: Pao_2 <80 mm Hg
Bulbar muscle weakness	Difficulty with secretions
Rapid decrease in VC	—

Abbreviation: VC, vital capacity.

idiopathic isolated phrenic neuropathy (BIPN) is also recognized as a rare cause of acute or subacute unexplained dyspnea, with especially prominent orthopnea.[30,32] BIPN usually has an acute, painless onset, without antecedent trigger, leading to hypercapnic respiratory failure. Patients demonstrate orthopnea, use of accessory respiratory muscles, and thoracoabdominal paradox. PFTs show an up to 50% decrease in VC between the supine and upright positions.[23] Chest radiographs show bilateral diaphragmatic elevation; electromyography demonstrates reduced or absent phrenic nerve conduction studies with active diaphragmatic denervation, and diaphragmatic ultrasound and fluoroscopy show reduced diaphragmatic excursion.[32]

Patients with both bilateral and severe unilateral IPN with coexisting pulmonary pathologic abnormalities are at high risk of SDB. Severe nocturnal hypoventilation and desaturation during REM sleep can occur, obviating polysomnographic evaluation. Patients suffer from fragmented sleep and consequently fatigue, morning headaches, and hypersomnia. Patients with unilateral diaphragmatic paralysis and concurrent ipsilateral pulmonary pathologic abnormalities often demonstrate worsened severity of disordered breathing with more profound oxyhemoglobin desaturation when they are positioned with the functioning, healthy diaphragm in recumbency during lateral non-supine sleep positions, due to worsened ventilation perfusion mismatch because the more restricted lung parenchyma is upright.[30] A minor contribution could also be due to lateral sleep on the side of the "healthy diaphragm," restricting hemithoracic expansion of the "healthy side" and exacerbating the ventilation perfusion (V/Q) mismatch.

During reinnervation of the diaphragm, which can be modest, partial, or complete, patients require NIPV to improve quality of life and prevent respiratory failure. NIPV often reduces sleep disruption and allows greater comfort and ease of resting in the recumbent position.[32,33] Diaphragmatic function can also be sustained by functional electrical stimulation of the phrenic nerve if there has not been substantial axonal degeneration.[34]

Neuromuscular Junction Disorders

Myasthenia gravis

Myasthenia gravis (MG) is an autoimmune disease characterized by fatigable weakness with antibodies directed against components of neuromuscular junction, most often against the postsynaptic nicotinic acetyl choline receptor. Muscle-specific tyrosine-kinase antibodies are also found in a subset of patients with MG. Most MG patients present with diplopia, ptosis, dysphagia, dysarthria, and weakness of limbs, neck extensors, and flexors, and facial and bulbar musculature, with involvement of the diaphragm leading to respiratory failure in severe cases. MG symptoms fluctuate and typically worsen with repeated use, especially in the evening.

Respiratory and sleep disturbances can be detected by subjective symptoms, such as nocturnal breathlessness, morning headache, fatigue, and daytime somnolence, or by objective testing demonstrating oxyhemoglobin desaturation or hypercapnia. SDB is especially prominent during REM sleep because of diaphragmatic weakness, with prominent obstructive, central, and mixed sleep apnea. OSA frequency is 15% to 20% higher in MG than in the normal population[35] because of oropharyngeal weakness. Daytime PFTs are usually normal when MG is in remission, or if there are no risk factors for respiratory compromise, such as older age, obesity, oropharyngeal weakness, or decreased total lung capacity.[36]

Although in stable disease there is no association with significant SDB,[37] myasthenic or iatrogenic cholinergic crisis (the latter resulting from excessive pyridostigmine treatment) may lead to pronounced SDB, respiratory insufficiency, and eventual respiratory failure. MG patients suspected of myasthenic or cholinergic crises require ICU monitoring, with frequent serial FVC and NIF monitoring. Intubation is indicated for FVC less than 20 mL/kg, NIF less than −20, or rapid respiratory decline with signs such as brow sweating, tachypnea, or accessory respiratory muscle use.

NIPV with BPAP can avert intubation and substantially decrease the duration of the hospitalization as compared with direct invasive ventilation.[38] BPAP should be initiated early, ideally before the development of hypercapnia, to maximize its chances of success.[38] As BPAP is being weaned off or after extubation, it is always safer to keep the patient on BPAP overnight, especially during the first 1 to 2 nights after daytime ventilation is removed.

Acute treatment of myasthenic crisis includes removing any precipitants (such as aggravating drugs, ie, β- or calcium-blocking antihypertensives, antiarrhythmics, certain antibiotics, or corticosteroids), intravenous cholinesterase inhibitor, plasma exchange, IVIg, NIPV, and steroids (which must be administered with caution and careful monitoring given propensity for temporary acute worsening of MG).

When needed, SDB is symptomatically treated by introduction of nasal continuous positive airway pressure (CPAP) or NIPV. Nocturnal hypoventilation and sleep apnea may be severe and occasionally require assisted ventilation.

Lambert-Eaton myasthenic syndrome and botulism

SDB in Lambert-Eaton myasthenic syndrome and botulism is much less frequent than in MG.[23] Significant muscle weakness can lead to severe respiratory impairment that may require assisted ventilation. Frequent clinical evaluation of the bulbar and cervical muscles can help identify segmental weakness that may assist in predicting diaphragmatic weakness and the need for NIPV or mechanical ventilation.

MYOPATHIES
Dystrophies

Duchenne muscular dystrophy

Duchenne muscular dystrophy (DMD) is a recessive X-linked muscle disease caused by mutation in dystrophin gene encoding the protein dystrophin. Clinical manifestations appear between 3 and 5 years of age, with progressive muscular weakness involving respiratory muscles ultimately causing respiratory failure, the most common cause of death (in 80%) by the third decade of life. Earlier in the course, especially in younger boys during the later first decade of life, OSA occurs commonly due to involvement of upper airway dilator muscles, and tonsillectomy alone is often sufficiently effective treatment. Progression of muscular weakness leads to musculoskeletal deformities of the rib cage in children.[10] As DMD advances, patients suffer from marked REM-related hypoventilation with profound oxyhemoglobin desaturations despite normal awake ventilation due to progressive weakness and kyphoscoliosis, especially when a state of wheelchair dependence is reached. Daytime predictors of sleep-related hypoventilation include a $Paco_2$ greater than 45 mm Hg and daytime symptoms of excessive sleepiness, morning headaches, and fatigue caused by sleep fragmentation and REM sleep deprivation.[5]

In patients suffering from sleep-related hypoventilation and daytime symptoms, polysomnography and NIPV should be considered. NIPV can improve sleep and quality of life and decrease daytime sleepiness, while improving pulmonary function and daytime gas exchange and increasing survival.[39,40] Significant nocturnal and later daytime respiratory insufficiency and ineffective coughing occur as weakness progresses, leading to complications, such as atelectasis and aspiration pneumonia, requiring 24-hour ventilatory support. Tracheostomy is indicated in patients with recurrent respiratory infections when direct airway suctioning is necessary, and in severely compromised chest wall compliance.[10]

Steroid use in children can slow progression of scoliosis and delay spinal corrective surgery.

Myotonic dystrophy

Myotonic dystrophy (DM) is an autosomal-dominant multisystem disorder affecting skeletal and cardiac muscle as well as the eye, endocrine functioning, and central nervous system. DM is divided into 2 subtypes. Myotonic dystrophy type 1 (Steinert disease, DM1) is caused by CTG trinucleotide repeat expansion of protein kinase (DMPK) gene.[41] DM1 is characterized by genetic anticipation, which results in increasingly severe phenotypic expression in successive generations. Myotonic dystrophy type 2 (DM2, proximal myotonic myopathy) results from CCTG repeat expansion within the zinc finger protein 9 (ZNF9) gene. DM2 is usually a milder phenotype with onset in middle adulthood, but may involve a different spectrum of sleep disturbances, including prominent restless legs syndrome.[41,42]

DM is characterized by muscle weakness and myotonia but may be associated with a wide variety of sleep disturbances[41–43] Interestingly, recent evidence shows extensive central nervous system white matter involvement in DM1 and DM2, while gray matter decrease (cortical areas, thalamus, putamen) was restricted to DM1.[44] In moderately advanced DM, hypersomnia, apathy, and mental decline have been linked to dysfunction of the dorsomedial thalamic nucleus.[10]

Sleep disturbances in DM may include prominent SDB with obstructive or CSA and sleep-related hypoventilation, central hypersomnia resembling narcolepsy or idiopathic hypersomnia, fatigue, insomnia, restless leg syndrome, and periodic limb movement disorder.[6,10,41,42,44,45] Because of severe diaphragmatic, intercostal, upper airway, and tongue muscle weakness, patients may demonstrate significant alveolar hypoventilation with hypoxemia and hypercapnia, especially during REM sleep. PFTs and arterial blood gases (ABGs) may underestimate the degree of nocturnal respiratory compromise, especially in DM1, where severe sleep hypoventilation may occur despite normal PFTs and ABGs while awake.[6]

In addition to prominent SDB, polysomnography in DM patients may show frequent arousals (associated with muscle pain/stiffness), decreased sleep efficiency, and frequent periodic leg movements. Central hypersomnia is especially frequent and prominent in DM1, has also been noted in DM2, and may result from decreased hypothalamic hypocretinergic and brainstem raphe serotonergic functioning and reduction of medullary reticular catecholaminergic neurons.[10] DM1 patients have been shown to demonstrate abnormal central REM sleep regulation with frequent sleep onset REM periods, increased REM density, and increased daytime and nighttime REM sleep propensity.[46]

Early PSG to evaluate for SDB may enable timely implementation of nocturnal CPAP for sleep apnea, or NIPV for sleep-related hypoventilation. If daytime somnolence persists despite effective therapy, then central nervous system stimulant drugs (eg, modafinil, methylphenidate, or dexamphetamine) may be considered,[10,43] and for significant restless legs symptoms, pharmacotherapy with a dopamine agonist drug (ie, pramipexole, ropinirole, rotigotine), or nondopaminergic agents (gabapentin, pregabalin, tramadol), may be considered.

Fascioscapulohumeral muscular dystrophy

Fascioscapulohumeral dystrophy (FSHD) is a slowly progressing myopathy resulting from macrosatellite repeat D4Z4 contraction on chromosome 4q35.[47] Polysomnography data suggest that FSHD patients are at risk for developing SDB because of pharyngeal muscle weakness, although respiratory muscles are spared. The risk is not dependent on the severity of disease, but is higher in the presence of weight gain, increased neck circumference, and kyphoscoliosis resulting from asymmetrical involvement of the trunk and scapular muscles.[47,48] Reduced nocturnal mobility also leads to poor sleep quality. Polysomnography shows longer sleep latency, frequent spontaneous arousals, reduced overall sleep time, and shortened REM sleep time.[47]

Limb-girdle muscular dystrophy
Limb-girdle muscular dystrophy (LGMD) is a descriptive term reserved for childhood-onset or adult-onset muscular dystrophy characterized by proximal skeletal muscle weakness and atrophy, with relative sparing of the bulbar muscles in most cases. Onset, progression, and distribution vary considerably among individuals and genetic subtypes, but overall LGMD is similar to Duchenne and Becker muscular dystrophy in sleep manifestations. SDB appears due to both CSA, on account of failure of respiratory control, and OSA, due to upper airway muscle weakness.[49] LGMD patients with SDB should be treated with nocturnal NIPV, and tracheostomy ventilation is rarely required.

Congenital muscular dystrophies
Congenital muscular dystrophy (CMD) is a clinically and genetically heterogeneous group of inherited muscle disorders with presentation between birth and early infancy, including laminin-α2–deficient CMD, Ullrich CMD, and muscle-eye-brain disease. Sleep is disrupted by CSA/hypopnea because of a central ventilatory control disorder, or by OSA/hypopnea resulting from upper airway muscle weakness.[49] Respiratory muscle atonia during REM sleep may cause nocturnal desaturation and hypoventilation. Early identification of SDB may prevent respiratory failure, so screening with polysomnography is recommended early in the course.[49]

Metabolic Myopathies

Metabolic myopathies are heterogeneous conditions that have common abnormalities of muscle energy metabolism, resulting in skeletal muscle dysfunction. The best known and most common example resulting in respiratory insufficiency is acid maltase deficiency, also known as Pompe disease, which is characterized by excessive accumulation of glycogen due to absence of acid maltase. The failure of diaphragmatic muscle function is most pronounced during REM sleep, resulting in SDB characterized by profound and long periods of sleep-related hypoventilation, substantial oxyhemoglobin desaturation, and hypercapnea. SDB and sleep-related hypoventilation may be predicted by diurnal PFTs.[50] To improve quality of life and prevent early respiratory failure, NIPV should be promptly instituted.[50–52] Recombinant enzyme replacement may improve survival and delay mechanical ventilation.[52]

Mitochondrial Myopathies

Mitochondrial encephalomyopathies are characterized by respiratory chain oxidative phosphorylation defects. These disorders result in reduced energy metabolism affecting the most energy-demanding tissues, primarily the muscles and brain. Prominent fatigue is typical, and various forms of nocturnal respiratory compromise have been reported.[6,51]

Inflammatory Myopathies

Inflammatory myopathies include dermatomyositis, polymyositis (PM), and inclusion-body myositis. These disorders lead to mobility impairment, loss of muscle tone, and weakness of respiratory muscles (particularly oropharyngeal muscles), leading to OSA and respiratory compromise.[53–55] PM is also associated with interstitial lung disease causing hypoxemia due to gas exchange abnormality.[53]

Critical illness neuromyopathy

Critical illness neuromyopathy (CINM) is an increasingly recognized complication of sepsis and multiorgan failure. Also known by the generic term ICU-acquired weakness, this condition can affect peripheral nerves (critical illness polyneuropathy) and muscles (critical illness myopathy). Often the disease manifests as combined signs of polyneuropathy and myopathy. Polyneuropathy is characterized by predominant motor nerve involvement, whereas myopathy is the product of myosin loss and occurs more commonly in patients treated with high-dose steroids and neuromuscular blocking.[44] CINM usually presents as unexplained, persistent diffuse weakness after respiratory support or neuromuscular paralysis, delaying weaning from mechanical ventilation.[45]

Preventive measures consist of early mobilization and reducing exposure to prolonged high-dose steroids and neuromuscular blocking agents. There is no specific treatment. Prolonged invasive ventilatory support is required given the diaphragmatic involvement. Duration of weaning can be increased 2 to 7 times, with continued supportive measures.[45] Full recovery has been reported in more than 50% of patients, although incomplete recovery remains unfortunately frequent in severe cases, and it is more common in patients with severe neuropathic involvement.[45]

DIAGNOSTIC ASSESSMENT AND APPROACH TO THE PATIENT WITH NEUROMUSCULAR DISEASE AND SLEEP-DISORDERED BREATHING

Assessment of sleep complaints is crucial in patients with neuromuscular disease for consideration of polysomnographic evaluation for OSA, CSA, or hypoventilation. A careful sleep history includes questioning about disruptive snoring, snort, or gasp arousals, witnessed pauses in breathing, and regular symptoms of morning headache, dry mouth, or sore throat. Inquiring about restless legs symptoms (uncomfortable urge to move the legs, rest onset/worsening, relief on movement or getting up to walk, and evening predominance) is also important, especially in DM patients.[42,43] However, some neuromuscular patients may still have significant SDB despite a paucity of clinical symptoms, so initial unattended screening studies such as portable oximetry should be considered to complement the history and physical examination.[43,56,57]

PFT may assist in evaluating for the likelihood of SDB, especially sleep-related hypoventilation, and may have prognostic value.[11] The most important PFT measures for prediction of SDB in neuromuscular patients are vital capacity (VC) in the upright and supine positions and maximal inspiratory and expiratory pressures. A decline in the VC between the sitting and supine positions by more than 20% is highly suggestive of diaphragmatic weakness and probable SDB and nocturnal hypoventilation. VC less than 50% and history of recurrent respiratory tract infections are frequent in patients with neuromuscular disease having nocturnal hypoventilation. Neuromuscular junction disorders, such as MG or Lambert-Eaton syndrome, lead to fluctuation of muscle weakness and VC, so caution in technique and interpretation is necessary, and declining or stable trends may be more reliable than single values. Sleep hypoventilation is especially likely when VC is less than 50% of the predicted value, or if a 20% or greater decline in VC between the upright and supine positions is seen. In such cases, polysomnography with prompt triage toward NIPV should be strongly considered.

Supine nasal inspiratory pressure (SNIP) measures inspiratory muscle function, especially diaphragmatic functioning. SNIP greater than 70 cm H_2O (in men) or greater than 60 cm H_2O (in women) essentially excludes significant respiratory muscle weakness. SNIP well predicts nocturnal hypoventilation and respiratory failure in ALS,[12] and NIPV should be initiated when SNIP is less than 40 cm H_2O.[58] Mouth pressures (maximal inspiratory pressure [MIP], maximal expiratory pressure [MEP], or bugle pressures) assess inspiratory and expiratory muscle functioning. Bugle pressure trends are very helpful in following respiratory functioning at the bedside in hospitalized neuromuscular patients, although caution is necessary in interpretation in patients with substantial facial muscle weakness, because this may lead to insufficient mouth sealing and consequently spuriously low measurements. Arterial blood gas (ABG) values remain in the normal range during wakefulness until later in the course of neuromuscular respiratory failure, and abnormal ABG values indicate significantly weak respiratory muscles, most often showing chronic, compensated respiratory acidosis with elevated $Paco_2$ and bicarbonate and normal or slightly reduced pH. Nocturnal hypoventilation is diagnosed by nighttime oxyhemoglobin desaturation (SpO_2 <88%) for 5 or more consecutive minutes, together with a morning ABG demonstrating daytime hypercapnia ($Paco_2$ >45 mm Hg) with raised pH values and bicarbonate.[6] When nocturnal hypoventilation is found, NIPV should be promptly initiated.

Portable screening devices are not very sensitive and are able to detect only moderate to severe OSA.[59] Polysomnography provides the most sensitive and specific assessment of sleep in patients with neuromuscular disorders and provide polygraphic data concerning not only respiratory function but also movement and sleep architecture. Absent REM sleep seems to correlate with a poor prognosis of neuromuscular disorders and suggests impending respiratory failure.

MANAGEMENT OF SLEEP-DISORDERED BREATHING IN NEUROMUSCULAR DISEASES

Prompt recognition and treatment of SDB in neuromuscular patients can significantly improve patient quality of life and survival. SDB may be the initial manifestation of impaired respiratory functions in neuromuscular patients. Optimizing lifestyle with weight loss for obese patients, sufficient nutrition, exercise, and rehabilitation of respiratory muscles, and ensuring adequate sleep hygiene with a regular sleep schedule and avoidance of caffeine, alcohol, or sedative drugs that may disturb sleep and suppress breathing is recommended for all patients. In acutely unstable hospital inpatients, respiratory failure can rapidly emerge, especially in AIDP/GBS, myasthenia, and high-level spinal cord injury.

For acutely deteriorating neuromuscular patients, invasive ventilation should be initiated in an ICU to avoid respiratory arrest. In most cases, endotracheal intubation with positive pressure ventilation is the preferred initial approach, although discussion concerning comorbidities, quality of life after extubation, and the patient's wishes must be rapidly considered. NIPV with BPAP is instead preferred in myasthenic crisis except in patients who have already developed severe hypercapnia, have excessive secretions (most myasthenic patients have increased respiratory secretions as a consequence of the use of pyridostigmine, but still most do well with the BPAP mask), or have such a degree of weakness and fatigue that demands controlled ventilation. Rapidly progressive bulbar and generalized muscle weakness, VC less than 20 mL/kg, Absolute MIP less than 30 cm H_2O, or MEP less than 40 cm H_2O predict impending respiratory failure and the need for invasive ventilation[60] in ALS. These numbers are sometimes extrapolated to other neuromuscular conditions, but their discriminatory value in these cases is less certain. Tracheostomy should be considered after 7 to 10 days of mechanical ventilation using endotracheal intubation because it permits better pulmonary toileting, is more comfortable to patients, reduces the risk of local complications (such as mucosal erosion and vocal cord stenosis), and might diminish the risk of infections.[61] Tracheostomy should also be considered in chronically treated neuromuscular patients when NIPV is failing, usually when bulbar muscle weakness or scoliosis progresses, for increasing patient safety when unable to clear secretions, and for prolonging survival.[12,58] Mechanical ventilation through the tracheostomy then provides positive pressure to reduce atelectasis and improves gas exchange to treat the hypercapnia from the ongoing hypoventilation. Tracheostomy impairs communication and swallowing, so is usually considered a last resort and requires careful discussion and advance planning with patients and their families.

NIPV is the preferred initial treatment of SDB and daytime ventilatory support in chronic, more stable neuromuscular patients. Two types of NIPV to consider are CPAP and BPAP. BPAP is a device that delivers a higher inspiratory than expiratory pressure that may increase tidal volume and improve alveolar ventilation, and a backup respiratory rate can be set in a BPAP spontaneous-timed mode device for patients with impaired respiratory drive or neuromuscular disease. BPAP is typically more effective for treatment of nocturnal hypoventilation, so CPAP should be initiated only when nocturnal ventilation is normal to avoid increasing burden on weak respiratory muscles. NIPV can be applied through a variety of interfaces, including nasal pillows or mask, or a full-face interface. NIPV may prevent declining lung function and improve sleep quality and quality of life.[13,15,60] NIPV should be initiated when patients become symptomatic from SDB or when FVC less than 50% is predicted, SNIP is less than 40 cm H_2O, $Paco_2$ is greater than 45 mm Hg, or when nocturnal oxyhemoglobin saturation is less than 88% for at least 5 minutes.[58,61,62] NIPV improves symptoms such as daytime sleepiness, fatigue, and morning headaches and helps sleep quality, daytime gas exchange, and nighttime oxygen saturation. It may also be used in palliative care settings when tracheostomy is not desired or is no longer needed.[1]

According to the American Academy of Sleep Medicine guidelines for NIPV, bilevel inspiratory/expiratory positive airway pressure setting titration should begin at 8/4 cm H_2O and titrated to a maximum of 30/20 cm H_2O.[6] NIPV success requires excellent patient adherence/compliance as well as interface comfort, fit, and seal. The earlier NIPV is initiated, the better tolerance may be achieved.[62] Barriers to NIPV efficacy include inability to clear secretions and neuromuscular weakness progression, Oxygen therapy can improve hypoxemia but could blunt hypoxic breathing drive if there is chronic hypercapnia, potentially leading to acute respiratory failure. Therefore, oxygen should only be used with NIPV.

Diaphragmatic pacing may replace long-term mechanical ventilation in some neuromuscular patients with intact phrenic nerve segments to stimulate the diaphragm, usually in the context of neuromuscular lesions involving failure of respiratory control centers in the brainstem, or malfunction of respiratory upper motor neurons, such as may be seen in spinal cord injury above C3 and in ALS. For ALS patients, diaphragmatic pacing may delay chronic NIPV or tracheostomy by up to 24 months.[16] Laparoscopic mapping of the diaphragm to identify optimal contractible motor points and daily diaphragmatic conditioning of weak or atrophic fibers is necessary before weaning of ventilatory support.[16]

SUMMARY

Sleep problems, especially SDB, are frequent in neuromuscular patients and contribute significantly to morbidity and mortality. SDB usually manifests before any daytime respiratory symptoms evolve in patients with neuromuscular disorders. Nocturnal hypoventilation is particularly common, and OSA and CSA are also common comorbidities in neuromuscular patients. During REM sleep, respiration depends on diaphragmatic effort, and REM-related hypoventilation and SDB are early manifestations in neuromuscular patients with evolving diaphragmatic weakness. Typical daytime symptoms of SDB include sleepiness, morning headaches, and orthopnea. Polysomnography should be considered when these symptoms emerge, or when supine abdominal paradox, daytime $Paco_2$ greater than 45 mg Hg, or impaired PFTs (VC <50% or MIP <40 cm H_2O) are seen. NIPV should then be promptly initiated because it may improve quality of life and delay mortality. In addition, other sleep problems in neuromuscular disorders may include central hypersomnia disorders similar to narcolepsy or restless legs syndrome in DM and other neuromuscular disorders, which may benefit from pharmacotherapy with stimulants or symptomatic therapies, respectively. A team approach involving critical care and sleep physicians is necessary to promptly identify and effectively treat SDB problems in patients with neuromuscular disorders.

REFERENCES

1. Perrin C, Unterborn JN, Ambrosio CD, et al. Pulmonary complications of chronic neuromuscular diseases and their management. Muscle Nerve 2004;29(1):5–27.
2. Kirk VG, Flemons WW, Adams C, et al. Sleep-disordered breathing in Duchenne muscular dystrophy: a preliminary study of the role of portable monitoring. Pediatr Pulmonol 2000;29(2):135–40.
3. Mellies U, Ragette R, Schwake C, et al. Daytime predictors of sleep disordered breathing in children and adolescents with neuromuscular disorders. Neuromuscul Disord 2003;13(2):123–8.
4. Labanowski M, Schmidt-Nowara W, Guilleminault C. Frequency of sleep-disordered breathing in a neuromuscular disease clinic population. Neurology 1996;47:1173–80.
5. Wagner MH, Berry RB. Disturbed sleep in a patient with Duchenne muscular dystrophy. J Clin Sleep Med 2008;4(2):173–5.
6. Sleep Hypoventilation in patients with neuromuscular diseases. Available at: https://www.clinicalkey.com/#!/ContentPlayerCtrl/doPlayContent/1-s2.0-S1556407X12001105. Accessed May 26, 2015.
7. Kühnlein P, Gdynia HJ, Sperfeld AD, et al. Diagnosis and treatment of bulbar symptoms in amyotrophic lateral sclerosis. Nat Clin Pract Neurol 2008;4(7):366–74.
8. Shoesmith CL, Findlater K, Rowe A, et al. Prognosis of amyotrophic lateral sclerosis with respiratory onset. J Neurol Neurosurg Psychiatry 2007;78(6):629.
9. Santos C, Braghiroli A, Mazzini L, et al. Sleep-related breathing disorders in amyotrophic lateral sclerosis. Monaldi Arch Chest Dis 2003;59(2):160–5.
10. Culebras A. Sleep-disordered breathing in neuromuscular disease. Sleep Med Clin 2008;3(3):377–86.
11. Gay PC, Westbrook PR, Daube JR, et al. Effects of alterations in pulmonary function and sleep variables on survival in patients with amyotrophic lateral sclerosis. Mayo Clin Proc 1991;66(7):686–94.
12. Benditt JO, Boitano LJ. Pulmonary issues in patients with chronic neuromuscular disease. Am J Respir Crit Care Med 2013;187(10):1046–55.
13. Annane D, Orlikowski D, Chevret S, et al. Nocturnal mechanical ventilation for chronic hypoventilation in patients with neuromuscular and chest wall disorders. Cochrane Database Syst Rev 2007;(4):CD001941.
14. Bourke SC, Tomlinson M, Williams TL, et al. Effects of non-invasive ventilation on survival and quality of life in patients with amyotrophic lateral sclerosis: a randomized controlled trial. Lancet Neurol 2006;5(2):140–7.

15. David WS, Bundlie SR, Mahdavi Z, et al. Polysomnographic studies in amyotrophic lateral sclerosis. J Neurol Sci 1997;152(Suppl 1):S29–35.

16. Onders RP, Elmo M, Khansarinia S, et al. Complete worldwide operative experience in laparoscopic diaphragm pacing: results and differences in spinal cord injured patients and amyotrophic lateral sclerosis patients. Surg Endosc 2009; 23(7):1433–40.

17. Chiò A, Calvo A, Ghiglione P, et al. Tracheostomy in amyotrophic lateral sclerosis: a 10-year population-based study in Italy. J Neurol Neurosurg Psychiatry 2010; 81(10):1141–3.

18. Mellies U, Dohna-Schwake C, Stehling F, et al. Sleep disordered breathing in spinal muscular atrophy. Neuromuscul Disord 2004;14(12):797–803.

19. Romigi A, Liguori C, Placidi F, et al. Sleep disorders in spinal and bulbar muscular atrophy (Kennedy's disease): a controlled polysomnographic and self-reported questionnaires study. J Neurol 2014;261(5):889–93.

20. Jubelt B. Post-polio syndrome. Curr Treat Options Neurol 2004;6(2):87–93.

21. Hsu AA, Staats BA. "Postpolio" sequelae and sleep-related disordered breathing. Mayo Clin Proc 1998;73(3):216–24.

22. Dean AC, Graham BA, Dalakas M, et al. Sleep apnea in patients with postpolio syndrome. Ann Neurol 1998;43(5):661–4.

23. Desai H, Mador MJ. Sleep in patients with respiratory muscle weakness. Sleep Med Clin 2008;3(4):541–50.

24. Giannoccaro M, Moghadam KK, Pizza F, et al. Sleep disorders in patients with spinal cord injury. Sleep Med Rev 2013;17(6):399–409.

25. Sankari A, Bascom A, Oomman S, et al. Sleep disordered breathing in chronic spinal cord injury. J Clin Sleep Med 2014;10(1):65–72.

26. Doorn P, Ruts L, Jacobs BC. Clinical features, pathogenesis, and treatment of Guillain-Barré syndrome. Lancet Neurol 2008;7(10):939–50.

27. Orlikowski D, Prigent H, Sharshar T, et al. Respiratory dysfunction in guillain-barré syndrome. Neurocrit Care 2004;1(4):415–22.

28. Karkare K, Sinha S, Taly AB, et al. Prevalence and profile of sleep disturbances in Guillain-Barre Syndrome: a prospective questionnaire-based study during 10 days of hospitalization. Acta Neurol Scand 2013;127(2):116–23.

29. Wijdicks EF, Roy TK. BiPAP in early guillain-barré syndrome may fail. Can J Neurol Sci 2006;33(1):105–6.

30. Khan A, Morgenthaler TI, Ramar K. Sleep disordered breathing in isolated unilateral and bilateral diaphragmatic dysfunction. J Clin Sleep Med 2014;10(5): 509–15.

31. Valls-Solé J, Solans M. Idiopathic bilateral diaphragmatic paralysis. Muscle Nerve 2002;25(4):619–23.

32. Jinnur P, Kumar N, Vassallo R, et al. Sleep pearls: a 51-year-old man with acute orthopnea and sleep-related hypoxia, with bilateral isolated phrenic neuropathy. J Clin Sleep Med 2014;10(5):595–8.

33. McCool FD, Solans M. Dysfunction of the diaphragm. N Engl J Med 2012; 366(10):932–42.

34. Grigg-Damberger MM, Wagner LK, Brown LK. Sleep hypoventilation in patients with neuromuscular diseases. Sleep Med Clin 2012;7:667–87.

35. Nicolle MW, Rask S, Koopman WJ, et al. Sleep apnea in patients with myasthenia gravis. Neurology 2006;67(1):140–2.

36. Martínez De Lapiscina EH, Erro ME, Ayuso T, et al. Myasthenia gravis: sleep quality, quality of life, and disease severity. Muscle Nerve 2012;46(2): 174–80.

37. Prudlo J, Koenig J, Ermert S, et al. Sleep disordered breathing in medically stable patients with myasthenia gravis. Eur J Neurol 2007;14(3):321–6.
38. Seneviratne J, Mandrekar J, Wijdicks EF, et al. Noninvasive ventilation in myasthenic crisis. Arch Neurol 2008;65(1):54–8.
39. Polat M, Sakinci O, Ersoy B, et al. Assessment of sleep-related breathing disorders in patients with duchenne muscular dystrophy. J Clin Med Res 2012;4(5): 332–7.
40. Simonds AK, Muntoni F, Heather S, et al. Impact of nasal ventilation on survival in hypercapnic Duchenne muscular dystrophy. Thorax 1998;53(11):949–52.
41. Schara U, Schoser BG. Myotonic dystrophies type 1 and 2: a summary on current aspects. Semin Pediatr Neurol 2006;13:71–9.
42. Lam EM, Shepard PW, St Louis EK, et al. Restless legs syndrome and daytime sleepiness are prominent in myotonic dystrophy type 2. Neurology 2013;81(2): 157–64.
43. Shepard P, Lam E, Dominik J, et al. Sleep disturbances in myotonic dystrophy type 2. Eur Neurol 2012;68:377–80.
44. Minnerop M, Weber B, Schoene-Bake JC, et al. The brain in myotonic dystrophy 1 and 2: evidence for a predominant white matter disease. Brain 2011;134(Pt 12): 3530–46.
45. Romigi A, Albanese M, Placidi F, et al. Sleep disorders in myotonic dystrophy type 2: a controlled polysomnographic study and self-reported questionnaires. Eur J Neurol 2014;21(6):929–34.
46. Yu H, Laberge L, Jaussent I, et al. Daytime sleepiness and REM sleep characteristics in myotonic dystrophy: a case-control study. Sleep 2011;34(2):165–70.
47. Della MG, Frusciante R, Dittoni S, et al. Sleep disordered breathing in facioscapulohumeral muscular dystrophy. J Neurol Sci 2009;285(1–2):54–8.
48. Tawil R. Facioscapulohumeral muscular dystrophy. Neurotherapeutics 2008;5: 601–6.
49. Pinard JM, Azabou E, Essid N, et al. Sleep-disordered breathing in children with congenital muscular dystrophies. Eur J Paediatr Neurol 2012;16(6):619–24.
50. Mellies U, Ragette R, Schwake C, et al. Sleep-disordered breathing and respiratory failure in acid maltase deficiency. Neurology 2001;57(7):1290–5.
51. Sharp LJ, Haller RG. Metabolic and mitochondrial myopathies. Neurol Clin 2014; 32(3):777–99.
52. Van der Ploeg AT, Clemens PR, Corzo D, et al. A randomized study of alglucosidase alfa in late-onset Pompe's disease. N Engl J Med 2010;362:1396–406.
53. Marie I, Hatron PY, Hachulla E, et al. Pulmonary involvement in polymyositis and in dermatomyositis. J Rheumatol 1998;25(7):1336–43.
54. Lacomis D, Zochodne DW, Bird SJ, et al. Critical illness myopathy. Muscle Nerve 2000;23:1785–8.
55. Hermans G, De Jonghe B, Bruyninckx F, et al. Clinical review: critical illness polyneuropathy and myopathy. Crit Care 2008;12:238.
56. St. Louis EK. Diagnosing and treating co-morbid sleep apnea in neurological disorders; part 2. Pract Neurol (Fort Wash Pa) 2010;9(5):26–31.
57. St. Louis EK. Diagnosing and treating co-morbid sleep apnea in neurological disorders; part 1. Pract Neurol (Fort Wash Pa) 2010;9(4):26–30.
58. Wolfe LF, Joyce NC, McDonald CM, et al. Management of pulmonary complications in neuromuscular disease. Phys Med Rehabil Clin N Am 2012;23(4): 829–53.
59. Kreitzer SM, Saunders NA, Tyler HR, et al. Respiratory muscle function in amyotrophic lateral sclerosis. Am Rev Respir Dis 1978;117(3):437–47.

60. Bourke SC, Bullock RE, Williams TL, et al. Noninvasive ventilation in ALS: indications and effect on quality of life. Neurology 2003;61:171–7.
61. Durbin CG. Indication for and timing of tracheostomy. Respiratory Care 2005; 50(4):483–7.
62. Atkeson AD, RoyChoudhury A, Harrington-Moroney G, et al. Patient-ventilator asynchrony with nocturnal noninvasive ventilation in ALS. Neurology 2011; 77(6):549–55.

Sleep in Traumatic Brain Injury

James Vermaelen, MD[a],*, Patrick Greiffenstein, MD[b],
Bennett P. deBoisblanc, MD[a]

KEYWORDS

- Traumatic brain injury • Critical care • Sleep disorders • Delirium • Melatonin

KEY POINTS

- Traumatic brain injury (TBI) is a common indication for ICU admission.
- Disruptions in sleep architecture are nearly ubiquitous in this population.
- The most commonly diagnosed sleep disturbances are insomnias, hypersomnias, and sleep-disordered breathing.
- The diagnosis of a sleep disturbance requires appropriate testing of patients for whom there is a high index of suspicion.

EPIDEMIOLOGY

There are 2 factors that challenge epidemiologic assessments of head injuries. First among them is the lack of consistency in defining the disease. TBI is defined as a functional derangement of the brain after traumatic injury. This derangement can be mild, as in a sports-related bell-ringing concussion, or it may be profound and associated with loss of consciousness and death. The use of various classification strategies makes comparisons across studies difficult. Second, there is a lack of consistency in selecting inclusion criteria for study. Some investigations include all patients who present to a hospital with a diagnosis of TBI, whereas others exclude patients managed solely in the outpatient setting or in an emergency department, even if TBI was fatal.

Despite these challenges, a couple of generalizations can be made. First, TBI is a common cause of hospitalization and ICU admission in the United States. Second, it has a trimodal age distribution, with peaks at ages 0 to 4 and 15 to 19 years and

Disclosures: None of the authors or their spouses has any commercial interests of any nature in any companies or products related to the subject matter in this article.

[a] Section of Pulmonary & Critical Care Medicine, Louisiana State University Health Sciences Center, 1901 Perdido Street, Suite 3205, New Orleans, LA 70112, USA; [b] Section of Trauma and Critical Care Surgery, Louisiana State University Health Sciences Center, 1542 Tulane Avenue, New Orleans, LA 70112, USA
* Corresponding author.
E-mail address: jverma@lsuhsc.edu

Crit Care Clin 31 (2015) 551–561
http://dx.doi.org/10.1016/j.ccc.2015.03.012
0749-0704/15/$ – see front matter Published by Elsevier Inc.

criticalcare.theclinics.com

a final upward slope over the age of 64 (**Fig. 1**).[1] The peak in early childhood is thought to be due to falls associated with increased independent activity when bipedalism is a new function. The second peak is found in adolescents and young adults who are society's greatest risk takers. The final rise is observed when sensory and motor abilities decline with advancing age.

In developed nations, the incidence of TBI requiring hospital admission is approximately 200 cases per 100,000 population per year. There has been a slight decrease in this incidence in recent years related to improved triaging after neuroimaging (**Fig. 2**).[2] In the United States, the Centers for Disease Control and Prevention estimates that approximately 25% of the nearly 2.4 million patients with TBI are hospitalized each year.[3]

There is no universal instrument for determining the severity of TBI. ICU admission is a poor surrogate for the severity of brain injury. Although mild TBI is characterized by minimal, temporary functional disability, a portion of such patients also have evidence of intracranial hemorrhage that requires close observation and frequent neurologic monitoring in an ICU. Many investigations default to the Glasgow Coma Scale score, which is often confounded by hemodynamic instability, intoxication, and preexisting conditions, such as deafness or dementia. Still others use radiographic classification, but when imaging is used alone it fails to reflect functional disturbances.

Nevertheless, up to 80% of TBI cases are classified as mild and require no further specific acute care.[2] The remaining cases are evenly divided between moderate and severe categories.[1,4] The most common mechanisms of injury among admitted patients are falls and motor vehicle collisions. Across all severities of TBI, the average ICU length of stay approximates 2 days, with an overall in-hospital mortality of 5.4%.[4] A percentage of these patients have ongoing or expanding hemorrhagic foci that subsequently have an impact on cerebral function and may lead to secondary brain injury. Patients with less severe TBI who warrant ICU admission are those with concomitant traumatic injuries of the torso, spine, or extremities and those who have suffered significant blood loss.

It has been well established that patients with TBI have a high incidence of sleep disorders, such as insomnia, hypersomnia, and sleep-disordered breathing.[5] Approximately 30% to 50% of patients complain of new-onset or worsening insomnia after

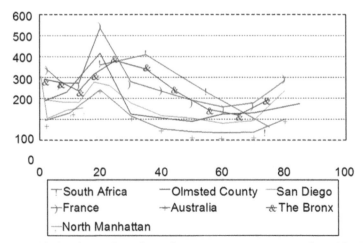

Fig. 1. Age-specific incidence of TBI. (*Data from* Bruns J Jr, Hauser WA. The epidemiology of traumatic brain injury: a review. Epilepsia 2003;44 (Suppl 10):2–10.)

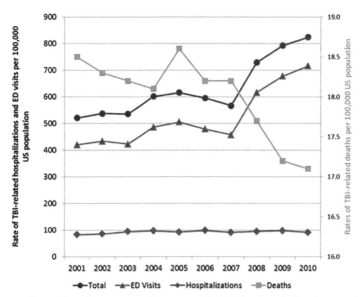

Fig. 2. Rates of TBI-related emergency department (ED) visits, hospitalizations, and deaths— United States, 2001–2010. (*From* Centers for Disease Control and Prevention. Rates of TBI-related emergency department visits, hospitalizations, and deaths — United States, 2001–2010. 2014. Available at: http://www.cdc.gov/traumaticbraininjury/data/rates.html. Accessed March 16, 2015.)

TBI. It is tempting to want to attribute insomnia to psychological conditions, such as posttraumatic stress disorder, but the incidence of insomnia after TBI has been reported to be higher than that of patients who have suffered orthopedic injuries alone.[6] Furthermore, there is a discrepancy between subjective and objective measures of insomnia after TBI, with patients overestimating the degree of insomnia experienced.

Several small cohort studies report the incidence of excessive daytime sleepiness as ranging from 25% to 52%.[6] Others estimate the incidence of posttraumatic hypersomnia to be 11% to 49%.[6] In the broader group of sleep-disordered breathing, central sleep apnea, obstructive sleep apnea, and upper airway resistance syndrome occur more commonly after TBI than in the general population.[6] In addition, there seems to be a complex interaction between brain injury, decreased arousal, impaired respiratory effort, and diminished executive functioning. Circadian rhythm disorders, movement disorders, and other parasomnias have also been reported after TBI, but their exact incidence is unclear.

PATHOPHYSIOLOGY

The pathophysiology of sleep disturbances after TBI is, for the most part, poorly understood. It is likely that many factors are involved, including

- Structural damage to sleep centers, such as the pineal gland
- Over- or underexpression of systemic neurohumoral mediators that can have an impact on sleep architecture in response to extracranial injury (eg, catecholamines)
- Impaired sleep hygiene in ICUs due to noise, artificial light, and procedures
- Administration of ICU medications that can affect sleep, such as sedatives, analgesics, and vasopressors

Direct damage can occur to the pineal gland, which synthesizes melatonin, a key regulator of normal sleep-wake cycles. Perturbations of melatonin production seem important after TBI. In an observational study, significantly lower levels of evening melatonin were found in neurotrauma patients than in age- and gender-matched controls. Furthermore, melatonin levels correlated with rapid eye movement (REM) sleep.[7] Building on these data, Yaeger[8] evaluated MRI in TBI patients. Longer tentorial length on T1-weighted imaging was shown to correlate with sleep-wake disturbance after mild TBI. In the same study, a smaller tentorial angle also correlated with sleep-wake disturbances and longer time to recovery. These data suggest that the location of the pineal gland within the tentorium and the length and angle of the tentorium itself can predict pineal gland injury and melatonin dyshomeostasis.

Axonal injury can contribute to sleep-wake disruption after TBI. In a rodent model of mild TBI, Hazra[9] demonstrated that the delayed formation of reactive astrocytes and activated microglia within the thalamus correlated with time to sleep disturbance. White matter changes also seem to play a role in sleep-wake disruption after TBI. In a retrospective study of patients with mild TBI and self-reported sleep-wake disturbances, Fakhran[10] showed significant differences in MRI fractional anisotropy in the parahippocampal regions of those patients with sleep disturbance compared with those without.

Functional changes in brain metabolism can also be seen in patients with sleep-wake disturbance after TBI. A recent study of military veterans with and without blast exposure identified decreased levels of glucose metabolism in multiple brain regions during wakefulness and REM sleep in those with TBI.[11] Other studies have also shown significantly impaired cerebral glucose metabolism in TBI patients, particularly in the thalamus.[12,13]

Hypocretin is an important mediator of wakefulness and the neurons that produce this peptide are found in the hypothalamus. The loss of hypocretin-expressing neurons may be a primary cause of narcolepsy and may contribute to sleepiness in Parkinson disease. Levels of hypocretin-1 are significantly decreased in the cerebrospinal fluid after TBI. Baumann[14] evaluated autopsy specimens of deceased patients with and without severe TBI and demonstrated that TBI patients had 27% fewer hypocretin-secreting neurons in the hypothalamus compared with controls. In another study, Nardone and colleagues,[15] using transcranial magnetic stimulation, identified decreased cortical excitability in TBI patients with excessive daytime sleepiness. They hypothesized that this was the result of dysfunction within the hypocretin neurotransmitter system.

The most plausible and best investigated pathophysiologic mechanism of sleep disturbance after TBI involves the neuropeptide melatonin. As discussed previously, melatonin is an important regulator of sleep. Although disruptions in melatonin production and regulation have been implicated in the sleep-wake disturbances of TBI, Seifman[16] demonstrated that non-TBI cohorts of ICU patients had similarly low levels of serum melatonin compared with those with TBI. This suggests that critical illness alone is enough to alter melatonin homeostasis. Both TBI and non-TBI cohorts did exhibit significantly lower levels of melatonin than normal healthy controls. Melatonin dyshomeostasis is likely involved in sleep disturbances in several illnesses.

Other physical and psychological factors can influence sleep after TBI. Sleep apnea is more prevalent in TBI population.[17] In several studies, levels of anxiety, depression, and pain in TBI patients have been shown to correlate with poor sleep quality when compared with noninjured control subjects.[18,19] Other studies have failed to show a correlation between injury severity and sleep changes.[5,18,19] Paradoxically, several investigations have shown more frequent sleep disturbances in mild TBI as opposed to moderate or severe TBI.[20,21] This may in part be due to difficulty in detecting differences in sleep quality in patients with more severe brain injury.

DIAGNOSIS

With a high prevalence of sleep disturbances in the TBI population, it is prudent for intensivists to have a high index of suspicion for these illnesses. Self-reporting instruments may be useful as screening tools, but they can be misleading, especially in the TBI population. Although there are a variety of screening tools for determining sleep disorders, only the Pittsburgh Sleep Quality Index (PSQI) has been validated in the TBI population.[22,23] Fichtenberg[22] studied 50 patients with TBI and found a 94% agreement between the PSQI and the *Diagnostic and Statistical Manual of Mental Disorders* (Fourth Edition) diagnoses of insomnia. Using a PSQI cutoff score of 8, sensitivity and specificity were 100% and 96%, respectively, and correctly distinguished 96% of insomnia cases. Some investigators, however, have reported a poorer performance of the PSQI.[23]

Although it is costly and time consuming, polysomnography (PSG) is the gold standard for evaluating sleep disorders, such as sleep apnea, narcolepsy, and periodic limb movements, all of which occur with increased frequency after TBI. Common PSG findings include longer sleep-onset latency, poor sleep efficiency, and shorter REM-onset latency.[24,25] Finally, PSG also provides added value in its ability to identify epileptiform activity in the traumatized brain.

Actigraphy, the noninvasive monitoring of human rest-activity cycles via strap-on accelerometers, is a useful method to obtain objective data when self-reporting tools are in doubt. Actigraphy correlates well with sleep duration defined by sleep diary in non-ICU populations. In the TBI population, however, this association weakens. Because of mobility impairment, actigraphy may miss arousals after sleep onset in this population.[26] If this occurs, sleep time can be overestimated.[27] In a small cohort of 16 ICU patients with TBI, actigraphs were placed for 10 days in patients who were medically stable and free from sedation. Patients who exhibited faster improvement in rest-activity cycles had lower disability at the time of hospital discharge. It remains unclear if interventions to improve this rest-activity cycle consolidation may improve outcomes.[28]

Additional testing of selected patients may be warranted after ICU discharge. The Multiple Sleep Latency Test and the Maintenance of Wakefulness Test are useful in the evaluation of patients whose ability to stay awake becomes a matter of safety. But these studies may have limited clinical utility in the TBI patient population.[29] Even after thorough testing, the cause of self-reported sleep disturbance can remain elusive. In a study of 65 patients 6-months after TBI, 43% remained without a specific diagnosis (other than TBI).[30]

NONPHARMACOTHERAPIES

There are few investigational studies of therapies that specifically target patients with TBI who have sleep disturbance. Most current recommendations have evolved from observations of unselected ICU patients. Whether studies of general ICU populations are applicable to TBI patients is unclear, but 2 general principles should apply:

1. Therapeutic interventions should be informed by the characteristics of the sleep disorder, (ie, insomnia, hypersomnia, sleep-disordered breathing, narcolepsy, and abnormalities in circadian rhythms).

2. Potential therapeutic targets should not be confined to the pathophysiologic sequelae of the injury itself but should also include preexisting neuropsychiatric conditions and the clinical treatment environment (noise, lighting, provider interruptions, drugs, and monitoring devices).

Improving sleep hygiene is the low-hanging fruit in ICUs. ICUs are noisy, artificially lighted environments that never sleep. Patient care is characterized by countless interruptions for vital signs checks, phlebotomies, radiographs, and procedures. It is intuitive that therapy for sleep disorders should start with attempts to optimize sleep hygiene. A few recent reports have described interventions that target environmental factors. In one report, a nursing-driven sleep hygiene protocol in the ICU was shown to significantly improve patient-reported sleep disruptions.[31] In a separate quality-improvement study of general ICU patients, a care bundle that focused on reducing nocturnal care activities and environmental noise and light led to reduced patient awakenings, reduced incidence and duration of delirium, and improved sleep efficiency. The reported compliance with these nonpharmacologic interventions was greater than 90%.[32] And in a third study, a provider checklist that targeted sleep hygiene in the ICU improved noise ratings and the incidence and prevalence of delirium and coma among unselected ICU patients. This intervention had no effect, however, on the results of a validated survey instrument for measuring sleep quality in ICU patients nor did it have an impact on secondary outcomes.[33]

Televisions in ICU rooms are misconceived as effective therapies for delirium. Some practitioners may even use televisions for coma stimulation. Available data do not support these practices. Instead, it is recommended that caregivers turn televisions off to improve sleep hygiene and reduce delirium.[33] Patient-directed music therapy delivered by noise-canceling headphones may, however, be useful. In a randomized study of 373 mechanically ventilated patients, self-initiated and self-terminated patient-directed music reduced anxiety and the need for sedation compared with usual care.[34] Selections were tailored by an experienced music therapist.

Sleep-disordered breathing is a common complication of TBI and is associated with a greater impairment of sustained attention and memory in TBI patients.[35] Sleep-disordered breathing is also predictive of higher all-cause mortality and recurrent vascular events after stroke and TIA.[36] Even in the absence of outcomes data, it seems prudent to identify and treat sleep apnea syndromes as early as possible in the course of TBI.

PHARMACOTHERAPY

Benzodiazepines were historically the most common class of drugs prescribed for agitation and sleep in ICUs because they have minimal cardiorespiratory side effects. Over the past decade, however, clinical investigations have highlighted the potential of benzodiazepines to be deliriogenic and prolong ICU lengths of stay.[37,38] It is still unclear if these data are applicable to TBI patients. Nevertheless, there has been reduced use of benzodiazepines and a broader use of dexmedetomidine and propofol in ICUs.

In a pilot study of 13 intubated but hemodynamically stable critically ill patients with various diagnoses, the effect of a continuous nocturnal infusion of the centrally acting α_2-agonist, dexmedetomidine, was assessed using PSG.[39] Dexmedetomidine improved sleep efficiency and reduced sleep fragmentation. The effects of dexmedetomidine on sleep architecture in TBI are unknown but it is clear that this drug can be used safely in the setting of TBI to control agitation and facilitate patient ventilator interactions.[40–43]

In experimental TBI, propofol has been shown to have both potentially beneficial and potentially harmful effects.[44,45] In patients with TBI, propofol had similar effects to midazolam on Glasgow Outcome Scale scores, mortality, intracranial pressure, and cerebral perfusion pressure.[46]

Antipsychotics are commonly used to control dissocial behaviors after TBI. Their use in ICUs is limited, however, by a paucity of clinical data. Antipsychotics have been associated with impaired neurologic recovery after experimental TBI.[47,48]

Dysautonomia may contribute to secondary brain injury in patients with severe TBI and β-adrenergic antagonists are increasingly used prophylactically to prevent this complication. A meta-analysis of cohort studies has suggested that β-blocker use may be associated with an up to 65% reduction in the adjusted odds of in-hospital death.[49] Because β-blockers are known to disrupt sleep architecture in outpatients,[50] the risks and benefits of this therapy in TBI should be tested in prospective, controlled clinical trials. One such trial, the DASH After TBI Study, is currently under way.

As discussed previously, patients with TBI have lower circulating plasma levels of melatonin, a neuropeptide involved in synchronization of circadian rhythms and sleep. Melatonin level was found significantly correlated with REM sleep in these patients.[7] Ramelteon is a highly selective melatonin type 1 and type 2 receptor agonist that can improve sleep architecture in subjects with transient insomnia.[51] In a study of hospitalized geriatric patients, ramelteon reduced the incidence of delirium by 90%.[52] Because sleep disruption and delirium often coexist in the critically ill,[53] it is intriguing to consider that therapies that target delirium in ICUs might also improve sleep architecture. Whether sleep disruption leads to delirium, whether delirium leads to sleep disruption, or whether both delirium and sleep disruption have a shared pathogenesis remains unknown. No major safety issues with ramelteon have been identified. **Table 1** summarizes the pros and cons of sedative hypnotics commonly used in ICUs in patients with TBI.

Table 1
Commonly used sedative hypnotics in the management of traumatic brain injury in ICUs

Drug	Pros	Cons
Benzodiazepines	• Antiepileptic • Minimal cardiorespiratory effects	• Can impair REM sleep • Can be deliriogenic • Prolong duration of mechanical ventilation
Dexmedetomidine	• Minimal effects of respiratory drive • Short acting • Does not adversely affect cerebral blood flow	• Requires continuous infusion • Occasionally causes bradycardia or hypotension
Propofol	• Allows control of patient ventilator dyssynchrony • Short half-life allows for easy neurochecks	• Can cause hypotension • Requires mechanical ventilation due to depression of respiratory drive • Rare propofol infusion syndrome
Ramelteon	• Improves sleep architecture • Reduces delirium	• Contraindicated with severe hepatic impairment • Some drug-drug interactions

To date there are no robust clinical data to support the use of the nonbenzodiazepine gabaergic drugs (zolpidem, zaleplon, and eszopiclone) in ICUs after TBI. Similarly, the use of antidepressants, antihistamines, and psychostimulants cannot be advocated for the treatment of sleep disorders in critically ill patients with TBI.

SUMMARY

TBI is a common indication for ICU admission. Disruptions in sleep architecture are nearly ubiquitous in this population. The most commonly diagnosed sleep disturbances are insomnias, hypersomnias, and sleep-disordered breathing. The pathophysiology of sleep disturbance after TBI may involve direct injury to sleep centers, neurohormonal responses to injury, poor ICU sleep hygiene, and side effects of medications. The diagnosis of a sleep disturbance requires appropriate testing of patients for whom there is a high index of suspicion. Therapy is focused on improving ICU sleep hygiene, treating sleep-disordered breathing, and the careful selection of sedative-hypnotics and anxiolytics.

REFERENCES

1. Bruns J Jr, Hauser WA. The epidemiology of traumatic brain injury: a review. Epilepsia 2003;44(Suppl 10):2–10.
2. Centers for Disease Control and Prevention. Rates of TBI-related emergency department visits, hospitalizations, and deaths — United States, 2001–2010. 2014. Available at: http://www.cdc.gov/traumaticbraininjury/data/rates.html. Accessed March 16, 2015.
3. McGuire L. CDC grand rounds: reducing severe traumatic brain injury in the United States. MMWR Morb Mortal Wkly Rep 2013;62:549–52.
4. Stead LG, Bodhit AN, Patel PS, et al. Emergency Medicine traumatic brain injury research network I. TBI surveillance using the common data elements for traumatic brain injury: a population study. Int J Emerg Med 2013;6:5.
5. Castriotta R. Prevalence and consequences of sleep disorders in traumatic brain injury. J Clin Sleep Med 2007;3:349–56.
6. Castriotta RJ, Murthy JN. Sleep disorders in patients with traumatic brain injury: a review. CNS Drugs 2011;25:175–85.
7. Shekleton JA, Parcell DL, Redman JR, et al. Sleep disturbance and melatonin levels following traumatic brain injury. Neurology 2010;74:1732–8.
8. Yaeger K. Evaluation of tentorial length and angle in sleep-wake disturbances after mild traumatic brain injury. Am J Roentgenol 2013;202:614–8.
9. Hazra A. Delayed thalamic astrocytosis and disrupted sleep-wake patterns in a preclinical model of traumatic brain injury. J Neurosci Res 2014;92:1434–45.
10. Fakhran S. Symptomatic white matter changes in mild traumatic brain injury resemble pathologic features of early alzheimer dementia. Radiology 2013;269:249–57.
11. Stocker R. Combat-related blast exposure and traumatic brain injury influence brain glucose metabolism during REM sleep in military veterans. Neuroimage 2014;99:207–14.
12. Garcia-Panach JA. Voxel-based analysis of FDG-PET in traumatic brain injury: regional metabolism and relationship between the thalamus and cortical areas. J Neurotrauma 2011;28:1707–17.
13. Nakayama N. Relationship between regional cerebral metabolism and consciousness disturbance in traumatic diffuse brain injury without large focal

lesions: an FDG-PET study with statistical parametric mapping analysis. J Neurol Neurosurg Psychiatry 2006;77:856–62.

14. Baumann C. Loss of hypocretin (orexin) neurons with traumatic brain injury. Ann Neurol 2009;66:555–9.

15. Nardone R, Bergmann J, Kunz A, et al. Cortical excitability changes in patients with sleep-wake disturbances after traumatic brain injury. J Neurotrauma 2011; 28:1165–71.

16. Seifman M. Measurement of serum melatonin in intensive care unit patients: changes in traumatic brain injury. Front Neurol 2014;5:237.

17. Mathias J. Prevalence of sleep disturbances, disorders, and problems following traumatic brain injury: a meta-analysis. Sleep Med 2012;13:898–905.

18. Makley M. Changes in sleep patterns following traumatic brain injury: a controlled study. Neurorehabil Neural Repair 2013;27:613–21.

19. Parcell D. Poor sleep quality and changes in objectively recorded sleep after traumatic brain injury: a preliminary study. Arch Phys Med Rehabil 2008;89: 843–50.

20. Mahmood O. Peuropsychological performance and sleep disturbance following traumatic brain injury. J Head Trauma Rehabil 2004;19:378–90.

21. Pillar G. Prevalence and risk of sleep disturbances in adolescents after minor head injury. Pediatr Neurol 2003;29:131–5.

22. Fichtenberg N. Insomnia screening in postacute traumatic brain injury: utility and validity of the Pittsburgh sleep quality index. Am J Phys Med Rehabil 2001;80: 339–45.

23. Masel BE, Scheibel RS, Kimbark T, et al. Excessive daytime sleepiness in adults with brain injuries. Arch Phys Med Rehabil 2001;82:1526–32.

24. Ouellet MC, Morin CM. Subjective and objective measures of insomnia in the context of traumatic brain injury: a preliminary study. Sleep Med 2006;7: 486–97.

25. Williams BR, Lazic SE, Ogilvie RD. Polysomnographic and quantitative EEG analysis of subjects with long-term insomnia complaints associated with mild traumatic brain injury. Clin Neurophysiol 2008;119:429–38.

26. Sinclair KL, Ponsford J, Rajaratnam SM. Actigraphic assessment of sleep disturbances following traumatic brain injury. Behav Sleep Med 2014;12:13–27.

27. Zollman FS, Cyborski C, Duraski SA. Actigraphy for assessment of sleep in traumatic brain injury: case series, review of the literature and proposed criteria for use. Brain Inj 2010;24:748–54.

28. Duclos C, Dumont M, Blais H, et al. Rest-activity cycle disturbances in the acute phase of moderate to severe traumatic brain injury. Neurorehabil Neural Repair 2013;28:472–82.

29. Bonnet M. ACNS clinical controversy: MSLT and MWT have limited clinical utility. J Clin Neurophysiol 2006;23:50–8.

30. Baumann C. Sleep-wake disturbances 6 months after traumatic brain injury: a prospective study. Brain 2007;130:1873–83.

31. Faraklas I, Holt B, Tran S, et al. Impact of a nursing-driven sleep hygiene protocol on sleep quality. J Burn Care Res 2013;34:249–54.

32. Patel J, Baldwin J, Bunting P, et al. The effect of a multicomponent multidisciplinary bundle of interventions on sleep and delirium in medical and surgical intensive care patients. Anaesthesia 2014;69:540–9.

33. Kamdar BB, King LM, Collop NA, et al. The effect of a quality improvement intervention on perceived sleep quality and cognition in a medical ICU. Crit Care Med 2013;41:800–9.

34. Chlan LL, Weinert CR, Heiderscheit A, et al. Effects of patient-directed music intervention on anxiety and sedative exposure in critically ill patients receiving mechanical ventilatory support: a randomized clinical trial. JAMA 2013;309: 2335–44.

35. Wilde MC, Castriotta RJ, Lai JM, et al. Cognitive impairment in patients with traumatic brain injury and obstructive sleep apnea. Arch Phys Med Rehabil 2007;88: 1284–8.

36. Birkbak J, Clark AJ, Rod NH. The effect of sleep disordered breathing on the outcome of stroke and transient ischemic attack: a systematic review. J Clin Sleep Med 2014;10:103–8.

37. Jakob SM, Ruokonen E, Grounds RM, et al. Dexmedetomidine for long-term sedation I. Dexmedetomidine vs midazolam or propofol for sedation during prolonged mechanical ventilation: two randomized controlled trials. JAMA 2012;307: 1151–60.

38. Fraser GL, Devlin JW, Worby CP, et al. Benzodiazepine versus nonbenzodiazepine-based sedation for mechanically ventilated, critically ill adults: a systematic review and meta-analysis of randomized trials. Crit Care Med 2013;41:S30–8.

39. Alexopoulou C, Kondili E, Diamantaki E, et al. Effects of dexmedetomidine on sleep quality in critically ill patients: a pilot study. Anesthesiology 2014;121: 801–7.

40. Hao J, Luo JS, Weng Q, et al. [Effects of dexmedetomidine on sedation and beta-endorphin in traumatic brain injury: a comparative study with propofol]. Zhonghua Wei Zhong Bing Ji Jiu Yi Xue 2013;25:373–6 [in Chinese].

41. Schoeler M, Loetscher PD, Rossaint R, et al. Dexmedetomidine is neuroprotective in an in vitro model for traumatic brain injury. BMC Neurol 2012;12:20.

42. Tang JF, Chen PL, Tang EJ, et al. Dexmedetomidine controls agitation and facilitates reliable, serial neurological examinations in a non-intubated patient with traumatic brain injury. Neurocrit Care 2011;15:175–81.

43. Wang X, Ji J, Fen L, et al. Effects of dexmedetomidine on cerebral blood flow in critically ill patients with or without traumatic brain injury: a prospective controlled trial. Brain Inj 2013;27:1617–22.

44. Rossaint J, Rossaint R, Weis J, et al. Propofol: neuroprotection in an in vitro model of traumatic brain injury. Crit Care (London, England) 2009;13:R61.

45. Thal SC, Timaru-Kast R, Wilde F, et al. Propofol impairs neurogenesis and neurologic recovery and increases mortality rate in adult rats after traumatic brain injury. Crit Care Med 2014;42:129–41.

46. Gu JW, Yang T, Kuang YQ, et al. Comparison of the safety and efficacy of propofol with midazolam for sedation of patients with severe traumatic brain injury: a meta-analysis. J Crit Care 2014;29:287–90.

47. Hoffman AN, Cheng JP, Zafonte RD, et al. Administration of haloperidol and risperidone after neurobehavioral testing hinders the recovery of traumatic brain injury-induced deficits. Life Sci 2008;83:602–7.

48. Kline AE, Hoffman AN, Cheng JP, et al. Chronic administration of antipsychotics impede behavioral recovery after experimental traumatic brain injury. Neurosci Lett 2008;448:263–7.

49. Alali AS, McCredie VA, Golan E, et al. Beta blockers for acute traumatic brain injury: a systematic review and meta-analysis. Neurocrit Care 2014;20: 514–23.

50. Betts TA, Alford C. Beta-blockers and sleep: a controlled trial. Eur J Clin Pharmacol 1985;28(Suppl):65–8.

51. Roth T, Stubbs C, Walsh JK. Ramelteon (TAK-375), a selective MT1/MT2-receptor agonist, reduces latency to persistent sleep in a model of transient insomnia related to a novel sleep environment. Sleep 2005;28:303–7 [Erratum appears in Sleep 2006;29(4):417 Note: Dosage error in article text].

52. Hatta K, Kishi Y, Wada K, et al. Preventive effects of ramelteon on delirium: a randomized placebo-controlled trial. JAMA Psychiatry 2014;71:397–403.

53. Weinhouse GL, Schwab RJ, Watson PL, et al. Bench-to-bedside review: delirium in ICU patients - importance of sleep deprivation. Crit Care (London, England) 2009;13:234.

Sedation in Critically Ill Patients

Mark Oldham, MD[a], Margaret A. Pisani, MD, MPH[b],*

KEYWORDS

- Sedation • Critically ill patients • Intensive care unit • Pain • Circadian rhythm
- Delirium

KEY POINTS

- Our understanding of the importance of sleep on recovery of patients who experience critical illness is still in its infancy.
- Although there is biological plausibility regarding the impact and importance of sleep in intensive care unit (ICU) patients especially related to immune dysfunction, infection risk, prolonged length of mechanical ventilation, and delirium development and duration, there are little published data.
- Despite the challenges of caring for critically ill patients, following the recommended guidelines for pain, agitation, and delirium, paying attention to early mobilization and sleep hygiene and individualizing patient care as needed, should lead to the best outcomes for patients.
- Future research studies should continue to inform our practice regarding treatment of pain, agitation, and delirium in the ICU.

INTRODUCTION

Sedation in the intensive care unit (ICU) is a topic that has been frequently researched, and debate still exists as to what are the best sedative agents for critically ill patients. There is increasing interest in sleep and circadian rhythm disturbances in the ICU and how they may impact on outcomes. In addition to patient-related and ICU environmental factors that likely impact sleep and circadian rhythm in the ICU, sedative and analgesic medications may also play a role. This article focuses on

- Current practice guidelines related to pain, sedation, and delirium in the ICU
- Effects of medications used for pain, sedation, and delirium on sleep stages
- Effects of medications used for pain, sedation, and delirium on circadian rhythm
- Conclusions on the interactions between medications, sleep, and circadian rhythm in the ICU

Disclosures: none.
[a] Department of Psychiatry, Yale-New Haven Hospital, 15 York Street, New Haven, CT 06510, USA; [b] Section of Pulmonary, Critical Care & Sleep Medicine, Yale University School of Medicine, PO Box 208057, TAC S425C, New Haven, CT 06520-8057, USA
* Corresponding author.
E-mail address: margaret.pisani@yale.edu

BACKGROUND

When patients are critically ill and admitted to an ICU, they are frequently intubated and mechanically ventilated. Historically when patients were placed on a ventilator they received large amounts of sedation. Work by Kress and colleagues[1] in 2000 demonstrated that you could safely stop sedation on a daily basis and allow patients to wake up. The benefits of this daily interruption of sedation and awakening has now been studied in several other trials and linked to spontaneous breathing trials in ventilated patients. Several recent reviews have summarized the importance of minimizing the amount of sedation in critically ill patients. **Fig. 1** presents a schematic of the interrelationship between critical illness, ICU care, and long-term outcomes.

Sedation in the Intensive Care Unit: Current Practice and Practice Guidelines

The Society of Critical Care Medicine released updated practice guidelines about the management of pain, agitation, and delirium (PAD) in 2013.[2] These guidelines used the GRADE methodology (Grading of Recommendations, Assessment, Development, and Evaluation) in their development. During the process of guideline development, the task force members posed clinically relevant questions that could be systematically evaluated using evidence in the literature. These questions were then transformed into descriptive clinical statements and actionable items. Each statement and recommendation included an assessment of the strength of the evidence based on the strength of the evidence and the relative risk or benefit of the treatment. Statements were defined as *weak* or *strong*; weak recommendations were worded as *we suggest*, and strong recommendations were worded as *we recommend*. No recommendation was made when there was a lack of sufficient evidence and consensus opinion was not used to make recommendations. In addition, an anonymous, online, iterative voting schema was used to achieve rapid and transparent consensus regarding the statements and recommendations. **Table 1** highlights the recommendations for PAD from the 2013 PAD guidelines.

Pain, agitation, and delirium assessments

The guidelines stress the importance of frequent evaluation of critically ill patients using validated measurement tools. For pain, using a patient self-report with a 1 to 10 numerical rating scale (NRS) is the preferred method for those patients who are able to respond. In those patients who are unable to use an NRS, a Behavioral Pain Scale (BPS) is recommended. Either the BPS[3] or Critical-Care Pain Observation Tool (CPOT)[4] can be used in the evaluation of critically ill patients. Both instruments are valid

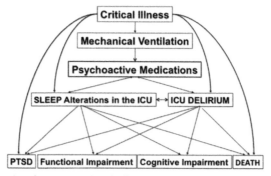

Fig. 1. The interaction between critical illness, ICU care, and patient outcomes. PTSD, posttraumatic stress disorder.

Table 1
PAD recommendations

	Pain	Agitation	Delirium
Assess	**≥4 Times Per Shift & prn**	**≥4 Times Per Shift & prn**	**Once a Shift & prn**
Assessment tools	• Self-report use the NRS • Unable to self-report use the BPS or CPOT	• RASS • SAS • With NMB use brain function monitoring	• CAM-ICU • ICDSC
Treat	Treat within 30 min *Nonpharmacologic:* relaxation therapy *Pharmacologic:* IV opioids: non-neuropathic pain Gabapentin or carbamazepine-neuropathic Epidural: postoperatively	Sedation should be targeted to a RASS (−2 to 0) or SAS (3–4) goal • *Agitation* (RASS >0, SAS >4): treat pain and with sedatives prn (propofol or dexmedetomidine preferred over benzodiazepines) • *Oversedated* (RASS <−2, SAS <3): hold sedatives until at target and then restart at 50% prior dose	Treat pain if present *Nonpharmacologic:* reorient, glasses, hearing aids *Pharmacologic:* no recommendation to treat delirium with medications *Suggest:* avoiding benzodiazepines, rivastigmine and avoiding antipsychotics if increased risk of Torsades de pointes
Prevent	Provide preprocedural analgesia and/or nonpharmacologic interventions Treat pain first and then provide sedation if needed	Daily SBT, early mobility when at goal sedation level, unless contraindicated EEG monitoring for those at seizure risk; treat burst suppression when there is an increased ICP	Identify delirium risk factors Early mobilization Sleep promotion Continue/restart baseline psychiatric medications if indicated

Abbreviations: BPS, Behavioral Pain Scale; CAM-ICU, Confusion Assessment Method for the ICU; CPOT, Critical, Care Pain Observation Tool; EEG, electroencephalography; ICDSC, Intensive Care Unit Delirium Screening Checklist; ICP, intracranial pressure; IV, intravenous; NMB, neuromuscular blockade; NRS, numeric rating scale; prn, as needed; RASS, Richmond Agitation Sedation Scale; SAS, Sedation Agitation Scale; SBT, spontaneous breathing trial.

Adapted from Barr J, Fraser GL, Puntillo K, et al. Clinical practice guidelines for the management of pain, agitation, and delirium in adult patients in the intensive care unit. Crit Care Med 2013;41(1):263–306.

and reliable. The use of observational pain scales that utilize vital signs are not reliable for the assessment of pain.[5,6] Pain should be assessed at least 4 times per a 12-hour nursing shift and more frequently if needed.

Assessing sedation in the ICU routinely is important for reducing oversedation and ensuring that patients are comfortable. The Richmond Agitation-Sedation Scale (RASS)[7] and the Sedation Agitation Scale[8] are the 2 instruments recommended by the PAD guidelines based on studies of their validity and reliability for assessing both the quality and depth of sedation in critically ill patients.[9,10] Sedation should also be assessed at least 4 times per a 12-hour nursing shift or more frequently if needed. Patients who are paralyzed with neuromuscular blocking agents cannot be assessed with sedation scales and should be monitored with objective measures of brain function, such as bispectral index or auditory evoked potentials.[11,12]

Delirium rates have been reported to be as high as 80% in research studies of critically ill patients, but it is frequently undiagnosed clinically.[13,14] Delirium has shown to increase length of mechanical ventilation, ICU and hospital length of stay, and mortality as well as increasing the risk for long-term cognitive dysfunction.[15–19] The PAD guidelines make a strong recommendation for delirium screening once each nursing shift and more frequently depending on patient status. The 2 recommended instruments for delirium screening are the Confusion Assessment Method for the ICU[20,21] and the Intensive Care Delirium Screening Checklist.[22]

Management of pain, agitation, and delirium

The PAD guidelines make several strong recommendations for treating pain in ICU patients. These recommendations include administering pain medications in the presence of significant pain determined by an NRS of 4 or greater, a BPS greater than 5, or a CPOT of 3 or greater and before performing any painful invasive procedure. Parenteral opioids should be the first-line treatment of non-neuropathic pain, and either gabapentin or carbamazepine can be given enterally for neuropathic pain either alone or in addition to opioids. Acetaminophen, nonsteroidal antiinflammatory drugs, or ketamine can be used as adjunctive pain medications in select patient populations to reduce dosing requirements and side effects from opioids.

Based on randomized controlled trials, the 2013 PAD guidelines emphasize the importance of minimizing sedation use that includes targeted sedation and daily sedative interruption.[2] The guidelines recommend treating pain first, that is, using analgesia first and then the sedative medication approach. Based on a meta-analysis performed during the development of the PAD guidelines that compared ICU outcomes in patients who received benzodiazepines versus nonbenzodiazepines (propofol or dexmedetomidine), there is a weak recommendation for preferential use of nonbenzodiazepines for sedation in critically ill patients.[2] Clearly the choice of a sedative agent needs to be tailored to the individual patient's clinical presentation; there is a role of benzodiazepines in patients with alcohol withdrawal, seizures, or severe anxiety and when there is a need for deep sedation.[23,24]

In a change from the 2002 guidelines, the 2013 PAD guidelines do not include a specific medication recommendation for treating delirium. Although haloperidol has been recommended to treat delirium in numerous reviews and guidelines, this is secondary to extrapolated data in its use for treating psychosis. There are no randomized controlled trials (RCTs) that have examined the use of haloperidol for treating delirium in critically ill patients. There are some small studies that have suggested that atypical antipsychotics may reduce delirium duration in critically ill patients, but they are not definitive.[25–27] Currently there is an ongoing multicenter RCT examining the use of haloperidol versus ziprasidone versus placebo, the MIND-USA (Modifying the Incidence of Neurologic Dysfunction-USA) study, which should answer questions regarding the use of these medications for delirium treatment. The one specific recommendation the PAD guidelines make regarding delirium treatment is against the use of rivastigmine secondary to high mortality rates observed during its use in ICU patients.[28] Two large RCTs demonstrated that the prevalence of delirium was lower in patients who were sedated with dexmedetomidine versus benzodiazepines.[29,30] Based on these two studies, the PAD guidelines recommend the avoidance of benzodiazepines in patients with delirium.

Although the PAD guidelines do not make any strong recommendations regarding the use of medications for delirium prevention in the ICU, they strongly recommend the use of early and progressive mobilization and the promotion of sleep hygiene. Sleep hygiene recommendations include reduction of noise and light at night and clustering of patient care activities to prevent sleep disruption. Both mobilization and sleep hygiene should help to maintain a normal circadian rhythm for ICU patients.

In summary, a key message of the PAD guidelines is the importance of integrated and patient-centered care for PAD in the ICU.

Sleep Physiology

Physiologic sleep architecture

Sleep is critical for health and well-being, particularly among the critically ill. From the late 1960s until just recently, the pioneering work of Rechtschaffen and Kales[31] has served as the standard for classifying sleep architecture. In this system, sleep stages are divided into rapid eye movement (REM) sleep and non-REM (NREM) sleep, with NREM being further subdivided into 4 stages numbered NREM 1 through NREM 4. More recently, the American Academy of Sleep Medicine (AASM) published new scoring criteria in which NREM is subdivided into 3 stages (N1, N2, N3). Effectively, NREM 3 and 4 are condensed into N3.[32] Polysomnography (PSG), which principally includes electroencephalography (EEG), electrooculography (EOG), and electromyography (EMG), is required for classification of sleep architecture with sleep/wake stages scored based on 30-second periods known as epochs.

The first stage of sleep is almost always N1, which represents the transition from wakefulness to other sleep stages. It comprises less than 5% of total sleep time (TST) and is characterized by EEG waves in the theta range (4–7 Hz). Additional features include slow, conjugate eye movements and vertex sharp waves.[32] N2 comprises roughly a half of TST and is defined by the presence of either K complexes (specifically those unassociated with arousals) or sleep spindles. A person is said to have entered N3, perhaps more commonly known as *slow wave sleep*, once slow, high-amplitude waves in the delta frequency (0.5–2.0 Hz) are seen over the frontal regions for at least 20% of an epoch. N3 seldom comprises more than 20% TST. REM sleep is characterized by an EEG similar to wakefulness (low amplitude, mixed frequency tracings), with the additional findings of REM on EOG and low tone on chin EMG. REM accounts for roughly a quarter of TST in healthy individuals.[33]

Physiologic sleep involves recurring 1- to 2-hour cycles of varying sleep depth. Initially, a person passes from wakefulness to N1 en route to N2. From here, sleep deepens to N3 then returns to N2 before entering REM. Most NREM sleep is achieved during the first few hours of a sleep period, with REM predominating toward the end of the sleep period. In the ICU, however, altered states of consciousness have been proposed because traditional sleep classification does not encompass findings from PSG among the critically ill.[34,35] Broadly, these proposals have included states of *pathologic wakefulness* and *atypical sleep*. In fact, in a recent PSG study of 37 ICU patients, 85% of all around-the-clock PSG data obtained could not be classified as *either* traditional wake or sleep based on AASM criteria.[35]

Two-process model of sleep

Borbély's[36] proposed 2-process model of sleep, which consists of a sleep-dependent homeostatic drive and a sleep-independent circadian component (Process S & C, respectively), remains the predominant model to explain sleep coordination. With prolonged sleep restriction, homeostatic drive (Process S) builds to create greater sleep propensity and ultimately deeper sleep; Process S may explain why deeper sleep occurs during the first third of the night. An independent circadian rhythm (Process C) is much more closely allied with the generation and timing of REM sleep.

In the following 2 sections, the authors take these two processes, S and C, in turn. First the effects of sedative agents on traditional sleep stages with an emphasis on NREM are discussed (see **Table 1**). Next the potential effects of sedatives on circadian rhythm with a broader consideration of 24-hour patterns of psychomotor activity are addressed.

Effects of Sedatives on Sleep Stages

Benzodiazepines

Since the introduction of chlordiazepoxide in 1957, the benzodiazepines have all but entirely supplanted the forerunning barbiturates and have found diverse utility in both inpatient and outpatient settings. Although often incorrectly described as γ-aminobutyric acid (GABA) agonists, benzodiazepines bind at a site distinct from GABA on a ligand-gated chloride ion channel. They serve as positive allosteric modulators of $GABA_A$ receptors because their binding facilitates the binding of GABA to $GABA_A$ receptors by way of a conformational change.[37] Indications for benzodiazepines include anxiety, panic disorder, alcohol withdrawal, preoperative apprehension, acute treatment of seizures, muscle spasms, short-term use for insomnia, and, in the case of midazolam, parenteral use for sedation. Common off-label uses include general sedation, acute management of agitation, adjunctive administration for mania, and treatment of acute catatonia. In particular, caution should be exercised in children, older patients, and those with acquired brain injury given the risk of delirium[38,39] and paradoxic agitation.[40] Later the authors discuss the 3 most common benzodiazepines used in the ICU: lorazepam, midazolam, and diazepam.[1]

Class effects on sleep stages

In general, benzodiazepines increase sleep efficiency (SE; ie, time asleep divided by time in bed), shorten sleep latency (SL; ie, time to fall asleep), suppress REM and N3, and cause a respective increase in percent of TST spent in N2.[41,42] Benzodiazepines constrict sleep to the theta-frequency range (4–7 Hz) at the expense of restorative slow wave (N3) sleep and memory-consolidating REM sleep. In fact, N3 suppression has been documented on drug-free nights even after one dose of midazolam, triazolam, or flurazepam the night prior.[43,44] Cerebral blood flow during benzodiazepine sedation differs from that seen with physiologic sleep.[45]

Benzodiazepines may also alter sleep in withdrawal. Sleep fragmentation is a common feature of benzodiazepine withdrawal that may persist for months after the last use.[37] A retrospective review of 28 mechanically ventilated ICU patients demonstrated that after only a few weeks of ICU-level care, patients may be at risk of developing acute withdrawal from sedatives, including benzodiazepines and opioids.[46]

Most deliria are characterized by diffuse slowing of brain waves on EEG, with triphasic waves and spindle comas perhaps representing unique clinical entities.[47] However, benzodiazepines, although deliriogenic, tend to increase the prevalence of fast, β waves and decrease the amplitude of the EEG tracing.[48] Such findings are consistent with their suppression of slow wave sleep.

Midazolam

Although available as an oral formulation outside the US, midazolam is restricted in the US to parenteral use for sedation of intubated or mechanically ventilated patients in the ICU, anesthesia induction, premedication before surgery, or procedural sedation. Studies of midazolam use for sedation in the ICU have uniformly revealed abnormal sleep architecture.[49–51] In particular, the effects of midazolam on sleep stages in mechanically ventilated patients has been studied comparing 2 different protocols: constant sedation (CS; $n = 11$) versus daily sedative interruption (DSI; $n = 11$).[49] In

---

[1] Although alprazolam is sometimes used in critical care settings, its short half-life and potent binding affinity mean that rebound anxiety, abuse liability, and potential for complicated withdrawal including seizures are all increased with this agent. It does not seem to offer significant benefits over the 3 agents discussed here.

this study, midazolam was titrated to achieve a RASS score of −4 to −5 during infusion. All subjects had abnormal sleep architecture, but 24-hour PSG revealed the DSI subjects had greater total duration of N3 (54 vs 0 minutes) and REM (6 vs 0 minutes) relative to CS subjects. The absence of *any* N3 or REM sleep among CS subjects is striking. Similarly, reportedly optimized midazolam infusion for sleep among 5 ICU subjects resulted in a median of 10-minute REM, no N3 sleep, and a median of 16 awakenings per hour.[50] Clearly, midazolam does not promote physiologic sleep.

Lorazepam

As with other benzodiazepines, lorazepam causes a shift toward N2 sleep and suppresses REM. Its sedative effects occur 10 to 40 minutes after peak plasma concentration because of the time required for entrance into the central nervous system,[52] and its half-life of 8 to 15 hours precludes minute-to-minute dose titration to achieve a narrowly defined sedation level. Although most of the evidence for lorazepam's effects on sleep is derived from outpatient settings, bolus lorazepam followed by infusion has been shown to increase β frequency on EEG.[53] In particular, cumulative daily lorazepam dose equivalents were found to be an independent predictor of severe REM reduction, defined as REM comprising less than 6% of TST, in a cohort of surgical ICU patients.[54]

In contradistinction to the division between REM and NREM sleep—collectively known as sleep macrostructure—studies have investigated subtle changes in brain wave patterns known as *sleep microstructure*. One such microstructural parameter, cyclic alternating pattern (CAP), seems to reflect instability of arousal and may detect the effects of ambient noise in situational insomnia.[55] In an outpatient study of healthy volunteers, lorazepam was only partly effective at blunting the effects of ambient noise on sleep disruption as reflected in CAP rate. Perhaps studies of sleep microstructure in the ICU would provide valuable information on how sedatives mediate the relationship between ambient stimuli in the ICU and sleep disruption.

Diazepam

Diazepam is seldom used as an infusion for continuous sedation because of its pharmacokinetic properties.[56] The parent compound diazepam has a half-life of roughly a day, but its principal metabolite nordazepam (also known as desmethyldiazepam) has a half-life of more than 120 hours in some individuals. Nordazepam accrues with repeated dosing, which precludes a reliable steady state. However, for the purposes of its intermittent use in the ICU, intravenous diazepam does exhibit rapid onset of sedative effects.[53] Although diazepam causes sleep architecture changes similar to other benzodiazepines, ICU studies of its influence on sleep when used for sedation are lacking.

Opioids

Opioids serve as agonists at the μ, δ, and/or κ opioid receptors; however, their principal mechanism for sedation and analgesia occurs via μ opioid agonism. A fairly limited literature describes the effects of opioids on sleep architecture,[57] and much of this literature has been conducted in prisoners with heroin addiction or in patients with chronic pain with an emphasis on cancer-related pain.[58] Studies of opioid-induced sleep changes generally do not attempt to disentangle intrinsic physiologic effects versus sleep changes effected by analgesia.

Studies before 1990 identified REM suppression as the most consistent effect of morphine, methadone, and heroin on sleep architecture.[57] Additional findings have included increased REM latency, decreased TST, and suppression of N3. However, these findings are difficult to interpret given that standardized Rechtschaffen and

Kales[31] sleep scoring was not performed in these studies, and all but one of these small studies was conducted in prisoners.

Beyond direct effects on sleep architecture, opioids may cause central sleep apnea (CSA) by way of respiratory suppression. Opioids cause dose-dependent reductions in central respiratory drive, which leads to hypoxia and hypercapnia,[59] an effect additive with benzodiazepines. It is unclear how clinically relevant CSA is in the ICU given the ready availability of ventilatory support; however, CSA may influence ventilator settings.

Morphine

In a rare placebo-controlled sleep study of opioids, Dimsdale and colleagues[60] investigated the PSG effects of single-dose sustained-release morphine and methadone in healthy subjects. In this 3-night crossover trial ($n = 46$), both sustained-release morphine 15 mg and methadone 5 mg at bedtime reduced N3 (7.6 minutes, 7.1 minutes, 11.7 minutes, respectively) and increased N2 (61.3 minutes, 63.8 minutes, 58.5 minutes, respectively) relative to placebo. This study did not reveal REM suppression or changes in either TST or wake after sleep onset.[60] An additional modern crossover placebo-controlled trial of 7 nonaddicted, pain-free subjects found that intravenous morphine 0.1 mg/kg reduced N3 *and* REM sleep while increasing the total time spent in NREM.[61] Data on whether morphine exerts significant effects on REM sleep remain equivocal.

Fentanyl

Fentanyl's lipophilic properties can lead to accumulation in fat stores with sustained use. Fentanyl may exert a more pronounced effect on consciousness than morphine, particularly at higher doses.[62] Clear conclusions on fentanyl's sleep-related effects in the ICU are typically confounded by coadministration of numerous other compounds. For instance, postoperative REM rebound has been documented in patients who received fentanyl in combination with thiopental, nitrous oxide, and isoflurane as anesthesia,[63] although the relative contribution of each anesthetic agent is difficult to differentiate. Additional analysis of postoperative nights supports an inverse relationship between morphine dose and REM sleep time.[63] Some studies convert fentanyl doses into morphine equivalents,[64] and others are unable to attribute independent effects of fentanyl given limited power.[65] Of note, a randomized study of fentanyl patient-controlled analgesia (PCA) versus alfentanil/morphine PCA found the latter regimen was better for analgesia only during the first 24 postoperative hours; but subjective reports of pain-related sleep disturbance was not statistically different between groups.[66]

Hydromorphone

Discussion of hydromorphone's effects on sleep is very limited in the literature. Like fentanyl, hydromorphone is often one of several sedatives included in a study of critical care patients[67]; but such studies do not allow for conclusions regarding its independent effects on sleep.

Propofol

Only recently was the propofol binding site on β_3 subunits of $GABA_A$ receptor-complexes described,[68] but additional findings suggest ancillary roles for glutamate modulation and cannabinoid activity in propofol's unique sedative properties.[69] Propofol may rarely cause a potentially fatal condition known as propofol infusion syndrome, characterized by refractory bradycardia plus at least one of the following: metabolic acidosis, rhabdomyolysis, hyperlipidemia, or hepatomegaly.[70]

Propofol causes regional, dose-dependent EEG effects. Unique among sedatives, it induces γ waves (35–55 Hz) on EEG,[71,72] which are faster than the β waves strengthened by benzodiazepines. Enhanced gamma power originating from the cingulate cortex seems to occur with low- and high-dose propofol, but dose-dependent emergence of slow wave activity resembling NREM sleep has been documented.[72] With escalating doses, propofol causes a burst-suppression pattern.[73,74] Propofol sedation to loss of consciousness is associated with a greater than 50% reduction in cerebral glucose metabolism, a metabolic change roughly twice as pronounced as seen in physiologic sleep.[75]

The effect of propofol on sleep has been studied using overnight EEG among the critically ill.[76] In this 2-night crossover study, 12 patients on assisted ventilation were administered either propofol titrated to a Ramsay scale score of 3 or no overnight sedation. During propofol nights, EEG revealed decreased REM sleep; but no differences were identified in SE, sleep fragmentation, or NREM sleep distribution. Although its applicability to critical care settings is unclear, 2-hour propofol infusions for 5 nights has been demonstrated to aid in normalization of sleep in patients with chronic primary insomnia.[77] Both on the first night following a 5-night propofol protocol and 6 months after therapy, subjects randomized to propofol had a greater proportion of N3 and REM than those who had received saline infusion.

Dexmedetomidine

The only α_2 agonist approved for parenteral use in the United States, dexmedetomidine has been of interest to intensivists because it causes sedation, anxiolysis,[78] and analgesia,[79] though not as effective as opioids,[80] without respiratory suppression.[81] It binds α_2-adrenergic receptors in the locus ceruleus, inhibiting norepinephrine release. This sympatholysis disinhibits the arousal-suppressing neurons in the ventrolateral preoptic area ultimately leading to sedation.[82] Its 2-hour half-life allows for effective dose titration, and its absence of active metabolites prevents accumulation with extended use. Devoid of GABAergic activity, dexmedetomidine is associated with less delirium risk than midazolam or propofol.[83]

In a 24-hour PSG study of ventilated ICU patients ($n = 10$), dexmedetomidine was associated with relative preservation of gross sleep–wake cycle, as 78% of sleep occurred overnight likely owing to DSI.[84] However, dexmedetomidine-induced sleep exhibited exclusively N1 and N2 stages and revealed significant fragmentation (9 arousals or awakenings an hour). In healthy subjects ($n = 11$), dexmedetomidine sedation induces a state similar to N2 sleep as evidenced by a similar prevalence of sleep spindles on EEG,[85] a conclusion further supported by functional MRI.[86]

Patients sedated with dexmedetomidine are more easily aroused than patients on most other sedatives.[87] In this regard, dexmedetomidine sedation is much more akin to physiologic sleep, which is defined as a state of reversible loss of consciousness. This feature likely explains how patients sedated with dexmedetomidine are more easily weaned off mechanical ventilation.[88] Nevertheless, patient reports seem to favor propofol over dexmedetomidine for sleep quality in critical care settings.[89]

Neuroleptics

This class of agents, also described with the terms typical and atypical antipsychotics, is perhaps best described as neuroleptics (from *lepsis*, Greek "to seize"), particularly because their use extends far beyond the management of psychosis. They are not sedatives in a traditional sense, but their historical designation as major tranquilizers speaks to their ataractic properties. They are commonly used in critical care settings for the management of agitation and hyperactive delirium. Data on the sleep-related effects of neuroleptics are derived principally from studies including patients with acute mental illness. Previously reviewed,[90] the impact of neuroleptics on the sleep architecture in schizophrenia may provide some insight into their global effects on sleep. They demonstrate relatively consistent improvements in sleep continuity, TST, and SE among patients with primary psychotic illness.

Haloperidol

In a 5-day crossover trial of healthy volunteers ($n = 20$), morning haloperidol increased NREM sleep, particularly N2, and enhanced SE[91]; but such findings are difficult to interpret because haloperidol was administered in the morning, more than 15 hours before sleep onset. As previously discussed, studies in patients with schizophrenia suggest that haloperidol may improve the shortened REM latency and sleep fragmentation typically seen in this condition[92]; but the effects of haloperidol on sleep vary with clinical status of psychotic symptoms.[93] Additionally, haloperidol may work synergistically with sleep deprivation in enhancing the phasic generation of saw tooth waves in REM sleep.[94] Overall, haloperidol does not seem to cause pronounced REM or N3 suppression.

Atypical neuroleptics

Atypical (or second generation) neuroleptics commonly used in critical care settings include risperidone, quetiapine, and olanzapine. Subjective sleep quality is generally more improved on atypical neuroleptics than on typicals,[95] and somnolence is a common feature of quetiapine and olanzapine in particular because of histamine (H_1) receptor antagonism.[96]

Olanzapine is often used in acute medical settings for its ability to mollify agitation.[97,98] Because sleepiness is a common side effect, it is often given at bedtime. In healthy male volunteers, bedtime olanzapine at 5 and 10 mg has been shown to *increase* N3 while suppressing REM sleep and increasing REM latency.[99] In a separate study of healthy volunteers, a single bedtime dose of olanzapine 10 mg *increased* N3 and prolonged REM latency, findings more pronounced in women ($n = 6$) than in men ($n = 7$), but caused insignificant effects on REM duration.[100] Additionally, in the crossover study of morning-dosed haloperidol cited earlier, subjects were also assigned to receive olanzapine and risperidone in random order on separate nights.[91] Morning olanzapine was associated with increased TST, SE, N3 sleep, and REM sleep on the night of administration, whereas risperidone led to decreased wake time, REM suppression, and a shift toward greater N2 sleep. Studies in patients with schizophrenia[101] and bipolar disorder who are manic[102] also attest to olanzapine's enhancement of NREM and overall sleep maintenance. Olanzapine seems to have a unique profile on sleep in that it enhances N3, and inconsistent data suggest that it may have limited effects on REM sleep.

Quetiapine is used in critical care settings for the management of agitation and delirium.[25] Like olanzapine, quetiapine also tends to cause sleep as a side effect. In a double-blind placebo-controlled study of healthy subjects, bedtime quetiapine at 25 or 100 mg increased TST, SE, percent in N2 sleep, and subjective sleep quality; however, the 100-mg dose was noted to worsen periodic leg movements during sleep.[103] Studies of quetiapine for the management of major depression,[104] bipolar depression,[105] and primary insomnia[106] have found quetiapine to also have hypnotic properties.

EFFECTS OF SEDATIVES ON CIRCADIAN RHYTHMS

Circadian rhythms describe recurring 24-hour cycles of psychomotor and physiologic activity; dozens of studies have investigated circadian rhythm disturbances among the critically ill, for which the authors use the term *circadian arrhythmias*. Common circadian arrhythmias in the ICU include pathologic wakefulness and nonrestorative daytime sleep, atypical sleep and nocturnal sleep fragmentation, near absence of REM or N3 sleep, blunted amplitude of circadian rhythms, and circadian phase delay. Unfortunately, most of these studies are not sufficiently powered or explicitly designed to isolate the effects of sedation, much less the effect of any particular agent on circadian rhythm. Such studies are generally observational and use a variety of sedation strategies: different sedative agents and doses, varying patient populations, and different timing (continuous vs intermittent; daytime sedation interruption or not). In this section, the authors turn to studies of circadian rhythm in critical care settings and extract from a limited evidence base regarding what is known about the effect of sedation on circadian rhythms.

Tables 2 and **3** present real-world observational ICU studies of circadian markers, such as core body temperature, blood pressure, actigraphy, cortisol, serum melatonin, and its metabolite 6-sulfatoxymelatonin (6-SMT), in which sedatives are *at the very least* listed. A surprising proportion of studies on circadian rhythm fail to provide any information on current medications despite the fact that many agents, sedatives in particular, not only influence sleep parameters (see earlier section) but also directly alter melatonin and other physiologic parameters often used to study circadian rhythms, such as core body temperature.

Effects of Sedatives on Melatonin

Both opioids and benzodiazepines influence melatonin release. Opioids are generally understood to increase melatonin perhaps by way of opioid receptors in the pineal gland.[121] In particular, studies of diazepam,[122] alprazolam,[123] and flunitrazepam[124] suggest that benzodiazepines decrease melatonin levels. The differential effects of opioids and benzodiazepines on melatonin levels leaves one to wonder what the resultant effect of concurrent opioids and benzodiazepines on melatonin release is, particularly because they are often used concurrently in the ICU. Further, one is left to speculate about the potential for a melatonin rebound after benzodiazepine washout or whether melatonin levels may dip after opioid use because of temporary pineal depletion. An additional pharmacologic consideration in studies of melatonin and 6-SMT derives from the fact that melatonin is released via β-agonism. Vasopressors, positive inotropes, and aerosolized β-agonists, such as albuterol, tend to increase melatonin levels; conversely, β-blockers may decrease melatonin secretion. All future ICU studies of circadian rhythm should report medications being used in study subjects.

Isolating the Effect of Sedatives on Circadian Rhythm

Even conscious, nonsedated ICU patients demonstrate very significant disruption in rest–activity cycles. In an observational study of using 24-hour actigraphy and urinary 6-SMT as an outcome measure, 14 conscious ICU subjects were found to be restless around the clock.[109] Subjects exhibited dramatic fragmentation of physiologic rest patterns: no subject experienced an hour of sustained rest over a period of up to 72 hours. Shilo and colleagues[109] specified that subjects were not on opioids, β-blockers, or other "drugs known to affect melatonin secretion."[109] Presuming that this includes benzodiazepines, these subjects reveal that even nonsedated ICU patients may often experience a circadian arrhythmia. Therefore, being able to isolate the effects of sedatives on circadian rhythm requires dedicated analysis.

Of the studies listed in **Table 1**, the study by Frisk and colleagues[113] may be the most illuminating. In this study of 16 ICU subjects, urinary 6-SMT and cortisol levels

Table 2
Effect of sedatives on sleep

Sedative Agent (Proprietary Name)	Dosing	Mechanism of Action	Pharmacokinetics	Effects on Sleep Architecture
Midazolam (Versed)	1–5 mg IVP 1–5 mg/h gtt	Positive allosteric modulator of-GABA$_A$ receptor	3–11 h $t_{1/2}$ 2- to 5-min onset Phase I metabolism Active metabolite	↓ REM, ↓ N3, ↑ %N2 Enhances β waves May ↑ SE and ↓ SL
Lorazepam (Ativan)	1–4 mg IVP 1–5 mg/h gtt		8- to 15-h $t_{1/2}$ ≥10-min onset Phase II (including extrahepatic) metabolism No active metabolites	
Diazepam (Valium)	1–5 mg IVP		24- to 120-h $t_{1/2}$ 5-min onset Phase I metabolism Nordazepam accrues	
Morphine (Roxanol; Duramorph)	1–5 mg/h gtt 2–5 mg IVP (for loading)	μ (κ and δ to lesser extent) opioid receptor agonists	3–7 h $t_{1/2}$ Slower onset than fentanyl Phase II metabolism	↓ N3, ↑ %N2 Likely ↓ REM May ↑ REM latency & ↓ TST
Fentanyl (Sublimaze)	20–100 μg/h gtt 50–100 μg IVP (for loading)		1.5- to 6.0-h $t_{1/2}$ <5-min onset Phase II metabolism Lipophilic: accrues in fat	
Hydromorphone (Dilaudid)	0.5–2 mg/h gtt 0.4–1.5 mg IVP (for loading)		1.5- to 3.5-h $t_{1/2}$ Phase II metabolism	

	Dose	Bind to β3 of GABAₐ; additional effects on glutamate and cannabinoid receptors		
Propofol (Diprivan)	50–200 mg/h gtt 1–3 mg/kg/h gtt		30- to 60-min $t_{1/2}$ <5-min onset Phase I & II metabolism Lipophilic: accrues in fat	↓ REM Enhances γ waves & dose-dependent burst suppression May not affect SE or NREM
Dexmedetomidine (Precedex)	0.2–1.5 µg/kg/h	$α_2$ agonist	2-h $t_{1/2}$ <5-min onset Phase I & II metabolism No active metabolites	↓ REM, ↓ N3 Enhances N2 spindle activity
Haloperidol[a] (Haldol)	1–10 mg IVP[b] 1–10 mg PO 1–10 mg IM	D_2 receptor antagonist	14- to 30-h $t_{1/2}$ Phase I metabolism Not given as an infusion	↑ N2, ↑ SE Limited effects on REM or N3
Risperidone[a] (Risperdal; Risperdal M-Tab)	1–6 mg PO 1–6 mg ODT	D_2 and 5-HT$_2$ receptor antagonists	20- to 30-h $t_{1/2}$ Phase I metabolism	↓ REM, ↑ %N2
Olanzapine[a] (Zyprexa; Zyprexa Zydis)	2.5–10 mg PO 5–10 mg ODT[c] 2.5–10 mg IM[d]		20- to 50-h $t_{1/2}$ Phase I metabolism	↑ N3, equivocal REM effects May ↑ TST and ↑ SE
Quetiapine[a] (Seroquel)	12.5–100 mg PO		6-h $t_{1/2}$ Phase I metabolism	↑ %N2, ↑ SE, ↑ TST

Abbreviations: %N2, percent of total sleep time spent in N2; gtt (guttae for drops), intravenous infusion; IM, intramuscular; IVP, (intravenous push), intravenous bolus; ODT, orally disintegrating tablet; PO, by mouth; $t_{1/2}$, half-life.

[a] All neuroleptics carry a black box warning for "increased mortality in elderly patients with dementia-related psychosis." Also, the use of neuroleptics for the management of general agitation, delirium, or sleep disturbances in the ICU is off-label.

[b] Haloperidol is not approved by the Food and Drug Administration for intravenous use; however, this route of administration is commonly used off-label in hospitals across the United States.

[c] Olanzapine is available as an orally disintegrating tablet under the brand name Zyprexa Zydis. The traditional 5-mg tablet can be broken in half to administer 2.5 mg, but the 5 mg ODT is too fragile for this purpose.

[d] Intramuscular olanzapine causes significant respiratory suppression and in general should not be administered with parenteral benzodiazepines unless a patient is on mechanical ventilation.

Table 3
Observational studies of circadian rhythms in the ICU in which sedative use is described

Reference	Population	Sedation	Comments
Dauch & Bauer,[107] 1990	31 ICU subjects with severe cerebral lesions	20 On sedation (no further description provided) 8 Received muscle relaxants	Nonexistence of physiologic CR measured by core body temperature associated with acute lesion, decreased level of consciousness, and neurologic findings No analysis of sedative effects on outcomes
Nuttall et al,[108] 1998	137 ICU subjects after thoracic or vascular operation: 17 with ICU psychosis and 120 without	All subjects: fentanyl epidural (plus midazolam during intubation for surgery) Specific sedatives listed only for ICU psychosis subjects	Cosinar rhythmometry of temperature and urinary output nadir randomly distributed around the clock for up to postoperative d 3 in most patients; no statistically significant difference between groups No analysis of sedative effects on outcomes
Shilo et al,[109] 1999	14 Conscious ICU subjects	No β-blockers, opiates, or other "drugs known to affect melatonin secretion"	24-h Actigraphy revealed no quiescent period longer than an h, and urine 6-SMT lacked physiologic nocturnal peak relative to non-ICU controls
Shiihara et al,[110] 2001	1 ICU subject	Midazolam and fentanyl over discrete period	Continuous monitoring of skin potentials; reduced skin conductance concurrent with sedation
Mundigler et al,[111] 2002	24 ICU subjects: 17 septic 7 nonseptic 23 rehab subjects	17 of 17 septic and 1 of 7 nonseptic subjects on sufentanil and midazolam No subject on β-blocker 17 of 17 septic and 3 of 7 nonseptic ICU subjects MV	Preserved CR (q4 h urinary 6-SMT): 1 of 17 septic ICU, 6 of 7 nonseptic ICU, and 18 of 23 controls ↓ Amplitude & delayed acrophase: septic ICU subjects more pronounced than nonseptic ICU and control subjects Conclusions confounded by co-occurrence of sepsis in 17 of 18 sedated subjects; also MV in all sedated subjects and only 2 of nonsedated
Olofsson et al,[112] 2004	8 ICU subjects: 5 of 8 septic	All sedated: most on midazolam/fentanyl; remainder on propofol/fentanyl	7 of 8 Without discernible CR of q4 h serum MT over 72 h No association of serum MT with sedation level
Frisk et al,[113] 2004	16 ICU subjects: 16 of 16 intubated	Use of benzodiazepines, propofol, opioids, cortisone,	75% Subjects lost CR (urinary 6-SMT and cortisol) periodically; 65% lost CR consistently

Source	Subjects	Medications	Conclusions
Paul & Lemmer,[114] 2007	24 ICU subjects: 11 cerebral injury, 13 without	adrenergic agents, and MV recorded during each urine collection. All: benzodiazepine/fentanyl, inotropic support; 23 of 24 MV, 1 of 24 assisted ventilation; No β-blockers or corticosteroids	Multiple regression analysis of factors on CR: MV (F = 66): decrease urinary 6-SMT; Benzodiazepine (F = 18): increase urinary 6-SMT; Adrenergic (F = 10): increase urinary 6-SMT; Cortisone (F = 39): increase urinary cortisol; Propofol (F = 5): decrease urinary cortisol. CR (measured by Chronos-Fit program),[127] including serum MT, serum cortisol, diurnal blood pressure & heart rate variation, actigraphy, and core body temperature, severely degraded, worse in cerebral injury group. Unable to isolate independent effect of sedation as all subjects sedated and ventilated
Perras et al,[115] 2007	15 ICU subjects: 5 high MT, 15 low MT	**High MT Low MT** Opioid 5 of 5 9 of 15 benzodiazepine 2 of 5 7 of 15 norepinephrine 2 of 5 8 of 15 Steroid 4 of 5 5 of 15 No β-blockers or clonidine	An h of 10,000 lux light overnight had limited effect on serum MT. Sample size precludes conclusions on medication effect
Riutta et al,[116] 2009	40 ICU nonseptic subjects	25 of 40: benzodiazepines; 14 of 40: other sedatives (mostly haloperidol); 20 of 40: opioids; 12 of 40: β-blockers; 20 of 40: MV; No adrenergics or steroids	Urinary 6-SMT q6 h were higher at night than during the d and serum cortisol at noon greater than at midnight, both suggesting gross CR preservation. Gross CR preservation (urinary 6-SMT & serum cortisol) among the 25 subjects receiving benzodiazepines, although doses and timing of administration not discussed; effect of other sedatives, opioids, and MV on CR not discussed
Lazreg et al,[117] 2011	22 ICU subjects: 12 comatose, 10 conscious	Limited information on sedatives; 4 of 12 comatose subjects on phenobarbital	Comatose subjects had greater preservation of CR in core body temperature and blood counts than noncomatose subjects. No analysis of sedative effects on outcomes

(continued on next page)

Table 3
(continued)

Reference	Population	Sedation	Comments
Verceles et al,[118] 2012	7 ICU subjects with severe sepsis	Medications that influence MT noted 2 of 7: propofol 1 of 7: dexmedetomidine 1 of 7: β-blocker 2 of 7: corticosteroid	Urinary 6-SMT revealed degradation of CR in all subjects No analysis of sedative effects on outcomes
Gehlbach et al,[119] 2012	22 ICU subjects	All sedated[a] on MV All: opioid 18 of 22: propofol 5 of 22: benzodiazepine	Urinary 6-SMT (16 subjects with data): grossly preserved CR in 13 of 16 but generally exhibited phase delay PSG (21 subjects with data): REM sleep in 2 of 21; slow wave sleep lack physiologic variation; spectral edge frequency 95% consistently low without diurnal variation (ie, around-the-clock low level of consciousness)
Yoshitaka et al,[120] 2013	40 Postoperative ICU subjects: 13 with delirium 27 no delirium	Delirium: 9 of 13 (69%) on MV (with continuous propofol) No delirium: 10 of 27 (37%) on MV (also with propofol) Non-MV subjects received morphine PCA	Change in MT 1 h after surgery predicted postoperative delirium (OR 0.5 [0.26, 0.99]). The point estimate OR of MV (hence, also of sedation) for postop delirium was 14.1, but a wide confidence interval (0.38, 519.2) precludes statistical significance

Abbreviations: CR, circadian rhythm; Benzo, benzodiazepines; MT, melatonin; MV, mechanical ventilation; OR, odds ratio; postop, postoperative; rehab, rehabilitation; 6-SMT, 6-sulfttatoxymelatonin.

[a] Daytime sedation interruption.

were obtained every 4 hours to evaluate for circadian rhythmicity. At the time of each measurement, researchers recorded whether that subject had received benzodiazepines, propofol, opioids, cortisone, adrenergic agents, or were on mechanical ventilation (MV) over the preceding 4 hours. These 342 data points served as the basis for a multiple regression analysis of factors affecting urinary 6-SMT or cortisol. They revealed that the single-most significant feature associated with 6-SMT level was MV, which was associated with decreased 6-SMT. Consistent with data in healthy subjects, benzodiazepines were independently associated with suppressed 6-SMT excretion; propofol was associated with a fairly weak but still statistically significant decrease in urinary cortisol. Opioids were not associated with significant alteration in urinary 6-SMT or cortisol (Frisk and colleagues,[113] 2004).

REM sleep is closely allied with circadian rhythms or the process C of sleep,[125] and as discussed previously benzodiazepines suppress REM sleep in healthy individuals. In fact, a dose-dependent relationship between benzodiazepine use and REM reduction has been documented in a surgical ICU.[54] In this study of overnight PSG, Trompeo and colleagues[54] stratified subjects into REM reduction or severe REM reduction based on whether REM sleep comprised greater or less than 6% of TST, respectively. REM sleep accounted for an average of 44 minutes in the REM reduction group ($n = 14$) versus a mean of 2.5 minutes in the severe REM reduction group ($n = 15$). A statistically significant, 10-fold difference in average daily lorazepam equivalents was identified between groups: 0.001 mg/kg/h (~1.8 mg in 24 hours presuming 70-kg subjects) among REM reduction subjects and 0.01 mg/kg/h among those with severe REM reduction.

Limitations of the Literature and Future Considerations

Although all ICU studies of circadian rhythms should include data regarding all potentially contributory factors (eg, medications, medical conditions, lighting and sound conditions, number of care interruptions, and so forth), enrollment of fairly small cohorts precludes statistically significant conclusions regarding the effects of sedatives on circadian rhythm.[107,108,110,117,120,126] For instance, an observational study of 40 nonseptic ICU subjects, half of whom were intubated, found that overnight urinary 6-SMT were generally higher than daytime values (Riutta and colleagues,[116] 2009), which is the expected circadian pattern. The authors further described that this pattern of elevated nightly urinary 6-SMT was seen among the 25 subjects on benzodiazepines concluding that "benzodiazepine treatment did not abolish the diurnal periodicity of [6-SMT] excretion."[116] However, in the absence of power calculations and appropriate statistical considerations of significance, such conclusions seem premature. Further, given that the effects of sedatives on circadian rhythm are likely to be dose related, correlational analysis that accounts for sedative dosing or sedation level on circadian rhythm outcomes would likely serve as meaningful outcomes.

On the other end of the spectrum are studies wherein all subjects are on continuous sedation with both opioids and GABAergic agents, that is, either benzodiazepines or propofol.[114] In such studies, providing information on cumulative doses and the timing of dose adjustments would further elucidate the effect of sedation on circadian rhythm. Finally, where sedatives are being administered, perhaps their administration based on categorical time blocks may be meaningful (eg, medications administered from 12–4 AM, 4–8 AM, 8 AM to 12 PM, and so forth). Such information would help to create correlations between medication administration and circadian rhythm outcomes because the timing of these outcomes is an inherently meaningful aspect of the assessment, namely, circadian rhythm.

The use of DSI deserves particular mention, particularly because its influence on circadian rhythms is at once both clinically apparent (patients are more alert and can be more participatory in care during the day and more restful at night) and likely confounding. For instance, Gehlbach and colleagues[119] conducted a study of 22 intubated ICU subjects who were all sedated using a DSI protocol. Gross preservation of circadian excretion of 6-SMT was observed in the 16 subjects for whom data were available; however, the degree to which a DSI protocol is directly responsible for circadian rhythm preservation remains unclear in the absence of a comparator group.

SUMMARY

Our understanding of the importance of sleep on recovery of patients who experience critical illness is still in its infancy. Although there is biological plausibility regarding the impact and importance of sleep in ICU patients, especially related to immune dysfunction, infection risk, prolonged length of MV, and delirium development and duration, there are little published data. Our understanding of how the medications we use in the ICU for pain, sedation, or delirium impact circadian rhythm is limited by several factors. The first challenge is our ability to easily and accurately measure circadian rhythm in an ICU setting. The second challenge is determining the impact of critical illness itself on circadian rhythm alterations. The third challenge is determining the impact various medications may have on circadian rhythm after adjusting for the multitude of confounding factors.

Despite the challenges of caring for critically ill patients, following the recommended guidelines for PAD, paying attention to early mobilization and sleep hygiene and individualizing patient care as needed, should lead to the best outcomes for patients. In addition future research studies should continue to inform our practice regarding treatment of PAD in the ICU.

REFERENCES

1. Kress JP, Pohlman AS, O'Connor M, et al. Daily interruption of sedative infusions in critically ill patients undergoing mechanical ventilation. N Engl J Med 2000; 342(20):1471–7.
2. Barr J, Fraser GL, Puntillo K, et al. Clinical practice guidelines for the management of pain, agitation, and delirium in adult patients in the intensive care unit. Crit Care Med 2013;41(1):263–306.
3. Payen JF, Bru O, Bosson JL, et al. Assessing pain in critically ill sedated patients by using a behavioral pain scale. Crit Care Med 2001;29(12):2258–63.
4. Gelinas C, Puntillo KA, Joffe AM, et al. A validated approach to evaluating psychometric properties of pain assessment tools for use in nonverbal critically ill adults. Semin Respir Crit Care Med 2013;34(2):153–68.
5. Arbour C, Gelinas C. Are vital signs valid indicators for the assessment of pain in postoperative cardiac surgery ICU adults? Intensive Crit Care Nurs 2010;26(2): 83–90.
6. Gelinas C, Arbour C. Behavioral and physiologic indicators during a nociceptive procedure in conscious and unconscious mechanically ventilated adults: similar or different? J Crit Care 2009;24(4):628.e7–17.
7. Sessler CN, Gosnell MS, Grap MJ, et al. The Richmond Agitation-Sedation Scale: validity and reliability in adult intensive care unit patients. Am J Respir Crit Care Med 2002;166(10):1338–44.
8. Riker RR, Picard JT, Fraser GL. Prospective evaluation of the Sedation-Agitation Scale for adult critically ill patients. Crit Care Med 1999;27(7):1325–9.

9. Ely EW, Truman B, Shintani A, et al. Monitoring sedation status over time in ICU patients: reliability and validity of the Richmond Agitation-Sedation Scale (RASS). JAMA 2003;289(22):2983–91.

10. Robinson BR, Berube M, Barr J, et al. Psychometric analysis of subjective sedation scales in critically ill adults. Crit Care Med 2013;41(9 Suppl 1):S16–29.

11. Deogaonkar A, Gupta R, DeGeorgia M, et al. Bispectral Index monitoring correlates with sedation scales in brain-injured patients. Crit Care Med 2004;32(12):2403–6.

12. Riker RR, Fraser GL, Simmons LE, et al. Validating the Sedation-Agitation Scale with the Bispectral Index and visual analog scale in adult ICU patients after cardiac surgery. Intensive Care Med 2001;27(5):853–8.

13. Pisani MA, Murphy TE, Van Ness PH, et al. Characteristics associated with delirium in older patients in a medical intensive care unit. Arch Intern Med 2007;167(15):1629–34.

14. Pisani MA. Delirium assessment in the intensive care unit: patient population matters. Crit Care 2008;12(2):131.

15. Pisani MA, Kong SY, Kasl SV, et al. Days of delirium are associated with 1-year mortality in an older intensive care unit population. Am J Respir Crit Care Med 2009;180(11):1092–7.

16. Ely EW, Gautam S, Margolin R, et al. The impact of delirium in the intensive care unit on hospital length of stay. Intensive Care Med 2001;27(12):1892–900.

17. Milbrandt EB, Deppen S, Harrison PL, et al. Costs associated with delirium in mechanically ventilated patients. Crit Care Med 2004;32(4):955–62.

18. Saczynski JS, Marcantonio ER, Quach L, et al. Cognitive trajectories after postoperative delirium. N Engl J Med 2012;367(1):30–9.

19. Girard TD, Jackson JC, Pandharipande PP, et al. Delirium as a predictor of long-term cognitive impairment in survivors of critical illness. Crit Care Med 2010; 38(7):1513–20.

20. Ely EW, Inouye SK, Bernard GR, et al. Delirium in mechanically ventilated patients: validity and reliability of the confusion assessment method for the intensive care unit (CAM-ICU). JAMA 2001;286(21):2703–10.

21. Ely EW, Margolin R, Francis J, et al. Evaluation of delirium in critically ill patients: validation of the Confusion Assessment Method for the Intensive Care Unit (CAM-ICU). Crit Care Med 2001;29(7):1370–9.

22. Bergeron N, Dubois MJ, Dumont M, et al. Intensive care delirium screening checklist: evaluation of a new screening tool. Intensive Care Med 2001;27(5): 859–64.

23. Wunsch H, Kahn JM, Kramer AA, et al. Use of intravenous infusion sedation among mechanically ventilated patients in the United States. Crit Care Med 2009;37(12):3031–9.

24. Fraser GL, Devlin JW, Worby CP, et al. Benzodiazepine versus nonbenzodiazepine-based sedation for mechanically ventilated, critically ill adults: a systematic review and meta-analysis of randomized trials. Crit Care Med 2013;41(9 Suppl 1):S30–8.

25. Devlin JW, Roberts RJ, Fong JJ, et al. Efficacy and safety of quetiapine in critically ill patients with delirium: a prospective, multicenter, randomized, double-blind, placebo-controlled pilot study. Crit Care Med 2010;38(2):419–27.

26. Girard TD, Pandharipande PP, Carson SS, et al. Feasibility, efficacy, and safety of antipsychotics for intensive care unit delirium: the MIND randomized, placebo-controlled trial. Crit Care Med 2010;38(2):428–37.

27. Skrobik YK, Bergeron N, Dumont M, et al. Olanzapine vs haloperidol: treating delirium in a critical care setting. Intensive Care Med 2004;30(3):444–9.

28. van Eijk MM, Roes KC, Honing ML, et al. Effect of rivastigmine as an adjunct to usual care with haloperidol on duration of delirium and mortality in critically ill patients: a multicentre, double-blind, placebo-controlled randomised trial. Lancet 2010;376(9755):1829–37.

29. Pandharipande PP, Pun BT, Herr DL, et al. Effect of sedation with dexmedetomidine vs lorazepam on acute brain dysfunction in mechanically ventilated patients: the MENDS randomized controlled trial. JAMA 2007;298(22): 2644–53.

30. Riker RR, Shehabi Y, Bokesch PM, et al. Dexmedetomidine vs midazolam for sedation of critically ill patients: a randomized trial. JAMA 2009;301(5):489–99.

31. Rechtschaffen A, Kales A. A manual for standardizing terminology, techniques and scoring systems for sleep stages of human subjects. Los Angeles (CA): UCLA Brain Information Service/Research Institute; 1968.

32. Iber C, Ancoli-Israel S, Chesson AL Jr, et al. The AASM manual for the scoring of sleep and associated events: rules, terminology and technical specifications. 1st edition. Westchester (IL): American Academy of Sleep Medicine; 2007.

33. Collop NA, Salas RE, Delayo M, et al. Normal sleep and circadian processes. Crit Care Clin 2008;24(3):449–60, v.

34. Drouot X, Roche-Campo F, Thille AW, et al. A new classification for sleep analysis in critically ill patients. Sleep Med 2012;13(1):7–14.

35. Watson PL, Pandharipande P, Gehlbach BK, et al. Atypical sleep in ventilated patients: empirical electroencephalography findings and the path toward revised ICU sleep scoring criteria. Crit Care Med 2013;41(8):1958–67.

36. Borbely AA. A two process model of sleep regulation. Hum Neurobiol 1982;1(3): 195–204.

37. Oldham M, Ciraulo D. Sedative, hypnotic, and anxiolytic drugs. In: McCrady B, Epstein E, editors. Addictions: a comprehensive guide book. New York: Oxford University Press; 2011. p. 155–73.

38. Pandharipande P, Shintani A, Peterson J, et al. Lorazepam is an independent risk factor for transitioning to delirium in intensive care unit patients. Anesthesiology 2006;104(1):21–6.

39. Marcantonio ER, Juarez G, Goldman L, et al. The relationship of postoperative delirium with psychoactive medications. JAMA 1994;272(19):1518–22.

40. Mancuso CE, Tanzi MG, Gabay M. Paradoxical reactions to benzodiazepines: literature review and treatment options. Pharmacotherapy 2004;24(9):1177–85.

41. Borbely AA, Mattmann P, Loepfe M, et al. Effect of benzodiazepine hypnotics on all-night sleep EEG spectra. Hum Neurobiol 1985;4(3):189–94.

42. Parrino L, Terzano MG. Polysomnographic effects of hypnotic drugs. A review. Psychopharmacology (Berl) 1996;126(1):1–16.

43. Borbely AA, Loepfe M, Mattmann P, et al. Midazolam and triazolam: hypnotic action and residual effects after a single bedtime dose. Arzneimittelforschung 1983;33(10):1500–2.

44. Borbely AA, Mattmann P, Loepfe M, et al. A single dose of benzodiazepine hypnotics alters the sleep EEG in the subsequent drug-free night. Eur J Pharmacol 1983;89(1–2):157–61.

45. Kajimura N, Nishikawa M, Uchiyama M, et al. Deactivation by benzodiazepine of the basal forebrain and amygdala in normal humans during sleep: a placebo-controlled [15O]H2O PET study. Am J Psychiatry 2004;161(4):748–51.

46. Cammarano WB, Pittet JF, Weitz S, et al. Acute withdrawal syndrome related to the administration of analgesic and sedative medications in adult intensive care unit patients. Crit Care Med 1998;26(4):676–84.

47. Kaplan PW, Sutter R. Seeing more clearly through the fog of encephalopathy. J Clin Neurophysiol 2013;30(5):431–4.
48. Breimer LT, Hennis PJ, Burm AG, et al. Quantification of the EEG effect of midazolam by aperiodic analysis in volunteers. Pharmacokinetic/pharmacodynamic modelling. Clin Pharmacokinet 1990;18(3):245–53.
49. Oto J, Yamamoto K, Koike S, et al. Effect of daily sedative interruption on sleep stages of mechanically ventilated patients receiving midazolam by infusion. Anaesth Intensive Care 2011;39(3):392–400.
50. Kim S, Park J, Lee YJ, et al. The optimal dose of midazolam for promoting sleep in critically ill patients: a pilot study. Korean J Crit Care Med 2014;29(3):166–71.
51. Feshchenko VA, Veselis RA, Reinsel RA. Comparison of the EEG effects of midazolam, thiopental, and propofol: the role of underlying oscillatory systems. Neuropsychobiology 1997;35(4):211–20.
52. Greenblatt DJ, Sethy VH. Benzodiazepine concentrations in brain directly reflect receptor occupancy: studies of diazepam, lorazepam, and oxazepam. Psychopharmacology (Berl) 1990;102(3):373–8.
53. Greenblatt DJ, von Moltke LL, Ehrenberg BL, et al. Kinetics and dynamics of lorazepam during and after continuous intravenous infusion. Crit Care Med 2000; 28(8):2750–7.
54. Trompeo AC, Vidi Y, Locane MD, et al. Sleep disturbances in the critically ill patients: role of delirium and sedative agents. Minerva Anestesiol 2011;77(6):604–12.
55. Parrino L, Boselli M, Spaggiari MC, et al. Multidrug comparison (lorazepam, triazolam, zolpidem, and zopiclone) in situational insomnia: polysomnographic analysis by means of the cyclic alternating pattern. Clin Neuropharmacol 1997;20(3):253–63.
56. Ochs HR, Greenblatt DJ, Lauven PM, et al. Kinetics of high-dose i.v. diazepam. Br J Anaesth 1982;54(8):849–52.
57. Moore P, Dimsdale JE. Opioids, sleep, and cancer-related fatigue. Med Hypotheses 2002;58(1):77–82.
58. Panagiotou I, Mystakidou K. Non-analgesic effects of opioids: opioids' effects on sleep (including sleep apnea). Curr Pharm Des 2012;18(37):6025–33.
59. Javaheri S, Randerath W. Opioid-induced central sleep apnea: mechanisms and therapies. Sleep Med Clin 2014;9(1):49–56.
60. Dimsdale JE, Norman D, DeJardin D, et al. The effect of opioids on sleep architecture. J Clin Sleep Med 2007;3(1):33–6.
61. Shaw IR, Lavigne G, Mayer P, et al. Acute intravenous administration of morphine perturbs sleep architecture in healthy pain-free young adults: a preliminary study. Sleep 2005;28(6):677–82.
62. Smith NT, Dec-Silver H, Sanford TJ Jr, et al. EEGs during high-dose fentanyl-, sufentanil-, or morphine-oxygen anesthesia. Anesth Analg 1984;63(4):386–93.
63. Knill RL, Moote CA, Skinner MI, et al. Anesthesia with abdominal surgery leads to intense REM sleep during the first postoperative week. Anesthesiology 1990; 73(1):52–61.
64. Cooper AB, Thornley KS, Young GB, et al. Sleep in critically ill patients requiring mechanical ventilation. Chest 2000;117(3):809–18.
65. Whitcomb JJ, Morgan M, Irvin T, et al. A pilot study on delirium in the intensive care unit: a creative inquiry project with undergraduate nursing students. Dimens Crit Care Nurs 2013;32(5):266–70.
66. Lee A, O'Loughlin E, Roberts LJ. A double-blinded randomized evaluation of alfentanil and morphine vs fentanyl: analgesia and sleep trial (DREAMFAST). Br J Anaesth 2013;110(2):293–8.

67. Friese RS, Diaz-Arrastia R, McBride D, et al. Quantity and quality of sleep in the surgical intensive care unit: are our patients sleeping? J Trauma 2007;63(6):1210–4.
68. Yip GM, Chen ZW, Edge CJ, et al. A propofol binding site on mammalian GABAA receptors identified by photolabeling. Nat Chem Biol 2013;9(11):715–20.
69. Guindon J, LoVerme J, Piomelli D, et al. The antinociceptive effects of local injections of propofol in rats are mediated in part by cannabinoid CB1 and CB2 receptors. Anesth Analg 2007;104(6):1563–9 table of contents.
70. Kam PC, Cardone D. Propofol infusion syndrome. Anaesthesia 2007;62(7):690–701.
71. Lee U, Mashour GA, Kim S, et al. Propofol induction reduces the capacity for neural information integration: implications for the mechanism of consciousness and general anesthesia. Conscious Cogn 2009;18(1):56–64.
72. Murphy M, Bruno MA, Riedner BA, et al. Propofol anesthesia and sleep: a high-density EEG study. Sleep 2011;34(3):283–291A.
73. Billard V, Gambus PL, Chamoun N, et al. A comparison of spectral edge, delta power, and bispectral index as EEG measures of alfentanil, propofol, and midazolam drug effect. Clin Pharmacol Ther 1997;61(1):45–58.
74. Herregods L, Rolly G, Mortier E, et al. EEG and SEMG monitoring during induction and maintenance of anesthesia with propofol. Int J Clin Monit Comput 1989;6(2):67–73.
75. Alkire MT, Haier RJ, Barker SJ, et al. Cerebral metabolism during propofol anesthesia in humans studied with positron emission tomography. Anesthesiology 1995;82(2):393–403 [discussion: 27A].
76. Kondili E, Alexopoulou C, Xirouchaki N, et al. Effects of propofol on sleep quality in mechanically ventilated critically ill patients: a physiological study. Intensive Care Med 2012;38(10):1640–6.
77. Xu Z, Jiang X, Li W, et al. Propofol-induced sleep: efficacy and safety in patients with refractory chronic primary insomnia. Cell Biochem Biophys 2011;60(3):161–6.
78. Paris A, Tonner PH. Dexmedetomidine in anaesthesia. Curr Opin Anaesthesiol 2005;18(4):412–8.
79. Guo TZ, Jiang JY, Buttermann AE, et al. Dexmedetomidine injection into the locus ceruleus produces antinociception. Anesthesiology 1996;84(4):873–81.
80. Cortinez LI, Hsu YW, Sum-Ping ST, et al. Dexmedetomidine pharmacodynamics: Part II: crossover comparison of the analgesic effect of dexmedetomidine and remifentanil in healthy volunteers. Anesthesiology 2004;101(5):1077–83.
81. Hsu YW, Cortinez LI, Robertson KM, et al. Dexmedetomidine pharmacodynamics: part I: crossover comparison of the respiratory effects of dexmedetomidine and remifentanil in healthy volunteers. Anesthesiology 2004;101(5):1066–76.
82. Nelson LE, Lu J, Guo T, et al. The alpha2-adrenoceptor agonist dexmedetomidine converges on an endogenous sleep-promoting pathway to exert its sedative effects. Anesthesiology 2003;98(2):428–36.
83. Pasin L, Landoni G, Nardelli P, et al. Dexmedetomidine reduces the risk of delirium, agitation and confusion in critically ill patients: a meta-analysis of randomized controlled trials. J Cardiothorac Vasc Anesth 2014;28(6):1459–66.
84. Oto J, Yamamoto K, Koike S, et al. Sleep quality of mechanically ventilated patients sedated with dexmedetomidine. Intensive Care Med 2012;38(12):1982–9.

85. Huupponen E, Maksimow A, Lapinlampi P, et al. Electroencephalogram spindle activity during dexmedetomidine sedation and physiological sleep. Acta Anaesthesiol Scand 2008;52(2):289–94.

86. Coull JT, Jones ME, Egan TD, et al. Attentional effects of noradrenaline vary with arousal level: selective activation of thalamic pulvinar in humans. Neuroimage 2004;22(1):315–22.

87. Hall JE, Uhrich TD, Barney JA, et al. Sedative, amnestic, and analgesic properties of small-dose dexmedetomidine infusions. Anesth Analg 2000;90(3): 699–705.

88. Torbic H, Papadopoulos S, Manjourides J, et al. Impact of a protocol advocating dexmedetomidine over propofol sedation after robotic-assisted direct coronary artery bypass surgery on duration of mechanical ventilation and patient safety. Ann Pharmacother 2013;47(4):441–6.

89. Corbett SM, Rebuck JA, Greene CM, et al. Dexmedetomidine does not improve patient satisfaction when compared with propofol during mechanical ventilation. Crit Care Med 2005;33(5):940–5.

90. Cohrs S. Sleep disturbances in patients with schizophrenia: impact and effect of antipsychotics. CNS Drugs 2008;22(11):939–62.

91. Gimenez S, Clos S, Romero S, et al. Effects of olanzapine, risperidone and haloperidol on sleep after a single oral morning dose in healthy volunteers. Psychopharmacology (Berl) 2007;190(4):507–16.

92. Maixner S, Tandon R, Eiser A, et al. Effects of antipsychotic treatment on polysomnographic measures in schizophrenia: a replication and extension. Am J Psychiatry 1998;155(11):1600–2.

93. Neylan TC, van Kammen DP, Kelley ME, et al. Sleep in schizophrenic patients on and off haloperidol therapy. Clinically stable vs relapsed patients. Arch Gen Psychiatry 1992;49(8):643–9.

94. Pinto LR Jr, Peres CA, Russo RH, et al. Sawtooth waves during REM sleep after administration of haloperidol combined with total sleep deprivation in healthy young subjects. Braz J Med Biol Res 2002;35(5):599–604.

95. Yamashita H, Mori K, Nagao M, et al. Effects of changing from typical to atypical antipsychotic drugs on subjective sleep quality in patients with schizophrenia in a Japanese population. J Clin Psychiatry 2004;65(11):1525–30.

96. Miller DD. Atypical antipsychotics: sleep, sedation, and efficacy. Prim Care Companion J Clin Psychiatry 2004;6(Suppl 2):3–7.

97. Meehan KM, Wang H, David SR, et al. Comparison of rapidly acting intramuscular olanzapine, lorazepam, and placebo: a double-blind, randomized study in acutely agitated patients with dementia. Neuropsychopharmacology 2002; 26(4):494–504.

98. Breier A, Meehan K, Birkett M, et al. A double-blind, placebo-controlled dose-response comparison of intramuscular olanzapine and haloperidol in the treatment of acute agitation in schizophrenia. Arch Gen Psychiatry 2002;59(5):441–8.

99. Sharpley AL, Vassallo CM, Cowen PJ. Olanzapine increases slow-wave sleep: evidence for blockade of central 5-HT(2C) receptors in vivo. Biol Psychiatry 2000;47(5):468–70.

100. Lindberg N, Virkkunen M, Tani P, et al. Effect of a single-dose of olanzapine on sleep in healthy females and males. Int Clin Psychopharmacol 2002;17(4): 177–84.

101. Goder R, Fritzer G, Gottwald B, et al. Effects of olanzapine on slow wave sleep, sleep spindles and sleep-related memory consolidation in schizophrenia. Pharmacopsychiatry 2008;41(3):92–9.

102. Moreno RA, Hanna MM, Tavares SM, et al. A double-blind comparison of the effect of the antipsychotics haloperidol and olanzapine on sleep in mania. Braz J Med Biol Res 2007;40(3):357–66.

103. Cohrs S, Rodenbeck A, Guan Z, et al. Sleep-promoting properties of quetiapine in healthy subjects. Psychopharmacology (Berl) 2004;174(3):421–9.

104. Trivedi MH, Bandelow B, Demyttenaere K, et al. Evaluation of the effects of extended release quetiapine fumarate monotherapy on sleep disturbance in patients with major depressive disorder: a pooled analysis of four randomized acute studies. Int J Neuropsychopharmacol 2013;16(8):1733–44.

105. Endicott J, Paulsson B, Gustafsson U, et al. Quetiapine monotherapy in the treatment of depressive episodes of bipolar I and II disorder: improvements in quality of life and quality of sleep. J Affect Disord 2008;111(2–3):306–19.

106. Tassniyom K, Paholpak S, Tassniyom S, et al. Quetiapine for primary insomnia: a double blind, randomized controlled trial. J Med Assoc Thai 2010;93(6):729–34.

107. Dauch WA, Bauer S. Circadian rhythms in the body temperatures of intensive care patients with brain lesions. J Neurol Neurosurg Psychiatry 1990;53(4): 345–7.

108. Nuttall GA, Kumar M, Murray MJ. No difference exists in the alteration of circadian rhythm between patients with and without intensive care unit psychosis. Crit Care Med 1998;26(8):1351–5.

109. Shilo L, Dagan Y, Smorjik Y, et al. Patients in the intensive care unit suffer from severe lack of sleep associated with loss of normal melatonin secretion pattern. Am J Med Sci 1999;317(5):278–81.

110. Shiihara Y, Nogami T, Chigira M, et al. Sleep-wake rhythm during stay in an intensive care unit: a week's long-term recording of skin potentials. Psychiatry Clin Neurosci 2001;55(3):279–80.

111. Mundigler G, Delle-Karth G, Koreny M, et al. Impaired circadian rhythm of melatonin secretion in sedated critically ill patients with severe sepsis. Crit Care Med 2002;30(3):536–40.

112. Olofsson K, Alling C, Lundberg D, et al. Abolished circadian rhythm of melatonin secretion in sedated and artificially ventilated intensive care patients. Acta Anaesthesiol Scand 2004;48(6):679–84.

113. Frisk U, Olsson J, Nylén P, et al. Low melatonin excretion during mechanical ventilation in the intensive care unit. Clin Sci (Lond) 2004;107(1):47–53.

114. Paul T, Lemmer B. Disturbance of circadian rhythms in analgosedated intensive care unit patients with and without craniocerebral injury. Chronobiol Int 2007; 24(1):45–61.

115. Perras B, Meier M, Dodt C. Light and darkness fail to regulate melatonin release in critically ill humans. Intensive Care Med 2007;33(11):1954–8.

116. Riutta A, Ylitalo P, Kaukinen S. Diurnal variation of melatonin and cortisol is maintained in non-septic intensive care patients. Intensive Care Med 2009;35(10): 1720–7.

117. Lazreg T, Naija W, Skhouri H, et al. Altered circadian rhythms in rectal temperature and circulating blood cells in intensive care unit patients. Biol Rhythm Res 2011;42(4):337–47.

118. Verceles AC, Silhan L, Terrin M, et al. Circadian rhythm disruption in severe sepsis: the effect of ambient light on urinary 6-sulfatoxymelatonin secretion. Intensive Care Med 2012;38(5):804–10.

119. Gehlbach BK, Chapotot F, Leproult R, et al. Temporal disorganization of circadian rhythmicity and sleep-wake regulation in mechanically ventilated patients receiving continuous intravenous sedation. Sleep 2012;35(8):1105–14.

120. Yoshitaka S, Egi M, Morimatsu H, et al. Perioperative plasma melatonin concentration in postoperative critically ill patients: its association with delirium. J Crit Care 2013;28(3):236–42.
121. Govitrapong P, Pariyanonth M, Ebadi M. The presence and actions of opioid receptors in bovine pineal gland. J Pineal Res 1992;13(3):124–32.
122. Djeridane Y, Touitou Y. Effects of diazepam and its metabolites on nocturnal melatonin secretion in the rat pineal and harderian glands. A comparative in vivo and in vitro study. Chronobiol Int 2003;20(2):285–97.
123. McIntyre IM, Norman TR, Burrows GD, et al. Alterations to plasma melatonin and cortisol after evening alprazolam administration in humans. Chronobiol Int 1993; 10(3):205–13.
124. Hajak G, Rodenbeck A, Bandelow B, et al. Nocturnal plasma melatonin levels after flunitrazepam administration in healthy subjects. Eur Neuropsychopharmacol 1996;6(2):149–53.
125. Aeschbach D. REM-sleep regulation: circadian, homeostatic, and non-REM sleep-dependent determinants. In: Mallick B, Pandi-Perumal S, McCarley R, et al, editors. Rapid eye movement sleep: regulation and function. Cambridge (United Kingdom): Cambridge University Press; 2011. p. 80–8.
126. Verceles AC, Liu X, Terrin ML, et al. Ambient light levels and critical care outcomes. J Crit Care 2013;28(1):110.e1–8.
127. Zuther P, Lemmer B. Chronos-Fit. Version 1.04, 2004. Available at: http://www.ma.uni-heidelberg.de/inst/phar/forschungLemmer.html.

Delirium in Critically Ill Patients

Peter Jackson, MD[a], Akram Khan, MD[b],*

KEYWORDS

- Delirium • Intensive care unit • Critically ill • Encephelopathy

KEY POINTS

- Delirium in the intensive care unit (ICU) is an extremely common and detrimental diagnosis, with a high incidence and effects including increases in mortality, longer duration of mechanical ventilation, and long-term cognitive dysfunction after discharge.
- There are trials suggesting that prophylaxis of postoperative delirium is possible with medications including haloperidol, atypical antipsychotics and ketamine; however, these trials are small and decisions should be made on a case-by-case basis.
- There are some promising studies, both pharmacologic and nonpharmacologic, for preventing delirium in nonoperative critically ill patients.
- Delirium is an acute mental disorder characterized by inattention, with varying causes, including medical illness and withdrawal from medications or substances.

INTRODUCTION

Delirium is an acute mental disorder characterized by inattention, with varying causes, including medical illness and withdrawal from medications or substances. Since the first use of the term delirium, researchers have used many different descriptors, such as intensive care unit (ICU) psychosis, ICU syndrome, encephalopathy, and even acute brain failure, to describe this condition.[1] In recent years, the critical care community has increasingly conformed to the term delirium, with the definition per the 4 criteria used in the *Diagnostic and Statistical Manual of Mental Disorders, Fifth Edition* (DSM-5) (**Box 1**).[2] It is generally accepted that not all 4 of these criteria need

Financial disclosure: This publication was made possible with support from the Oregon Clinical and Translational Research Institute (OCTRI), grant number UL1 RR024140 from the National Center for Advancing Translational Sciences (NCATS), a component of the National Institutes of Health (NIH), and NIH Roadmap for Medical Research.
Author contributions: P. Jackson and A. Khan were involved in the conception, delineation, design, and writing of the article and in its revision before submission.
[a] Division of Pulmonary and Critical Care Medicine, Department of Internal Medicine, School of Medicine, Oregon Health & Science University, 3181 Southwest Sam Jackson Park Road, Portland, OR 97239, USA; [b] Division of Pulmonary and Critical Care Medicine, Department of Internal Medicine, School of Medicine, Oregon Health & Science University, 3181 Southwest Sam Jackson Park Road, UHN67, Portland, OR 97239-3098, USA
* Corresponding author.
E-mail address: khana@ohsu.edu

Crit Care Clin 31 (2015) 589–603
http://dx.doi.org/10.1016/j.ccc.2015.03.011
0749-0704/15/$ – see front matter © 2015 Elsevier Inc. All rights reserved.

Box 1
Criteria used to define delirium based on DSM-5

Disturbance in attention

Change in cognition

Development over a short interval and fluctuating course

Evidence from history, physical examination, or laboratory findings that the disturbance is a physiologic consequence of another medical condition, substance intoxication, or withdrawal

---

to be present to reach the diagnosis and that the severity and manifestations of delirium can vary significantly.[3]

EPIDEMIOLOGY AND SUBTYPES OF DELIRIUM

Delirium in the ICU is extremely common, with an incidence ranging between 45% and 87%.[4–7] A study by Milbrandt and colleagues[8] in 2004 evaluated the cost of delirium to the US health care system and estimated the economic burden to be $4 to $16 billion annually. This wide range in incidence and costs is likely caused by differences in prevalence estimates from different subspecialty ICUs (eg, surgical versus medical) as well as differing ICU populations with a variable severity of illness.[7]

Delirium is being increasingly recognized as a significant contributor to the morbidity and mortality of critically ill patients. Recent studies have shown an increase in total ventilator days, ICU length of stay, need for chemical sedation, and long-term cognitive impairment.[9–11] In 1 study that followed 821 surgical and medical ICU patients,[10] 34% who suffered from delirium had cognitive impairment at 12 months compared with only 6% at baseline. In a 2004 article in the *Journal of the American Medical Association*,[11] a cohort of 224 critically ill patients on mechanical ventilation were prospectively evaluated for development of delirium. After controlling for clinical variables including age, severity of illness, comorbid conditions, coma, and use of sedatives or analgesic medications, delirium was independently associated with a 3.2-fold increase in 6-month mortality.

In an effort to yield prognostic information, delirium has been classified into motoric subtypes of hyperactive, hypoactive, and mixed.[4–6] This situation has at times led to

---

Table 1
Hyperactive, hypoactive, and mixed subtypes of delirium

Characteristic	Hyperactive	Hypoactive	Mixed
Percentage in ICU	1.6	43.5	54.1
Psychomotor	Agitation, restlessness, emotional lability	Decreased responsiveness, apathy, withdrawal	Combination of both
Hallucinations/ delusions	Common	Rare	Variable
Prognosis	Better	Worse	Variable
Age	Younger	Older	All
Sleep-wake cycle disturbance	More common	Less common	More common

Data from Meagher DJ, Trzepacz PT. Motoric subtypes of delirium. Semin Clin Neuropsychiatry 2000;5:75–85; and Peterson JF, Pun BT, Dittus RS, et al. Delirium and its motoric subtypes: a study of 614 critically ill patients. J Am Geriatr Soc 2006;54:479–84.

subjectivity in identification and classification. The characteristic patterns of the 3 subtypes of delirium are listed in **Table 1**, with the differences in the incidence, clinical features, and prognosis of the 3 subtypes.

RISK FACTORS FOR DELIRIUM IN THE INTENSIVE CARE UNIT

Given the significant impact of delirium on patient outcomes and its high prevalence, multiple studies evaluating causes and contributors to delirium in the ICU have been performed. In 2008, a systematic review[12] identified 25 contributing factors but called for more research into factors that may pose risk for delirium. Researchers have also tried to develop models to predict the development of delirium using clinical findings and laboratory values. In the PRE-DELIRIC (Prediction of Delirium in ICU Patients) trial, published in the *British Medical Journal* in 2012, van den Boogard and colleagues[13] examined 1613 consecutive patients in a single hospital in the Netherlands and developed a prediction model for the development of delirium using 10 risk factors: age, APACHE-II (Acute Physiology and Chronic Health Evaluation II) score, admission group, coma, infection, metabolic acidosis, use of sedatives and morphine, urea concentration, and urgent admission (**Box 2**). The scoring system was temporally validated at the same center and externally validated with 894 other patients at 4 additional centers within the Netherlands. The model using 10 risk factors that are readily available within 24 hours of ICU admission was shown to have a high predictive value, with an area under the receiver operating curve of 0.85 (0.84–0.87) after external validation, which was superior to nurse and doctor prediction of 0.59 (0.49–0.70).[13]

Box 2
PRE-DELIRIC equation of prediction model for the development of delirium using 10 identified risk factors that are readily available within 24 hours of ICU admission

Risk of delirium = $1/(1 + exp[-(-6.31 + 0.04 \times$ age $+ 0.06 \times$ APACHE-II score + 0 for noncoma or 0.55 for drug-induced coma or 2.70 for miscellaneous coma or 2.84 for combination coma + 0 for surgical patients or 0.31 for medical patients or 1.13 for trauma patients or 1.38 for neurology/neurosurgical patients + 1.05 for infection + 0.29 for metabolic acidosis + 0 for no morphine use or 0.41 for 0.01–7.1 mg/24 h morphine use or 0.13 for 7.2–18.6 mg/24 h morphine use for 0.51 for >18.6 mg/24 h + 1.39 for use of sedatives + 0.03 $\times$ urea concentration (mmol/L) + 0.40 for urgent admission)])

The intercept of the scoring system is expressed as –6.31; the other numbers represent the shrunken regression coefficients (weights) of each risk factor.

From van den Boogaard M, Pickkers P, Slooter AJ, et al. Development and validation of PRE-DELIRIC (Prediction of Delirium in ICU Patients) delirium prediction model for intensive care patients: observational multicentre study. BMJ 2012;344:e420; with permission.

A recent meta-analysis by Zaal and colleagues identified 1626 unique studies of risk factors for delirium in the period between 2000 and 2013 and evaluated 33 after screening for quality and bias. The study reported 11 variables that were considered to have moderate or strong evidence for contributing to delirium in both ICU and general inpatient settings. Furthermore, the investigators found that dexmedetomidine use seemed to be protective.

1. Age	2. Dementia	3. Hypertension
4. Coma	5. APACHE score	6. Delirium previous day
7. Emergency surgery	8. Mechanical ventilation	9. Organ failure
10. Polytrauma	11. Metabolic acidosis	

A significant portion of risk factors noted by Zaal and colleagues[14] are indications for ICU admission, which helps to further explain the prevalence of delirium within in the critical care setting. However, there were some specific risk factors that, although they did not show a strong association in this analysis, have been associated with delirium in other studies focussed in the ICU (eg, PRE-DERILIC).[13]

In one prospective analysis of the ICU population, additional risk factors that were identified were as follows[3,15]:

- Use of centrally acting medications (ie, benzodiazepines, opioids, anticholinergics)
- Physical restraints
- Foley catheters, arterial catheters, gastric tube
- Number of intravenous (IV) infusions
- ICU length of stay
- Lack of sunlight
- Lack of visitors

Sleep deprivation is another risk factor that has been associated with delirium in the ICU. ICU patients experience poor sleep with fragmentation, with lack of rapid eye movement (REM) and stage IV or deep sleep being characteristic.[16,17] It has also been suggested that REM deprivation can lead to delirium, and it is known that sleep deprivation can manifest in ways that are similar to delirium (eg, decreased attention, somnolence).

In summary, studies have shown that a combination of fixed characteristics (ie, age, chronic illnesses), illness severity, and iatrogenic or preventable factors have been associated with the development of delirium. Many of these risk factors are specific to the critical care setting and may represent targets for interventions to decrease patients risk of delirium (**Fig. 1**).

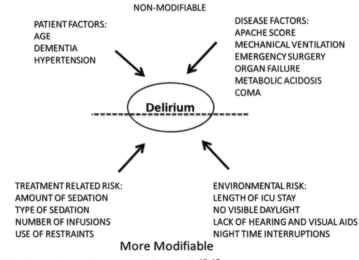

Fig. 1. Risk factors for delirium. *Data from* Refs.[13–15]

PATHOPHYSIOLOGY AND CAUSE OF DELIRIUM IN THE INTENSIVE CARE UNIT

Given the burden of delirium on the health care system, there has been increasing interest in better defining the pathophysiology of this disorder. It has been difficult to elucidate a definitive pathogenesis, because of the multiple insults that could lead to the final pathway of neuronal cell apoptosis and decreases in synaptic plasticity, which may lead to delirium. In this section, the pathogenesis of delirium is discussed. The final cause is likely to be a combination of these factors (**Box 3**).

Box 3
Proposed mechanisms of delirium in the ICU

Alterations in cerebral blood flow

Cerebral hypoperfusion

Degradation of blood-brain barrier

Endothelial dysfunction

Activation of microglia

Acetylcholine depletion

Monoamine (dopamine, norepinephrine, and serotonin) depletion

---

Theories on pathogenesis of delirium are based on the risk factors discussed in the previous section. One of the most consistent associations is with severity of illness and sepsis. Encephalopathy associated with sepsis is common, with a recent multicenter trial[18] estimating its prevalence as 32.3%. Delirium in sepsis is often believed to be mediated through inflammatory cytokines and endotoxin.[19] Higher systemic inflammatory markers in patients with sepsis, including C-reactive protein, cortisol, and interleukin 8 (IL-8), are associated with an increased incidence of delirium.[20–22] The pathway by which inflammation can cause delirium is complex. The pathway includes degradation of the blood-brain barrier (BBB), activation of microglia, endothelial dysfunction, and alterations in cerebral blood flow (CBF), as well as changes in neurotransmitter levels.[23–28] Data regarding breakdown in the BBB have been reported in animal models. Alteration of the BBB allows for infiltration of leukocytes and cytokines into the central nervous system, leading to microvascular thrombosis and apoptosis.[21,27] A rat abdominal sepsis model[23] showed derangement in amino acid transport across the BBB that was similar to that seen in hepatic encephalopathy. Similarly, in a pig model of sepsis with fecal peritonitis,[24] areas of the frontal cortex showed increase in perimicrovascular edema and disruption of astrocytic end-feet via electron microscopy. Further associations have been made in the absence of bacteria, where interferon γ or IL injections alone in animal models have been shown to increase vascular permeability and cause electroencephalographic findings that are similar to those seen in sepsis, even in the absence of bacteria.[25] In humans, a retrospective review of 652 patients receiving IL-2 given for chemotherapy[26] reported that 30% of patients develop delirium during treatment. This finding again suggests a link to inflammation as a trigger event for delirium, even in the absence of frank sepsis.

Inflammation has also been shown to activate microglia, which have a phagocytic role during homeostasis that allows clearance of dysfunctional neurons. The excitation of microglia by inflammatory mediators results in a self-activating cascade that leads to increases in reactive oxygen species and nitric oxide synthase.[27,28] This positive feedback loop then leads to further inflammatory mediator influx, apoptosis, and γ-aminobutyric acid upregulation. Patients with baseline poor cognition are likely primed for this response by having more reactive microglial response. This response globally leads to a depressed level of synaptic activity and the phenotype of delirium.[29]

An additional mechanism that may be at play in delirium, both in sepsis and in other states, is that of decreased CBF.[30,31] Changes in CBF are associated with inflammation, given the known microvascular perturbations present in sepsis and disease states with high inflammatory activity. There have been numerous studies with neuroimaging techniques that have shown a decrease in CBF in delirious patients, both in sepsis and in other disease states.[31,32] In one study in 2003 by Yokota and colleagues,[31] computed tomography (CT) showed a 43% reduction in CBF in patients during delirious states and even more reduction in the frontal lobes. Further research using neuroimaging modalities to evaluate CBF[32] also showed reduction in CBF in alcohol withdrawal delirium, making a decrease in CBF a possible common pathway for delirium.

Other hypotheses for delirium in the ICU involve alterations in neurotransmitter levels within the central nervous system. Some of the neurotransmitters implicated are acetylcholine and the monoamines (dopamine, norepinephrine, and serotonin) or their precursors.[33] The hypothesis that acetylcholine mediates the development of delirium is supported by the clinical finding that anticholinergic medications commonly cause alterations in consciousness.[33,34] Many of the risk factors, such as anesthetics and opiates, are known to affect the release of acetylcholine and the availability of postsynaptic receptors.[34] Dedicated neuroimaging has also shown that areas of high acetylcholine synthesis have lesions during delirium, indicating decreased ability for the brain to synthesize adequate levels of acetylcholine. Inflammation within the brain promotes a cholinergic deficit through various pathways, including ischemia, as well as more direct effects of inflammatory mediators.[34] Trials with cholinesterase inhibitors to prevent and treat delirium[35,36] have been conducted, with negative results, indicating the complex and multifactorial nature of this disorder.

Dopamine is considered the monoamine most likely to be involved with the development of delirium.[37] This hypothesis is supported by the observation that dopamine agonists, like anticholinergics, increase the risk of delirium and that haloperidol and atypical antipsychotics that antagonize dopamine have been used to treat delirium effectively.[38] Genetic research into polymorphisms of the dopamine transport gene (DAT) in a European meta-analysis[39] suggests that alterations in certain DAT genotypes are protective against developing delirium.

EVALUATION AND MONITORING OF DELIRIUM IN THE INTENSIVE CARE UNIT

There has been some research into development of biomarkers for delirium, but currently, there is no blood test as a gold standard for diagnosis.[20,21] The diagnosis of delirium is therefore clinical and can be complex given its waxing and waning nature as well as its various phenotypes (hyperactive, hypoactive, and mixed). Given this difficulty, there has been interest in monitoring for delirium, to identify it early and evaluate and treat reversible causes, because screening for delirium has been shown to increase the rate of its diagnosis to 64%.[40] It is difficult to assess for delirium in the ICU, because patients are often sedated, being given high amounts of analgesics, or may be intubated, all of which make verbal communication difficult. Although several tools may be used to monitor for delirium, the most common in the ICU are the confusion assessment method for the ICU (CAM-ICU) and the intensive care delirium screening checklist (ICDSC), both of which are recommended by the most recent guidelines on pain and sedation in the ICU.[41]

The CAM-ICU is validated to detect delirium in nonverbal ventilated patients and is the most studied of the monitoring instruments.[42] The CAM-ICU assigns scores to 4 different features: acute onset or fluctuating course, inattention, altered level of consciousness, and disorganized thinking. The sensitivity and specificity vary between studies, with reported sensitivity of 93% to 100% and specificity of 98% to 100% in a single-center study.[43] Subsequent studies have shown a less robust detection rate, with a sensitivity as low as 47% but specificity that remains higher than 80% in most trials.[44] These differences in sensitivity are usually attributed to implementation processes and time spent teaching evaluators about the CAM-ICU algorithm, which often differ between many of the trials.

The ICDSC is a more recent tool, first created in 2001.[45] The tool evaluates 8 different items all based on the DSM criteria. It differs from the CAM-ICU in that the observation occurs over a longer period and the scores are not dichotomous but represent a range. Furthermore, this tool does not elicit verbal responses but relies on observational methods to detect the changes detailed in **Table 2**. In the first study evaluating the new tool, 93 patients were studied in a single center, with a score of 4 or greater indicating delirium. The ICDSC was shown to have a sensitivity of 99% but specificity slightly lower than the CAM-ICU, at 64%.[45]

Table 2
Scoring systems for the diagnosis of delirium in the ICU

CAM-ICU	ICDSC
Scoring is positive or negative according to the following criteria	Score of 4 or greater indicates delirium. 1-3 is designated sub-syndromal delirium
Patient must be sufficiently awake (RASS score, −3 or more) for assessment according to the following criteria:	Patient must show at least a response to mild or moderate stimulation. Then, score 1 point for each of the following features, as assessed in the manner believed appropriate by the clinician:
Must have an acute change from mental status at baseline or fluctuating mental status during the past 24 h and Must have >2 errors on a 10-point test of attention to voice or pictures If the RASS is not 0 and the above 2 criteria are positive, the patient is delirious If the RASS is 0 and the above 2 criteria are positive: Disorganized thinking using 4 yes/no questions and a 2-step command is assessed; >1 error means the patient is delirious; ≤1 error excludes delirium	Deviation from normal wakefulness Inattention Disorientation Hallucination Psychomotor agitation Inappropriate speech or mood Disturbance in sleep or wake cycle Fluctuation in symptoms
Sensitivity: 80% in pooled analysis Specificity: 95.9% in pooled analysis	Sensitivity: 74% in pooled analysis Specificity: 81.9% in pooled analysis

Abbreviation: RASS, Richmond agitation–sedation scale.[46]
    Data from Refs.[41,43,45,47]

SCORING SYSTEMS FOR THE DIAGNOSIS OF DELIRIUM IN THE INTENSIVE CARE UNIT

Given the number of different tools and the differences in the various methods for screening, there have been investigations to attempt to evaluate and to compare them with each other and clinician evaluation alone. A recent meta-analysis[47] showed a pooled sensitivity and specificity for CAM-ICU of 80% and 95.9% and a pooled sensitivity and specificity for ICDSC of 74% and 81.9%, validating both as good measures of delirium in ICU. In choosing one or the other, it may be useful to use CAM-ICU in patients in whom ensuring that the patient diagnosed with delirium does have the condition (high specificity) is important. The ICDSC, by nature of its more continuous scoring system, may be useful for identifying subsyndromal delirium, which may have prognostic implications.

Data are less clear on the usefulness of these tools outside research settings. In 1 study,[48] researchers measured CAM-ICU in a clinical setting, in which delirium experts assessed 181 noncomatose patients and provided a diagnosis, which was then compared with the CAM-ICU scores. CAM-ICU showed a sensitivity of 47% and a specificity of 98%, with a positive predictive value of 95% and a negative predictive value of 72%. There have not been similar trials regarding the use of ICDSC in pragmatic settings, but it would not be surprising if the ability to detect delirium was less than reported in research settings.

Prevention of Delirium in the Intensive Care Unit

Delirium can be associated with infection, pain, metabolic derangements, and hypoxemia, among other conditions, which should be evaluated for and adequately treated to decrease its risk. Given the prevalence, known risk factors, and complications of delirium, there has been increasing interest in preventing delirium. Clinical studies of delirium prevention can be divided into pharmacologic and nonpharmacologic prevention.[9,16,49–54]

Nonpharmacologic interventions

Trials evaluating nonpharmacologic interventions usually seek to eliminate potentially modifiable risk factors either one at a time or in bundles of multiple risk factors. In one of the earlier bundled trials,[54] 852 non-ICU, general medicine patients aged 70 years or older underwent either protocol-driven screening and management of risk factors for delirium, including cognitive impairment, sleep deprivation, immobility, impairments in vision and hearing, and dehydration or usual care. The intervention group had a delirium rate of 9.9% versus 15% in the group receiving usual care. Similarly, implementation of a bundle of nonpharmacologic interventions, consisting of environmental noise and light reduction designed to reduce disturbing patients during the night, was associated with improved sleep and a reduced incidence of delirium in the ICU.[50]

Immobility as a risk factor for delirium was evaluated in ventilated ICU patients by Shweickert and colleagues.[55] The study evaluated 104 ventilated patients assigned to either daily sedation interruption with or without physical and occupational therapy and found a statistically significant improvement in functional status at discharge (59% vs 35%) and shorter median duration of delirium (2 vs 4 days), as well as a reduction in ventilator days. A subsequent quality improvement study[56] confirmed the results and applicability in clinical settings.

Sleep deprivation is known to be a risk factor for delirium, with interruptions in REM sleep being the most significant.[17] ICU patients sleep poorly and have limited REM and slow-wave or deep sleep.[16] Studies have evaluated improvement in sleep quality and its effect on the development of delirium. In 1 study by Van Rompaey and colleagues,[57] earplugs were given to 69 patients within the ICU, with 67 controls. The study found higher reported sleep quality in the intervention group and a hazard ratio of 0.47 for the emergence of confusion. Furthermore, there was a delay in the time to development of delirium in those patients given earplugs, if the condition developed at all. A trial in 2013 by Kamdar and colleagues[58] sought to provide a multifaceted approach to improve sleep quality, which entailed reducing ambient noise, nighttime procedures, and so forth, and resulted in a 20% decrease in the incidence of delirium and shorter time of delirium. However, there was no improvement in sleep quality. This finding was confirmed in a secondary analysis by the investigators.[59] This finding suggests that reductions in noise, procedures, and so forth may decrease delirium regardless of effect on sleep quality.

Bundled practices
Recently, there have also been trials of bundled practices to prevent delirium in the ICU (eg, ABCDE bundles [awakening and breathing coordination, delirium monitoring/management, and early exercise/mobility]).[9] These bundles seek to create an opt-out rather than opt-in method for performing interventions. This strategy ensures that a greater percentage of patients have limited amounts of sedation, early mobility, and delirium monitoring. A recent multicenter trial of 296 patients (146 before and 150 after implementation)[9] noted an odds ratio of 0.55 for the development of delirium after implementation. The study also showed a decrease by 3 ventilator days in mechanical ventilation and an improvement in mobilization (**Box 4**).

Box 4
Nonpharmacologic delirium prevention methods

Early mobility

Measures to improve sleep (earplugs, reduce ambient noise, reduce nighttime procedures and sleep interruption)

Protocolized bundles of sedation interruption, spontaneous breathing trials, early mobilization, and delirium monitoring

---

Pharmacologic Interventions

Limiting sedation and choice of sedative
Sedative use in the ICU is often necessary, but studies have shown that deep sedation with any agent leads to more time on the ventilator as well as an increase in mortality.[59–61] Decrease in the use of medications, particularly sedatives and benzodiazepines, can also lead to a decrease in the incidence of delirium.[41,59,62] Several studies have suggested that benzodiazepines may have a higher risk of delirium than other sedatives.[41,63] Agitation caused by pain may cause more sedatives to be given, which could lead to increases in delirium, as shown by post hoc analysis that showed shorter duration of mechanical ventilation and decreased use of sedatives with daily pain assessment.[64] Pain management with ketamine before cardiac surgery showed a decrease in delirium rates to 3% versus 31% in 1 trial,[65] although the effects of ketamine may have been pleiotropic.

Sedation with dexmedetomidine, an α_2-adrenoreceptor antagonist, may decrease the risk of delirium when used in place of benzodiazepines or possibly other sedatives, as shown in the 2007 MENDS (Maximizing the Efficacy of Targeted Sedation and Reducing Neurologic Dysfunction) trial.[66] In this study, patients were randomized to either lorazepam or dexmedetomidine and had 4 more days alive or free of delirium.

Another trial evaluating dexmedetomidine versus propofol or midazolam[67] showed an increase in a score quantifying patient interaction with dexmedetomidine in both groups. The study evaluated a composite end point of neurocognitive adverse events including delirium that was significantly lower in dexmedetomidine versus propofol (18% vs 29%) but not different versus midazolam. No obvious decrease in delirium as measured by CAM-ICU at 1 time point 48 hours after cessation of sedation was noted in either group. These results suggest a possible benefit of dexmedetomidine, which has been recommended in recent guidelines for patients with risk factors for delirium.[41]

Pharmacologic prophylaxis for delirium

Studies of delirium prophylaxis have had mixed results. Trials of the cholinesterase inhibitor rivastigmine were negative, with a trend toward harm.[35,36] Statins have recently gained interest as agents for delirium prevention, because a recent prospective cohort trial showed an association between delirium-free days and statin administration. If statins were administered, patients had an odds ratio of 2.28 of being delirium free the following day after controlling for illness severity.[51]

Typical antipsychotics have been used in preventing delirium in the postoperative population. In a large trial, Wang and colleagues[52] evaluated 457 patients after noncardiac surgery and gave the 229 in the intervention group a bolus of 0.5 mg IV and then 0.1 mg/h of haloperidol after surgery for 12 hours. The incidence of delirium was 15.3% in the treatment arm versus 23.2% in the control arm. The time to delirium development was longer in the intervention group, who also had increased delirium-free days as well as a shorter ICU stay. The MIND (Modifying the Impact of ICU-Associated Neurological Dysfunction) study randomized nonsurgical intubated ICU patients to haloperidol, ziprasidone (an atypical antipsychotic), or placebo and found no difference in time of delirium or incidence of delirium in the 3 treatment arms.[68] This was a pilot study, the results of which should be used with caution. Atypical antipsychotics such as risperidone have also had promising results in postoperative cardiac surgery patients, with a reduction in delirium from 31.7% to 11.1 % in the medication group.[69] There have been no high-quality trials that are positive for delirium prevention with antipsychotics outside the postoperative period.

The melatonin agonist ramelteon was used in a recent study in 67 elderly Japanese ICU patients for the prevention of delirium.[49] Patients were 65 to 89 years old and able to take oral medication. Only 3% of the treatment group developed delirium during their 7-day trial period compared with 32% of the control arm. These results suggest a large treatment effect; however, given the small sample size and larger than expected reduction, further studies are needed in this area. Studies of melatonin have had mixed results, for example, rates of 11% in treatment group in 1 study,[70] and another study[71] showed no benefit (**Table 3**).

Table 3
Evidence on haloperidol, risperidone, and ramelteon prevention for delirium

Haloperidol	Risperidone	Ramelteon
Evidence in postoperative patients. Incidence 15.3% vs 23.2%	Evidence in cardiac postoperative patients. Incidence 11.1% vs 31.7%	Evidence in case series and outpatients as well as ICU elderly patients. 3% vs 32%
Negative trial in nonoperative ICU patients (MIND study)	Limited or no trials in nonoperative patients	No evidence for postoperative patients

Treatment of Delirium in the Intensive Care Unit

Treatment of delirium is multifaceted and involves treatment of the agitation that may cause harm to the patient from self-extubation, falls, and so forth, as well as treatment of delirium with the intention of faster resolution. Management of agitation from delirium frequently utilizes the antipsychotic haloperidol, despite the lack of large randomized controlled trials and limited evidence of benefit for expediting the resolution of delirium.[68,72] Unfortunately, alternative agents such as benzodiazepines or other sedatives are associated with more harm, as discussed earlier, making the management of agitation in delirium difficult.

There are relatively few trials evaluating the treatment of delirium once it starts. The MIND trial, for example, showed no difference in delirium-free days in patients given haloperidol, ziprasidone, or placebo with 14 versus 15 versus 12.5 delirium-free days, respectively.[68] Trials evaluating Haldol versus atypical antipsychotics such as olanzapine or risperidone have been undertaken, and a meta-analysis determined that there was no significant difference in treatment effect and perhaps fewer side effects in the atypical antipsychotics.[73] There is only 1 trial[71] to our knowledge that evaluated treatment of delirium and showed reduction in duration of delirium after it began. This trial evaluating quetiapine, an atypical antipsychotic, in 36 ICU patients who could also receive haloperidol as needed showed a reduction in duration of delirium to 36 versus 120 hours and less agitation. In addition, patients were more likely to be discharged home rather than to a skilled nursing facility. Despite the positive findings, this was a small trial and there was no effect on mortality or duration of stay within the ICU. There is an ongoing trial by Ely and colleagues, the MIND-USA study (ClinicalTrials.gov Identifier: NCT01211522), which will likely shed light on this issue, with plans for results in 2017.

SUMMARY

Delirium in the ICU is an extremely common and detrimental diagnosis, with a high incidence and effects, including increases in mortality, longer duration of mechanical ventilation, and long-term cognitive dysfunction after discharge. There are trials suggesting that prophylaxis of postoperative delirium is possible with medications, including haloperidol, atypical antipsychotics, and ketamine; however, these trials are small and decisions should be made on a case-by-case basis. There are some promising studies, both pharmacologic and nonpharmacologic, for preventing delirium in nonoperative critically ill patients. Medications such as ramelteon as well as nonpharmacologic care bundling practices involving early mobility, awakening, daily spontaneous breathing trials, and screening for delirium are safe methods by which we may be able to reduce delirium in the ICU. Decreasing depth of sedation and considering dexmedetomidine in high-risk populations may be a useful strategy and is now included in national guidelines.

Despite the advances in monitoring and some promise in methods for prevention, our ability to treat delirium after it begins remains limited. There has been only one small trial showing a truly positive effect with quetiapine added to haloperidol on delirium duration after it begins, and this requires a larger validation before becoming standard practice. Perhaps the most promising aspect of delirium research is the increasing recognition of it as a serious and debilitating condition and the new trials that will be coming soon, which include a trial planned to enroll 876 patients with delirium to evaluate treatment with haloperidol and ziprasidone with a placebo control, the MIND-USA study, and trials evaluating prevention with haloperidol for nonsurgical patients, as well as larger trials of melatonin and ramelteon. Through these studies, it is hoped that management strategies can be developed that not only reduce delirium incidence and its duration but also lead to a reduction in the mortality and morbidity associated with it.

REFERENCES

1. McGuire BE, Basten CJ, Ryan CJ, et al. Intensive care unit syndrome: a dangerous misnomer. Arch Intern Med 2000;160:906–9.
2. American Psychiatric Association and American Psychiatric Association, DSM-5 Task Force. Diagnostic and statistical manual of mental disorders: DSM-5. Washington, DC: American Psychiatric Association; 2013.
3. Ouimet S, Kavanagh BP, Gottfried SB, et al. Incidence, risk factors and consequences of ICU delirium. Intensive Care Med 2007;33:66–73.
4. Pandharipande P, Cotton BA, Shintani A, et al. Motoric subtypes of delirium in mechanically ventilated surgical and trauma intensive care unit patients. Intensive Care Med 2007;33:1726–31.
5. Meagher DJ, Trzepacz PT. Motoric subtypes of delirium. Semin Clin Neuropsychiatry 2000;5:75–85.
6. Peterson JF, Pun BT, Dittus RS, et al. Delirium and its motoric subtypes: a study of 614 critically ill patients. J Am Geriatr Soc 2006;54:479–84.
7. Cavallazzi R, Saad M, Marik PE. Delirium in the ICU: an overview. Ann Intensive Care 2012;2:49.
8. Milbrandt EB, Deppen S, Harrison PL, et al. Costs associated with delirium in mechanically ventilated patients. Crit Care Med 2004;32:955–62.
9. Balas MC, Vasilevskis EE, Olsen KM, et al. Effectiveness and safety of the awakening and breathing coordination, delirium monitoring/management, and early exercise/mobility bundle. Crit Care Med 2014;42:1024–36.
10. Pandharipande PP, Girard TD, Ely EW. Long-term cognitive impairment after critical illness. N Engl J Med 2013;369:1306–16.
11. Ely EW, Shintani A, Truman B, et al. Delirium as a predictor of mortality in mechanically ventilated patients in the intensive care unit. JAMA 2004;291:1753–62.
12. Van Rompaey B, Schuurmans MJ, Shortridge-Baggett LM, et al. Risk factors for intensive care delirium: a systematic review. Intensive Crit Care Nurs 2008;24:98–107.
13. van den Boogaard M, Pickkers P, Slooter AJ, et al. Development and validation of PRE-DELIRIC (Prediction of Delirium in ICU patients) delirium prediction model for intensive care patients: observational multicentre study. BMJ 2012;344:e420.
14. Zaal IJ, Devlin JW, Peelen LM, et al. A systematic review of risk factors for delirium in the ICU. Crit Care Med 2015;43:40–7.
15. Van Rompaey B, Elseviers MM, Schuurmans MJ, et al. Risk factors for delirium in intensive care patients: a prospective cohort study. Crit Care 2009;13:R77.
16. Cooper AB, Thornley KS, Young GB, et al. Sleep in critically ill patients requiring mechanical ventilation. Chest 2000;117:809–18.
17. Trompeo AC, Vidi Y, Locane MD, et al. Sleep disturbances in the critically ill patients: role of delirium and sedative agents. Minerva Anestesiol 2011;77:604–12.
18. Salluh JI, Soares M, Teles JM, et al. Delirium epidemiology in critical care (DECCA): an international study. Crit Care 2010;14:R210.
19. Marshall JC. Inflammation, coagulopathy, and the pathogenesis of multiple organ dysfunction syndrome. Crit Care Med 2001;29:S99–106.

20. Zhang Z, Pan L, Deng H, et al. Prediction of delirium in critically ill patients with elevated C-reactive protein. J Crit Care 2014;29:88–92.
21. Alexander SA, Ren D, Gunn SR, et al. Interleukin 6 and apolipoprotein E as predictors of acute brain dysfunction and survival in critical care patients. Am J Crit Care 2014;23:49–57.
22. McGrane S, Girard TD, Thompson JL, et al. Procalcitonin and C-reactive protein levels at admission as predictors of duration of acute brain dysfunction in critically ill patients. Crit Care 2011;15:R78.
23. Jeppsson B, Freund HR, Gimmon Z, et al. Blood-brain barrier derangement in sepsis: cause of septic encephalopathy? Am J Surg 1981;141:136–42.
24. Papadopoulos MC, Lamb FJ, Moss RF, et al. Faecal peritonitis causes oedema and neuronal injury in pig cerebral cortex. Clin Sci (Lond) 1999;96:461–6.
25. Krueger JM, Walter J, Dinarello CA, et al. Sleep-promoting effects of endogenous pyrogen (interleukin-1). Am J Physiol 1984;246:R994–9.
26. Rosenberg SA, Lotze MT, Yang JC, et al. Experience with the use of high-dose interleukin-2 in the treatment of 652 cancer patients. Ann Surg 1989;210: 474–84 [discussion: 84–5].
27. Westhoff D, Witlox J, Koenderman L, et al. Preoperative cerebrospinal fluid cytokine levels and the risk of postoperative delirium in elderly hip fracture patients. J Neuroinflammation 2013;10:122.
28. Cerejeira J, Firmino H, Vaz-Serra A, et al. The neuroinflammatory hypothesis of delirium. Acta Neuropathol 2010;119:737–54.
29. Sanders RD. Hypothesis for the pathophysiology of delirium: role of baseline brain network connectivity and changes in inhibitory tone. Med Hypotheses 2011;77:140–3.
30. Bowton DL, Bertels NH, Prough DS, et al. Cerebral blood flow is reduced in patients with sepsis syndrome. Crit Care Med 1989;17:399–403.
31. Yokota H, Ogawa S, Kurokawa A, et al. Regional cerebral blood flow in delirium patients. Psychiatry Clin Neurosci 2003;57:337–9.
32. Kitabayashi Y, Narumoto J, Shibata K, et al. Neuropsychiatric background of alcohol hallucinosis: a SPECT study. J Neuropsychiatry Clin Neurosci 2007;19:85.
33. Hshieh TT, Fong TG, Marcantonio ER, et al. Use of medications with anticholinergic effect predicts clinical severity of delirium symptoms in older medical inpatients. Arch Intern Med 2001;161:1099–105.
34. Hshieh TT, Fong TG, Marcantonio ER, et al. Cholinergic deficiency hypothesis in delirium: a synthesis of current evidence. J Gerontol A Biol Sci Med Sci 2008;63: 764–72.
35. van Eijk MM, Roes KC, Honing ML, et al. Effect of rivastigmine as an adjunct to usual care with haloperidol on duration of delirium and mortality in critically ill patients: a multicentre, double-blind, placebo-controlled randomised trial. Lancet 2010;376:1829–37.
36. Gamberini M, Bolliger D, Lurati Buse GA, et al. Rivastigmine for the prevention of postoperative delirium in elderly patients undergoing elective cardiac surgery–a randomized controlled trial. Crit Care Med 2009;37:1762–8.
37. Trzepacz PT. Is there a final common neural pathway in delirium? Focus on acetylcholine and dopamine. Semin Clin Neuropsychiatry 2000;5:132–48.
38. Skrobik YK, Bergeron N, Dumont M, et al. Olanzapine vs haloperidol: treating delirium in a critical care setting. Intensive Care Med 2004;30:444–9.
39. van Munster BC, de Rooij SE, Yazdanpanah M, et al. The association of the dopamine transporter gene and the dopamine receptor 2 gene with delirium, a meta-analysis. Am J Med Genet B Neuropsychiatr Genet 2010;153B:648–55.

40. van Eijk MM, van Marum RJ, Klijn IA, et al. Comparison of delirium assessment tools in a mixed intensive care unit. Crit Care Med 2009;37:1881–5.
41. Barr J, Fraser GL, Puntillo K, et al. Clinical practice guidelines for the management of pain, agitation, and delirium in adult patients in the intensive care unit. Crit Care Med 2013;41:263–306.
42. Wei LA, Fearing MA, Sternberg EJ, et al. The confusion assessment method: a systematic review of current usage. J Am Geriatr Soc 2008;56:823–30.
43. Ely EW, Inouye SK, Bernard GR, et al. Delirium in mechanically ventilated patients: validity and reliability of the confusion assessment method for the intensive care unit (CAM-ICU). JAMA 2001;286:2703–10.
44. Pun BT, Gordon SM, Peterson JF, et al. Large-scale implementation of sedation and delirium monitoring in the intensive care unit: a report from two medical centers. Crit Care Med 2005;33:1199–205.
45. Bergeron N, Dubois MJ, Dumont M, et al. Intensive care delirium screening checklist: evaluation of a new screening tool. Intensive Care Med 2001;27:859–64.
46. Sessler CN, Gosnell MS, Grap MJ, et al. The Richmond agitation-sedation scale: validity and reliability in adult intensive care unit patients. Am J Respir Crit Care Med 2002;166:1338–44.
47. Gusmao-Flores D, Salluh JI, Chalhub RÁ, et al. The confusion assessment method for the intensive care unit (CAM-ICU) and intensive care delirium screening checklist (ICDSC) for the diagnosis of delirium: a systematic review and meta-analysis of clinical studies. Crit Care 2012;16:R115.
48. van Eijk MM, van den Boogaard M, van Marum RJ, et al. Routine use of the confusion assessment method for the intensive care unit: a multicenter study. Am J Respir Crit Care Med 2011;184:340–4.
49. Hatta K, Kishi Y, Wada K, et al. Preventive effects of ramelteon on delirium: a randomized placebo-controlled trial. JAMA Psychiatry 2014;71:397–403.
50. Patel J, Baldwin J, Bunting P, et al. The effect of a multicomponent multidisciplinary bundle of interventions on sleep and delirium in medical and surgical intensive care patients. Anaesthesia 2014;69:540–9.
51. Page VJ, Davis D, Zhao XB, et al. Statin use and risk of delirium in the critically ill. Am J Respir Crit Care Med 2014;189:666–73.
52. Wang W, Li HL, Wang DX, et al. Haloperidol prophylaxis decreases delirium incidence in elderly patients after noncardiac surgery: a randomized controlled trial. Crit Care Med 2012;40:731–9.
53. Brummel NE, Girard TD. Preventing delirium in the intensive care unit. Crit Care Clin 2013;29:51–65.
54. Inouye SK, Bogardus ST Jr, Charpentier PA, et al. A multicomponent intervention to prevent delirium in hospitalized older patients. N Engl J Med 1999;340:669–76.
55. Schweickert WD, Pohlman MC, Pohlman AS, et al. Early physical and occupational therapy in mechanically ventilated, critically ill patients: a randomised controlled trial. Lancet 2009;373(9678):1874–82.
56. Needham DM, Korupolu R, Zanni JM, et al. Early physical medicine and rehabilitation for patients with acute respiratory failure: a quality improvement project. Arch Phys Med Rehabil 2010;91:536–42.
57. Van Rompaey B, Elseviers MM, Van Drom W, et al. The effect of earplugs during the night on the onset of delirium and sleep perception: a randomized controlled trial in intensive care patients. Crit Care 2012;16:R73.
58. Kamdar BB, King LM, Collop NA, et al. The effect of a quality improvement intervention on perceived sleep quality and cognition in a medical ICU. Crit Care Med 2013;41:800–9.

59. Kamdar BB, Niessen T, Colantuoni E, et al. Delirium transitions in the medical ICU: exploring the role of sleep quality and other factors. Crit Care Med 2015; 43:135–41.
60. Girard TD, Kress JP, Fuchs BD, et al. Efficacy and safety of a paired sedation and ventilator weaning protocol for mechanically ventilated patients in intensive care (awakening and breathing controlled trial): a randomised controlled trial. Lancet 2008;371:126–34.
61. Shehabi Y, Bellomo R, Reade MC, et al. Early intensive care sedation predicts long-term mortality in ventilated critically ill patients. Am J Respir Crit Care Med 2012;186:724–31.
62. Patel SB, Poston JT, Pohlman A, et al. Rapidly reversible, sedation-related delirium versus persistent delirium in the intensive care unit. Am J Respir Crit Care Med 2014;189:658–65.
63. Pandharipande P, Shintani A, Peterson J, et al. Lorazepam is an independent risk factor for transitioning to delirium in intensive care unit patients. Anesthesiology 2006;104:21–6.
64. Payen JF, Bosson JL, Chanques G, et al. Pain assessment is associated with decreased duration of mechanical ventilation in the intensive care unit: a post hoc analysis of the DOLOREA study. Anesthesiology 2009;111:1308–16.
65. Hudetz JA, Patterson KM, Iqbal Z, et al. Ketamine attenuates delirium after cardiac surgery with cardiopulmonary bypass. J Cardiothorac Vasc Anesth 2009; 23:651–7.
66. Pandharipande PP, Pun BT, Herr DL, et al. Effect of sedation with dexmedetomidine vs lorazepam on acute brain dysfunction in mechanically ventilated patients: the MENDS randomized controlled trial. JAMA 2007;298:2644–53.
67. Jakob SM, Ruokonen E, Grounds RM, et al. Dexmedetomidine vs midazolam or propofol for sedation during prolonged mechanical ventilation: two randomized controlled trials. JAMA 2012;307:1151–60.
68. Girard TD, Pandharipande PP, Carson SS, et al. Feasibility, efficacy, and safety of antipsychotics for intensive care unit delirium: the MIND randomized, placebo-controlled trial. Crit Care Med 2010;38:428–37.
69. Prakanrattana U, Prapaitrakool S. Efficacy of risperidone for prevention of postoperative delirium in cardiac surgery. Anaesth Intensive Care 2007;35:714–9.
70. Al-Aama T, Brymer C, Gutmanis I, et al. Melatonin decreases delirium in elderly patients: a randomized, placebo-controlled trial. Int J Geriatr Psychiatry 2011; 26:687–94.
71. Devlin JW, Roberts RJ, Fong JJ, et al. Efficacy and safety of quetiapine in critically ill patients with delirium: a prospective, multicenter, randomized, double-blind, placebo-controlled pilot study. Crit Care Med 2010;38:419–27.
72. Flaherty JH, Gonzales JP, Dong B. Antipsychotics in the treatment of delirium in older hospitalized adults: a systematic review. J Am Geriatr Soc 2011; 59(Suppl 2):S269–76.
73. Lonergan E, Britton AM, Luxenberg J, et al. Antipsychotics for delirium. Cochrane Database Syst Rev 2007;(2):CD005594.

Index

Note: Page numbers of article titles are in **boldface** type.

Crit Care Clin 31 (2015) 605–619
http://dx.doi.org/10.1016/S0749-0704(15)00039-1
0749-0704/15/$ – see front matter © 2015 Elsevier Inc. All rights reserved.

criticalcare.theclinics.com

Printed and bound by CPI Group (UK) Ltd, Croydon, CR0 4YY

03/10/2024

01040492-0007